Adult CCRN® Certification Review

Kendra Menzies Kent, MS, RN-BC, CCRN, CNRN, SCRN, TCRN, is currently a staff nurse in the intensive care unit at St. Mary's Hospital, West Palm Beach, Florida. She is a highly experienced critical care nurse and an accomplished critical care registered nurse (CCRN) instructor, with multiple specialty certifications within critical care. She also has extensive clinical experience in the majority of these specialty areas. She is an accomplished clinician and nurse educator and manager, having worked as a staff nurse, unit manager, nurse educator, and director of critical care at Parkland Hospital in Dallas, as well as at other notable acute care facilities. She received her BSN degree from University of Texas, Arlington, and her MSN as a clinical nurse specialist in medical–surgical nursing from Texas Women's University. She is currently an educational consultant for Med Ed Seminars in Charlotte, North Carolina, having served as a speaker for Health and Sciences Television Network (HSTN) and HSTN videos. An accomplished author, Kendra has edited or contributed to various books on critical care.

Adult CCRN® Certification Review

Think in Questions, Learn by Rationales

Kendra Menzies Kent, MS, RN-BC, CCRN, CNRN, SCRN

SPRINGER PUBLISHING COMPANY

NEW YORK

Springer Publishing Company, LLC
11 West 42nd Street
New York, NY 10036
www.springerpub.com

Acquisitions Editor: Elizabeth Nieginski
Composition: Newgen Imaging

ISBN: 978-0-8261-9833-4
e-book ISBN: 978-0-8261-9834-1
14 15 16 17 / 5 4 3 2 1

Publisher's Acknowledgments
Springer Publishing Company recognizes that the Adult CCRN® Certification Exam is a registered service mark of the American Association of Critical-Care Nurses (AACN) and has applied this service mark to the first mention of the exam in each of the chapters in this book and on its cover.

The publisher sincerely thanks and acknowledges Bimbola F. Akintade PhD, ACNP-BC, MBA, MHA, and Liza Marmo RN-BC, MSN, CCRN, ANP-C, for their careful and thoughtful review of the manuscript.

Library of Congress Cataloging-in-Publication Data

CIP data is available from the Library of Congress.

Special discounts on bulk quantities of our books are available to corporations, professional associations, pharmaceutical companies, health care organizations, and other qualifying groups. If you are interested in a custom book, including chapters from more than one of our titles, we can provide that service as well.

For details, please contact:
Special Sales Department, Springer Publishing Company, LLC
11 West 42nd Street, 15th Floor, New York, NY 10036–8002
Phone: 877-687-7476 or 212-431-4370; Fax: 212-941-7842
E-mail: sales@springerpub.com

Printed in the United States of America by Bradford & Bigelow.

To my wonderful husband, Robby, and to my parents, Sid and Judy,
for all the love and support they have given me.

Contents

Introduction

Welcome to the journey toward certification. This book was written to help guide the reader on the pathway of the journey. It is written in a question/answer format to encourage you to think in questions when studying for the examination. When you study, I encourage you to ask yourself, "What can be asked about this particular topic?" "What would be a good question?" "What is important in this disease?" "What makes it different from other disorders?" This prepares you to anticipate the kinds of questions that might be asked and not just attempt to memorize content for the certification examination.

The book also provides multiple-choice questions similar to the questions that are found on the Adult Critical-Care Registered Nurse (CCRN®) examination. These questions allow the nurse to practice taking an examination and also assist the nurse in determining areas that require further study prior to taking the CCRN examination. The answers and rationale, including some test-taking skills, are provided for each question, further preparing the nurse for the real examination.

WHY CERTIFICATION?

The most important reason for certification is to do it for yourself (Box I.1). Certification is viewed as a mark of excellence in an area of specialty. It is an achievement and qualification that can be seen by peers, physicians, leaders of health care institutes, and patients/families. Becoming certified takes a certain dedication to critical care nursing and demonstrates a level of competency. The CCRN examination is developed to verify knowledge in critical care nursing.

Box I.1 Reasons to Become Certified

Validates your knowledge of critical care to your hospital and peers
Validates your knowledge of critical care to the patients
Validates your knowledge of critical care to the physician
Promotes continuing excellence in the nursing profession
Demonstrates competency
Assists with hospital credentialing
Provides monetary benefit (from some hospitals)

ADULT CCRN EXAMINATION INFORMATION

The CCRN examination follows the blueprint developed by the American Association of Critical Care Nurses (AACN). The test is developed and reviewed by experts in critical care. The *CCRN Application Handbook* can be accessed from the website www.certcorp.org. The examination application may be completed online or can be printed and mailed or faxed to the AACN Certification Corporation. The Adult CCRN provides a 3-year certification for critical care nurses.

EXAMINATION

The Adult CCRN examination consists of 150 multiple-choice questions, of which 25 questions will not count for or against you. These 25 questions are being tested for use in future examinations. You will not know which questions count, so complete all 150 questions as if they count. The test is not arranged per system, and it is randomized. You may have one question on the renal system and the next one is on the cardiovascular system. The time allowed to complete the examination is 3 hours (50 questions per hour).

Eligibility requirements to take the Adult CCRN examination are RN licensure and 1,750 hours of direct bedside care of critically ill patients during the previous 2 years with 875 of those hours obtained in the year preceding application to take the examination. Or, one must have been practicing as an RN for 5 years with a minimum of 2,000 hours of direct care of critically ill patients with 144 of those hours logged during the preceding year. Nurse educators and managers in the adult critical care areas may apply hours spent at the bedside supervising nurses and nursing students.

The Adult CCRN examination is offered year-round as a computer-based test (CBT) and is also given as paper–pencil in certain circumstances. Once AACN receives your application and approves it, they send a confirmation e-mail and postcard. Once confirmed, there is a 90-day window to take the examination. You will need to schedule your examination at an approved testing center. These centers can be found at www.goAMP.com. Immediate test results with score breakdown are available with the CBT. Obtaining scores from a paper–pencil test will take 3 to 4 weeks. Following successful completion of the exam (which everyone will have done), a certificate will be sent by mail within 3 to 4 weeks.

> **❯ HINT**
> Do not schedule your exam at the end of the 90-day window. If for some reason you are unable to take the examination on the scheduled date, you will have to pay an extra $100 to reschedule.

Renewal of your CCRN license can be made through continuing education recognition points (CERPs) or retaking the examination. The CERP requirement is 100 hours in various categories (A, B, & C). For more details on renewal, use the AACN's website for renewal by the CERPs brochure.

TEST PLAN

The Adult CCRN test plan is a blueprint for the exam content. Each major system is divided into subheadings and topics, and clinical judgment, professional caring, and ethical practice.

The amount of coverage in each of the systems is:

- Cardiovascular, 20%
- Pulmonary, 18%
- Endocrine, 5%
- Hematology/Immunology 2%
- Neurology, 12%
- Gastroenterology, 6%
- Renal, 6%
- Multisystem, 8%
- Behavioral/Psychosocial, 4%
- Professional Caring Practice, 20%

The CCRN blueprint also has a list of "testable nursing actions," which are nursing actions under each body system that may be tested. Nursing assessment, monitoring, and pharmacology are included in each body system and should be reviewed in preparation for the examination.

For additional, detailed information, please consult the Adult CCRN Exam Handbook (www.aacn.org).

PREPARATION

Be positive!! Avoid any negative thoughts about passing the examination. These thoughts can cause a self-fulfilling prophecy. Set the test date, then establish a realistic schedule for preparing for the examination. Set your priorities; study those areas you are less familiar with first. Look at the percentage of each body system and establish timelines based on the largest to smallest percentage. Know how you study best, by yourself or in study groups. Study in a manner that works best for you. There are flash cards, practice questions, review courses, and study books in outline format and narrative format available for studying. Practice your test questions within a set time limit to familiarize yourself with the time limitations. Allow 2 minutes or less per question (remember the 50-questions-per-hour rule).

When using the practice test questions to study, determine several things when the answers and rationale are being reviewed. Analyze why you missed the question: Did you simply not know the content? Go back and restudy this section. Did you misread the question? Did you misread the answers? Did you miss an important element in the question or scenario? Was there a clue based on age, timeline, or symptoms?

Study those areas that you are least comfortable with, or those that are not in your specialty area. As adult learners, we tend to want to read and study what we like, or what we can use on a daily basis. For this examination, do not spend as much time in your area of specialty (you already know it) but focus on other areas you are not familiar with in your clinical practice.

DAY OF THE TEST

Before the examination eat a healthy meal and limit the amount of liquids (to avoid the need for breaks during the exam). Remember, restroom breaks are allowed but the testing time does not stop!

Do not try to cram immediately before the test; this will increase your anxiety. After the exam, make plans to do something special for yourself.

Know where you have to go for the test before the actual day of the test, and also know how long it will take you to get there at the appointed time. Running late and feeling hurried will increase your anxiety and can poorly affect your test-taking skills. Remember, if you are more than 15 minutes late, you will not be allowed to take the examination.

Bring your letter of approval and two forms of identification (one picture ID). You cannot bring any personal effects into the testing room, so leave everything in the car or at home (usually a locker is provided for you to put your personal items in).

You are allowed to do a tutorial on the computer before you start your exam if you need some assistance with CBT. The test time begins as soon as you start the first question of the actual exam. Leaving the testing site without authorization results in an automatic voiding of the test. You will be allowed only 3 hours from the time the test is started.

Results of the examination will be presented onsite at the completion of your exam following a test evaluation.

TEST-TAKING SKILLS

Frequently, the difference between pass or fail depends on one's test-taking skills. An important reminder: Do not read into the questions; take the question and information provided at face value. Answer all questions; do not leave any questions blank. A blank answer will be counted against you. Answering the question, even if it is an "educated" guess, will give you a one out of four chance of being correct.

Key words are important phrases or words used to focus attention on what the question is specifically asking. Examples include *always, earliest, first, on admission, best, least, immediately,* and *initial.*

> ❯ HINT
> If the question asks for the "best" response, this is an indication that all answers are probably correct and you will have to determine the best answer for that particular scenario.

Eliminate incorrect options first. Sometimes, you will immediately see an answer that is incorrect. Mark through it to narrow down your choices and improve your odds. Frequently you can get the choices down to two that are more correct than others.

> **HINT**
> Eliminating options gives a 50/50 chance for an educated guess of the correct answer.

Avoid those answers with words such as "always" or "never." There is rarely a time in the medical field in which you will always or never take a particular action. If three of the four answers are similar, choose the answer that does not sound similar.

Do not change answers unless absolutely sure. You can "bookmark" a question that you are not sure about and return to it at the end of the test. Sometimes, you will feel more comfortable with the answer after you come back to it.

> **HINT**
> First impressions are usually good! Do not spend too much time on any one question.

Do not let it worry you if you do not know all the answers. Take a deep breath and keep going. Rejoice in those answers you know and find easy!

> **HINT**
> You are not really supposed to know all the answers.

Do not try to establish patterns, such as using "two As in a row" for answers.

If there is a long scenario with a large amount of data, read the question first, then read the scenario, then reread the question. Sometimes there will be erroneous data that is not required to answer the question. Too much time may be spent on trying to comprehend the whole scenario.

> **HINT**
> Do not forget to reread the question to make sure you read it correctly the first time.

Read all answers before you make a choice; there may be more than one correct answer, but one will be the better answer for the question.

> **HINT**
Do not choose the first one that appears to be correct. Use the *most* correct answer.

Read the question carefully and answer only the question asked. Do not read into the question or think you need more information/data to answer the question.

> **HINT**
The question will provide you with all the information needed to correctly answer the question.

Time frame questions are frequently used in the test. Use the time frame to assist with making the correct choice. Example: Which complication of subarachnoid hemorrhage is seen 7 to 10 days after the bleed?

> **HINT**
All answers may be correct, but only one will occur more commonly during the time frame provided in the question.

Questions may be worded using the lead-in, "What is the gold standard ...?" This is not asking what is the most common routine but what is the most reliable and accurate.

Scenarios: Read the patient's description, word for word. Read the question, then formulate an answer. Read answers and choose the one closest to your formulated answer. Reread the question after answering to ensure you understood the question correctly.

> **HINT**
When the question is answered, you are done. Move on to the next question. Do not second-guess yourself.

Look for answers that facilitate the care of the patient. Facilitative words include *nurture, aid, support, reinforce, encourage,* and *assist.*

SUMMARY

Certification is a great path toward personal growth and professionalism. You have taken the first step and are on your way to a great journey. Learning is an amazing thing and you will learn new information, remember things you may have previously learned, and apply this to your practice while studying for this examination. Good luck on your journey, and stay positive and excited about the learning process.

Cardiovascular System Review

In this chapter, you will review:

■ Acute coronary syndrome
■ Cardiogenic shock
■ Arrhythmias associated with acute myocardial infarction (AMI)
■ Heart failure
■ Dissecting thoracic and abdominal aorta aneurysms
■ Cardiac trauma
■ Cardiomyopathies
■ Hypertensive crisis
■ Valvular heart disease
■ Peripheral artery disease
■ Hypovolemic shock
■ Cardiac surgeries
■ Hemodynamic monitoring
■ Intra-aortic balloon pump counterpulsation
■ Pacemakers

ACUTE CORONARY SYNDROME

■ *What are acute coronary syndromes (ACSs)?*
■ **Unstable angina (UA), ST-segment elevation myocardial infarction (STEMI), and non-ST-segment elevation myocardial infarction (NSTEMI)**

UA, STEMI, and NSTEMI are typically considered to be complications of ACS (Box 1.1).

Box 1.1 Acute Coronary Syndromes (ACSs)

ACS	Echocardiogram Findings	Cardiac Enzyme Results
Unstable angina	Normal or nonspecific T-wave changes	Normal
Non-ST-segment elevation myocardial infarction (MI)	Normal or new onset ST-segment depression	Elevated
ST-segment elevation MI	Elevated ST-segment in two or more contiguous leads	Elevated

> **HINT**
The findings on the 12-lead electrocardiogram (ECG) make the initial differentiation between STEMI and NSTEMI/UA. It is important to obtain an ECG immediately when there is chest pain.

PATHOPHYSIOLOGY

- ◼ *What are the characteristics of a "vulnerable" plaque in the coronary artery?*
- ◼ **Large lipid-rich core, thin fibrous cap over the lipid core, and activated smooth muscle cells and macrophages**

Vulnerable plaque, also called "unstable plaque," is more likely to cause ACS. It is more likely to rupture than a "stable plaque." The stable plaque has a thinner lipid-rich core and a thicker fibrous cap.

> ❭ HINT
>
> A patient presents with UA but is ruled out for an AMI. The patient is then typically referred for a cardiac catheterization. The most common finding will be a near-complete obstruction of the involved coronary artery. This is a stable plaque. The patient did not have an AMI.

- ◼ *What is plaque erosion?*
- ◼ **The endothelium erodes, exposing the intimal layer to the components of the circulating blood**

Plaque rupture is the most common cause of ACS, but erosion of the plaque can also initiate AMI. Both the rupture and erosion lead to the release of tissue factor, proinflammatory factors, and procoagulants, causing intracoronary thrombosis (Box 1.2).

Box 1.2 Other Causes of AMI

Coronary artery spasm	Pulmonary hypertension
Coronary artery embolism	Coronary vasculitis
Hypertrophic cardiomyopathy	Congenital coronary abnormalities
Dilated cardiomyopathy	Trauma
Restricted cardiomyopathy	

PREVENTION OF ACS

- ◼ *What is a commonly prescribed cholesterol-lowering drug?*
- ◼ **Statin**

Statins are HMG-CoA reductase inhibitors and are commonly prescribed to lower cholesterol. Other cholesterol-lowering therapies include omega-3 fatty acids, fibrates, and lifestyle changes (Box 1.3).

Box 1.3 Prevention of ACS

Lifestyle changes	Smoking cessation
	DASH-like diet
	Regular physical activity
	Weight management
Class I recommendation	Blood pressure control
	Low-density lipoprotein (LDL)-C lowering therapy
	β-blocker
	Angiotensin-converting enzyme (ACE) inhibitor/ angiotensin receptor blocker (ARB)

(continued)

Box 1.3 Prevention of ACS *(continued)*

Class II recommendation	Glycemic control in diabetes mellitus
	Aspirin (ASA)/antiplatelet agent
	Omega-3 fatty acids
Other	Influenza vaccination

SYMPTOMS/ASSESSMENT

■ *What is a positive Levine sign?*

■ **Clenched fist held over the chest wall in association with angina chest pain**

The chest pain is described as a pressure, heaviness, squeezing, burning, or choking sensation. Typical locations for radiation of pain are the arms, shoulders, and neck. The intensity of angina does not change with respiration, cough, or change in position.

■ *What is the most common atypical sign of ACS?*

■ **Shortness of breath**

These include epigastric discomfort, nausea and vomiting, diaphoresis, dyspnea, and generalized weakness.

> **> HINT**
> A question on nontypical symptoms would most likely involve a woman
> in the scenario because women often experience the nontypical
> symptoms of AMI.

■ *Which abnormal heart sound accompanies chest pain caused by AMI?*

■ **S₄ gallop**

An S_4 gallop is caused by a resistant ventricle during the late diastolic phase. The S_4 is typically present with chest pain and disappears when chest pain is alleviated. An S_3 gallop is associated with congestive heart failure (CHF) or volume overload. It occurs during the early diastolic phase (Box 1.4).

Box 1.4 Associated Symptoms of Angina

Cool, clammy skin	Heart rate changes (tachy or brady)
S_3 gallop	Arrhythmias
S_4 gallop	Diaphoresis
Blood pressure changes (hyper- or hypo-)	

> **> HINT**
> An S_3 or S_4 may be used in the scenario as a hint for the answer.
> Remember, S_3 is CHF and S_4 is angina.

■ *Which patient population may have a "silent" MI?*

■ **Diabetics**

Patients with diabetes mellitus may experience an MI without significant chest pain. This may be attributed to their autonomic neuropathy leading to sensory denervation.

■ *Which two locations for an AMI may result in bradycardia?*
■ **Inferior wall AMI and posterior wall AMI**

The SA node is perfused by the proximal right coronary artery (RCA) in 55% of the population and by the proximal circumflex artery (LCX) in 45% of the population. A loss of blood flow through the RCA or the LCX, depending on the dominance, will result in bradycardia. The presence of a first-degree heart block (prolongation of the PR interval) indicates ischemia at the level of the atrioventricular (AV) node, which is mostly supplied by RCA.

DIAGNOSIS

■ *What is the initial diagnostic test obtained with the onset of chest pain?*
■ **12-lead ECG**

A 12-lead ECG is performed and interpreted within 10 minutes of arrival in the emergency department (ED) with chest pain. If the initial 12-lead shows ST-segment elevation in two contiguous leads, then reperfusion strategies are initiated. If the initial 12-lead does not show significant finding but if the patient continues to have chest pain, then an ECG may be obtained as often as every 10 minutes.

> ❯ HINT
> Remember that a person can be having an AMI without elevating ST segments. The differentiation between UA and NSTEMI is cardiac enzymes.

■ *The finding of ST-segment elevation in leads II, III, and a ventricular fibrillation (VF) indicates the need for what follow-up ECG?*
■ **Right precordial lead placement (right-sided ECG)**

An inferior wall AMI (leads II, III, and aVF) may also involve the wall of the right ventricle (RV). The best diagnostic for RV involvement is to obtain a right precordial ECG and look for ST-segment changes in V_{3R} and V_{4R}. Another change in lead placement may be to extend the left precordial leads laterally toward the left posterior chest to better view the posterior-lateral infarction.

> ❯ HINT
> The best ECG lead placement for the diagnosis of a posterior wall AMI is on the back even though this is not commonly performed. Typically, look for reciprocal changes in the anterior leads. The changes include tall R waves and ST depression in V_1 and V_2 (sometimes V_3). This is a reciprocal change of ST-segment elevation and Q waves (or loss of R wave height). Posterior infarcts are mirror images of anterior infarcts.

■ *Which leads are used to recognize lateral wall ischemia and infarction?*
■ **Leads I, aVL, V_5, V_6**

Leads I, aVL, V_5 and V_6 all view the lateral aspect of the left ventricle. ST elevation in leads I and aVL only indicate a high lateral STEMI (Box 1.5).

Box 1.5 Localizing the Infarct

Wall Involvement	Leads of Monitor	Involved Coronary Artery
Anterior wall myocardial infarction (AWMI)	V3–V4 or loss of R-wave progression	Left anterior descending (LAD)
Septal wall	V1–V2	LAD
Lateral wall MI (LWMI)	I, aVL, V5, V6	Left circumflex (LCX)
Inferior wall MI (IWMI) or RV infarct	II, III, aVF	Right coronary artery (RCA)

■ *Which ECG change indicates an acute injury?*

■ **An elevated ST segment**

An elevated ST segment indicates a potentially reversible injury. An ST-segment elevation of ≥1 mm is considered significant. ST segments return to normal after reperfusion.

> **HINT**
>
> Q wave without ST-segment changes indicate a previous MI and are usually noted to be of an "undetermined" age. It is important to compare a patient's ECG with an old one, if available, to evaluate for old or new changes.

■ *What is considered to be a "significant" Q wave?*

■ **A Q wave of 2 mm or more in depth or longer than 0.04-second duration or greater than a third of the height of the QRS complex**

Significant Q waves indicate irreversible myocardial damage (infarction). Q waves may develop within several hours of injury or may take up to several days to weeks to occur. Q waves can persist for the lifetime of a patient.

> **HINT**
>
> Inferior leads typically have small Q waves but are not significant.

■ *Which of the cardiac enzymes is the preferred biomarker for diagnosing an AMI?*

■ **Troponin levels**

Troponin levels are more sensitive and specific to AMI than creatine phosphokinase-MB (CPK-MB). There are other causes of elevated troponin levels, which may include chronic heart failure (HF), acute cardiomyopathy, cardiac contusions, myocarditis, and chronic kidney disease.

■ *How long after the onset of myocardial injury will an increase in cardiac enzymes occur?*

■ **4 to 6 hours**

CPK-MB and troponin increase within 4 to 6 hours after ischemia. To rule out MI, cardiac enzymes are commonly drawn every 8 hours for 24 hours. CPK-MB levels return to baseline within 36 to 40 hours. Troponin levels remain elevated for up to 10 days.

- ■ *Which cardiac protein elevates first?*
- ■ **Myoglobin**

Myoglobin levels elevate within 1 hour of ischemia and return to normal within 24 hours. Myoglobin is a sensitive marker for muscle damage but is not specific to myocardial muscle.

> ❯ HINT
> Elevated myoglobin increases suspicion of AMI in patients presenting with anginal-type chest pain.

MANAGEMENT OF AMI

- ■ *Name two emergency treatments for STEMI.*
- ■ **Emergency coronary balloon angioplasty with stenting and intravenous (IV) thrombolytic agent**

Primary percutaneous coronary intervention (PCI) is the recommended therapy for STEMI, but thrombolytic therapy remains an important option for treatment in hospitals without PCI capabilities.

> ❯ HINT
> IV thrombolytics is only indicated in a STEMI and is not a treatment for NSTEMI or UA.

- ■ *What is the standard for "door-to-balloon" time?*
- ■ **Less than 90 minutes**

Current standards mandate that the time to primary PCI should be less than 90 minutes. PCI includes angioplasty, aspiration thrombectomy, and/or stent placement. Stents are either bare-metal stents (BMS) or drug-eluting stents (DES).

- ■ *For which types of ACS is PCI indicated?*
- ■ **STEMI, NSTEMI, and UA**

PCI is indicated if ischemic symptoms started less than 12 hours ago, clinical evidence of ongoing ischemia is between 12 and 24 hours after onset of symptoms, or if there is cardiogenic shock/severe HF regardless of time delay from onset.

> **HINT**
> PCI should not be performed in a noninfarct artery at the time of
> primary PCI in patients with STEMI who are hemodynamically stable.

High-risk MIs have better outcomes with primary PCI therapy (Box 1.6).

Box 1.6 High-Risk Myocardial Infarctions

Elderly patients	Systolic blood pressure (BP) < 100
Anterior wall STEMI	Signs of acute heart failure or low
Serious ventricular arrhythmias	cardiac output (CO)
	Cardiogenic shock

■ *Which drug therapy is recommended to support primary PCI?*

■ **Anticoagulant and/or antiplatelet agent**

Aspirin (ASA) and thienopyridine (clopidogrel, prasugrel, or ticagrelor) should be given as early as possible or at the time of the PCI. A GP IIb/IIIa receptor antagonist may also be used at the time of the primary PCI if receiving unfractionated heparin (UFH). These include abciximab, tirofiban, and eptifibatide. Bivalirudin monotherapy may be used instead of the combination of UFH and a GP IIb/IIIa receptor antagonist.

> **HINT**
> Prasugrel should not be administered to patients with a history of prior
> stroke or transient ischemic attack (TIA).

■ *What is the minimal time required for dual antiplatelet drug therapy in DES?*

■ **1 year**

A dual antiplatelet therapy is recommended for a minimum of 1 year after a DES and 1 month (4–6 weeks) after placement of a BMS. A BMS is recommended for:

1. High risk of bleeding
2. Predicted compliance issues
3. Known need for a surgical procedure

The dual antiplatelet is an aspirin and a thienopyridine (P2Y$_{12}$ receptor inhibitor). Thienopyridines include clopidogrel (Plavix), prasugrel (Effient), or ticagrelor.

■ *What are the clinical indications for fibrinolytic therapy?*

■ **STEMI, hyperacute T wave, posterior infarction (reciprocal ST-segment depression V$_1$–V$_3$), and new-onset left bundle branch block (LBBB)**

> **HINT**
> Peaked T waves are tall and narrow and develop at the onset of the
> infarction. These are called "peaking" or "hyperacute" T waves. Rule
> out peaked T waves due to hyperkalemia.

Fibrinolytic therapy is a treatment option and should be given, if not contraindicated, within 12 hours of onset of ischemic symptoms if PCI cannot be performed within 120 minutes.

■ *What is the recommendation for "door-to-needle" time when administering a fibrinolytic agent?*

■ **30 minutes or less**

If fibrinolytic therapy is used, the goal for "door-to-needle" time is less than 30 minutes from presentation to medical facility.

■ *When would a fibrinolytic agent be administered to a patient with STEMI beyond the 12-hour window?*

■ **Ongoing signs of ischemia**

A fibrinolytic agent may be administered when PCI is not available and the patient has clinical evidence of ongoing ischemia (symptoms and/or ECG changes), hemodynamic instability, or when a large area of myocardium is at risk. This should still occur within 12 to 24 hours of the onset of symptoms.

> **HINT**
> If the scenario is a STEMI patient in cardiogenic shock or acute severe HF, immediate transfer is recommended to a hospital with PCI capabilities, irrespective of the time of onset of symptoms.

■ *Which ACS patients would not be a candidate for fibrinolytic therapy?*

■ **NSTEMI and UA**

Fibrinolytic therapy is not indicated in NSTEMI or UA, and transfer to a hospital with PCI capabilities is mandated (Boxes 1.7 and 1.8).

Box 1.7 Absolute Contraindications of Fibrinolytic Therapy

Prior intracranial hemorrhage	Suspected aortic dissection
Known intracranial vascular lesion (e.g., aneurysm, arteriovenous malformation [AVM])	Active bleeding
Known malignant intracranial tumor	Ischemic stroke within 3 months
Significant traumatic brain injury within 3 months	

Box 1.8 Fibrinolytic Agents

	Streptokinase	Alteplase (tPA)	Reteplase (rPA)	Tenecteplase (TNK)
Dose	1.5 million units over 30–60 minutes	15 mg bolus followed by 0.75 mg/kg given over 30 minutes, then 0.5 mg/kg over 1 hour	Two 10 U boluses given 30 minutes apart	Based on kilograms of body weight
Half-life	20 minutes	4–6 minutes	18 minutes	20 minutes
90-minute patency	50%	75%	60%–70%	75%
Fibrin specificity	− −	++	+	+++

❯ HINT
A patient with an NSTEMI or ST depression (unless confirmed posterior MI) is not a candidate for thrombolytic therapy.

■ *Following the administration of a fibrinolytic agent, what medications should be given to prevent early reinfarction?*

■ **Aspirin (ASA), clopidogrel (Plavix), and an anticoagulation drug**

Early reinfarction following thrombolytic therapy may be prevented with the administration of antiplatelet and anticoagulation medications. An ASA (81–325 mg) should continue indefinitely. Clopidogrel (Plavix) should be continued for at least 14 days and up to 1 year. Anticoagulation therapy is recommended for a minimum of 48 hours and may continue throughout hospitalization (up to 8 days). Anticoagulation therapy can include one of the following: UFH, enoxaparin (Levenox), or fondaparinux.

❯ HINT
Clopidogrel (Plavix) is administered initially as a loading dose except in patients older than 75 years of age.

■ *What are the four signs of reperfusion following the administration of a fibrinolytic agent or PCI?*

■ **Relief of chest pain, ST-segment return to baseline, abrupt onset of ventricular arrhythmias, and increased levels of cardiac enzymes (washout effect)**

When the coronary artery is reperfused, there is a relief of chest pain and return of ST-segment toward baseline due to the reversal of the ischemic injury. Reperfusion of the previously obstructed coronary artery allows the washout of cardiac enzymes accumulated distal to the obstruction with accompanying ventricular arrhythmias and short runs of ventricular tachycardia (VT).

❯ HINT
The most important sign is the relief of chest pain and ST-segment improvement of more than 50%.

■ *What is the most sensitive continuous monitor used to recognize MI or efficacy of treatment for STEMI?*

■ **ST-segment monitoring**

ST-segment monitoring is recommended for patients with ACS. If the patient suffered a STEMI, use the best lead with the ST elevation as the "fingerprint" to monitor for changes in the elevation of the ST segment. If the patient does not have ST-segment elevation, monitor leads III and V_5. ST-segment monitoring can also recognize a "silent MI" and may be more sensitive than a patient reporting chest pain in some situations.

> **HINT**
>
> High-risk surgical patients may also benefit from continuous ST-segment monitoring. Lead V_5 is the most valuable for identifying demand-related ischemia.

■ *What is the indication of a coronary artery bypass graft (CABG) in a patient with a STEMI?*

■ **Coronary artery anatomy not amendable by PCI**

An urgent CABG is indicated in patients with a STEMI experiencing ongoing or recurrent ischemia, cardiogenic shock, and severe HF, and when coronary artery anatomy is not amendable by PCI. Another indication is a patient who presents within 6 hours of onset of symptoms and is not considered to be a candidate for PCI or fibrinolytic therapy.

■ *What is the primary intervention for an RV infarction?*

■ **Fluid bolus**

The RV pumps differently from the left ventricle (LV). The LV has both spiral and circular muscles. The spiral muscles wrap around in such a manner that contribute to the contraction or "wringing" out of the blood of the heart. Volume overload worsens LV HF. In patients with LV involvement, fluid intake is limited, and venodilators such as nitrates and morphine are administered to lower the preload. The RV pumps using a bellows-type mechanism with the free wall moving toward the septum. Volume in the RV is required to produce an adequate stroke volume (SV). With RV involvement, fluid boluses are indicated.

> **HINT**
>
> Nitrates should not be used in RV infarction. Inotropic agents and intra-aortic balloon counterpulsations may also be indicated.

■ *Which class of anticoagulation therapy is not recommended in UA or NSTEMI?*

■ **Vitamin K antagonist**

An aspirin is recommended immediately and must be continued indefinitely. Clopidogrel (Plavix) may also be used as a substitute or as dual antiplatelet therapy. Glycoprotein IIb/IIIa inhibitors may also be administered to patients at higher risk and may be used as a third antiplatelet drug. UFH has been found to be beneficial for patients with UA. Factor Xa inhibitors have been shown to produce favorable outcomes in UA/NSTEMI and direct thrombin inhibitors may be an alternative. Warfarin (Coumadin), a vitamin K antagonist, has shown no benefit and may increase bleeding risk.

■ *What two drugs administered after ACS have been found to reduce LV remodeling?*

■ **β-blockers and ACE inhibitors**

β-blockers blunt the effects of the sympathetic nervous system, thereby reducing heart rate, blood pressure (BP), and contractility. They may also reduce the risk of serious arrhythmia by preventing maladaptive remodeling of the LV. ACE inhibitors can also prevent the adverse remodeling of the LV following an MI. They should be initiated during hospitalization and continued long term (unless contraindicated).

> **HINT**
β-blockers are contraindicated if signs of cardiogenic shock or severe HF are present.

■ *Which medication is indicated within the first 24 hours of AWMI with a ventricular ejection fraction (EF) of less than 40%?*
■ **ACE inhibitor**

This is an American College of Cardiology (ACC) and American Heart Association (AHA) Class I recommendation for AWMI. An ACE inhibitor may also be indicated for other types of AMI within the first 24 hours in the absence of hypotension. ACE inhibitors function as arterial vasodilators, decreasing LV afterload, lowering BP, and preventing adverse LV remodeling. Following an AMI, ventricular remodeling can result in sudden cardiac death (SCD) from ventricular arrhythmias.

> **HINT**
High-intensity statin therapy should be administered in all patients with STEMI (unless contraindicated).

■ *Which clinical situations would be contraindicated to administer an aldosterone blocker?*
■ **Elevated serum creatinine levels and hyperkalemia**

Inspra (Eplerenone) is an aldosterone blocker used in acute MIs and HF with an LVEF less than 40%. Contraindications include serum creatinine levels greater than 2.5 mg/dL in men and greater than 2.0 mg/dL in women. It is also contraindicated to administer if potassium levels are greater than 5.0 mEq/L.

■ *Acute pulmonary edema following an inferior MI with new onset holosystolic murmur indicates which complication?*
■ **Acute severe mitral regurgitation**

Acute severe mitral regurgitation usually occurs within 24 hours of the infarction but may occur up to 3 to 5 days later. Early recognition and management with inotropic therapy, intra-aortic balloon counterpulsation, and surgery can improve outcomes. Urgent surgical repair of the mitral valve is a Class I recommendation by the ACC/AHA.

> **HINT**
Mitral regurgitation causes a holosystolic murmur. Look at the type of murmur given as a hint in the scenario.

■ *What is the recommended treatment for pericarditis after STEMI?*
■ **ASA**

ASA is the recommended drug therapy following a STEMI. If ASA—even at higher doses—is ineffective, then administration of acetaminophen, colchine, or opioid analgesics may be ordered.

> ❯ **HINT**
> If pericarditis is due to STEMI, do not administer glucocorticoids and nonsteroidal anti-inflammatory drugs. These are potentially harmful in this situation.

COMPLICATIONS

■ *Which type of AMI is most likely to result in development of an LV mural thrombus?*
■ **AWMI**

A large AWMI develops LV regional wall akinesia or dyskinesia with blood stasis. The contributing factors of a thrombus include inflammation of the endocardium and a hypercoagulable state. The presentation is an embolic stroke and symptoms depend on the location of the embolus. An echocardiogram can be used to identify the thrombus in the LV. Anticoagulation therapy is used to manage the thrombus (heparin followed by warfarin for 3–6 months).

> ❯ **HINT**
> This complication of an LV mural thrombus typically occurs within the first 10 days of AMI.

■ *Following ventricular septal rupture (VSR), what type of murmur does the patient suddenly develop?*
■ **Loud, harsh holosystolic murmur**

The other symptoms of VSR include shortness of breath, biventricular failure, chest pain, and hypotension. This complication may occur within 24 hours of the AMI and then peaks again 3 to 5 days after the AMI. Very rarely would it present after 2 weeks. Treatment would be to manage the patient with vasodilators (reduce afterload), inotropic agents, diuretics, or mechanical support with an intra-aortic balloon pump (IABP) until the defect can be repaired surgically.

> ❯ **HINT**
> The complication of cardiogenic shock does not produce a murmur and mitral regurgitation has a soft systolic murmur.

■ *What is the most common arrhythmia or cause of death in an LV free wall rupture?*
■ **Pulseless electrical activity (PEA)**

LV free wall rupture may occur with large, transmural infarctions. Clinical presentation may include sudden, severe chest pain with abrupt hemodynamic collapse and PEA. This is due to the rapid development of pericardial tamponade (Box 1.9).

Box 1.9 Complications of AMI

Cardiogenic shock	Arrhythmias
Pericarditis	Ventricular free wall rupture
Post–myocardial infarction syndrome (Dressler's syndrome)	Cardiac tamponade
Left ventricular aneurysm	Ventricular septal rupture
Papillary muscle rupture/mitral regurgitation	Left ventricular mural thrombus

CARDIOGENIC SHOCK

- **What is the most severe form of HF?**
- **Cardiogenic shock**

Cardiogenic shock is the most severe form of HF and requires emergency management. Cardiogenic shock and pericardial tamponade are life-threatening conditions.

PATHOPHYSIOLOGY

- **What is the primary cause of cardiogenic shock?**
- **Ischemia**

Cardiogenic shock remains the leading cause of mortality in AMI. Ischemic cardiomyopathy is the primary cause of cardiogenic shock. Cardiogenic shock is defined as hypoperfusion due to cardiac failure (Box 1.10).

Box 1.10 Other Causes of Cardiogenic Shock

Hypertrophied cardiomyopathy	Stress-induced cardiomyopathy (takotsubo cardiomyopathy)
Aortic dissection with aortic insufficiency	Acute valvular regurgitation (endocarditis or chordal rupture)
Aortic or mitral stenosis (increases myocardial stress)	Cardiac tamponade
Acute myopericarditis	Massive pulmonary embolism

- **Which type of AMI is most likely associated with cardiogenic shock?**
- **AWMI**

Risk factors for the development of cardiogenic shock following an AMI include AWMI, multiple-vessel disease, older age, hypertension, prior MI, STEMI, and the presence of LBBB.

> **HINT**
> May use these risk factors as hints in a scenario to assist with
> recognizing cardiogenic shock.

SYMPTOMS/ASSESSMENT

▪ *What are the characteristic hemodynamic parameters of cardiogenic shock?*
▪ **Low cardiac output (CO)/cardiac index (CI), high systemic vascular**
  resistance (SVR), and high filling pressures

Cardiogenic shock demonstrates persistent hypotension with severe reduction in CO/CI and
adequate or elevated filling pressures. Compensatory mechanisms for low CO/CI include
vasoconstriction (elevates SVR) and tachycardia, which actually worsen the CO/CI due to high
resistance and increased workload of the heart, causing a vicious cycle to develop (Box 1.11).

> **HINT**
> Severe reduction of CI is defined as less than 1.8 L/min/m² without
> support and less than 2.0 to 2.2 L/min/m² with support.

Box 1.11 Other Symptoms of Cardiogenic Shock

Tachycardia	Altered mental status
Cool, clammy skin	Tachypnea
Pale nail beds with delayed capillary refill	Presence arrhythmias
Decreased urine output	

DIAGNOSIS

▪ *What monitoring device may be used to assist with the diagnosis*
  of cardiogenic shock?
▪ **Pulmonary artery catheter (PAC)**

A PAC provides information on the CO/CI, filling pressures and enables the calculation of
SVR. These readings are used to define and recognize cardiogenic shock. Newer hemodynamic monitors that are minimally invasive and that use the arterial waveform may also
be used to assist with the diagnosis.

> **HINT**
> An echocardiogram may be used to confirm the diagnosis of high filling
> pressures and to rule out other causes of hypotension following an AMI.

MEDICAL MANAGEMENT

▪ *What is the greatest concern when administering an inotropic agent to a*
  patient in cardiogenic shock?
▪ **Increase in myocardial workload and oxygen consumption**

Inotropic agents are frequently needed to increase CO and reduce filling pressures in the RV and LV, but they can increase the oxygen demand in a heart with limited oxygen supply. This may increase the ischemic injuries to the myocardium. Inotropes are recommended in hypoperfusion states with or without pulmonary congestion, but may be initiated at a lower dose in cardiogenic shock to limit complications.

> ❯ **HINT**
> Inotropes can also induce arrhythmias in ischemic hearts and should be closely monitored.

■ *What is a first-line intervention in managing hypotension in cardiogenic shock?*
■ **Inotropes**

Vasoconstrictors (e.g., norepinephrine) should not be used initially to treat hypotension in cardiogenic shock due to the presence of increased SVR. Other interventions for managing hypotension in cardiogenic shock include a combination of inotropic agents with vasodilators, fluid challenges with inotropic agents, and mechanical assistance (IABP, left ventricular assist device [LVAD]).

> ❯ **HINT**
> If vasoconstrictors are needed, it is recommended that norepinephrine be used with caution instead of dopamine.

SURGICAL MANAGEMENT

■ *What is the surgical procedure for managing cardiogenic shock?*
■ **Revascularization**

Emergency revascularization with a CABG procedure is indicated to improve survival. It may not improve the 30-day survival but it has been shown to improve long-term survival (6-month and 6-year outcome studies).

> ❯ **HINT**
> Mechanical devices (e.g., IABP) may be used as a bridge to stabilize the patient prior to surgery.

ARRHYTHMIAS ASSOCIATED WITH AMI

PATHOPHYSIOLOGY

■ *What is the most common reason for atrial arrhythmias following an AMI?*
■ **Left atrial (LA) distension**

LA distention is frequently caused by high pressure in the LV. Atrial arrhythmias (PACs, atrial flutter, atrial fibrillation [AF]) are frequently a result of LA distention following an AMI.

DIAGNOSIS

■ *What is the ECG finding of a first-degree heart block?*
■ **PR interval prolonged greater than 0.20**

A prolonged PR interval without loss of ventricular conduction indicates that the block is above the bundle of His. Calcium channel blockers and β-blockers may exacerbate the prolonging of the PR interval but should only be stopped if hemodynamically unstable or a higher degree of block occurs.

■ *What ECG change determines whether the block is above or below the nodal area?*
■ **Width of the QRS**

Supranodal or intranodal blocks produce a narrow QRS pattern. Blocks that occur below the nodal area produce a wide QRS complex.

MEDICAL MANAGEMENT

■ *Are rate-control drugs more effective in atrial flutter or AF?*
■ **Atrial fibrillation**

Atrial flutter is managed similarly to AF except ventricular rate control in the atrial flutter is not as responsive to rate-control drugs. A patient who develops an atrial flutter and is hemodynamically compromised requires synchronized electrical cardioversion.

■ *What complication of AMI would limit the use of IV diltiazem in the treatment of AF?*
■ **Moderate to severe HF**

The use of IV diltiazem in managing ventricular rate should be done cautiously following an AMI due to the complication of HF.

> **❭ HINT**
> Remember that some calcium channel blockers have negative inotropic effects.

COMPLICATIONS

■ *Following an inferior AMI, the patient presents with heart rate less than 40 bpm and hypotension. If BP is unresponsive to atropine, what complication may be the cause?*
■ **RV infarction and/or volume depletion**

An RV infarction can be present with an inferior wall MI. The presence of RV involvement and/or volume depletion will frequently result in continued hypotension, despite treatment with atropine. Obtain right-sided 12-lead ECG and administer fluids for RV involvement to correct the hypotension.

> **HINT**
> Bradycardia does not require treatment if the patient is hemodynamically stable (Box 1.12). Review Advanced Cardiovasular Life Support (ACLS) certification.

Box 1.12 Arrhythmias

Arrhythmia	Causes	Treatment/Management
Paroxysmal supraventricular tachycardia (PSVT)	Left atrial (LA) distention from elevated left ventricular (LV) pressures Inflammation (pericarditis)	Adenosine when hypotension not present If hypotensive, may use intravenous (IV) diltiazem or β-blocker If severe hypotension, perform synchronized electrical cardioversion
Atrial flutter	Sympathetic overstimulation of LA (usually transient)	Similar to AF except not responsive to rate-control drugs If symptomatic, perform synchronized electrical cardioversion If refractory medical management, may overdrive atrial pace
Atrial fibrillation	LV failure Ischemia to atria Right ventricular (RV) infarction Pericarditis	If unstable, immediate synchronized electrical cardioversion If stable, control the ventricular rate IV amiodarone or digoxin β-blocker may be used if not hypotensive Anticoagulation therapy
Bradycardia	Inferior or posterior wall myocardial infarction Vagal stimulation	If unstable, administer atropine 0.5 to 1 mg External or transvenous pacing
First-degree atrioventricular block	Inferior wall myocardial infarction	No treatment required
Second-degree Mobitz Type I AV block	Inferior wall myocardial infarction	No treatment required if hemodynamically stable
Second-degree Mobitz Type II AV block	Anterior wall myocardial infarction	Transcutaneous or transvenous pacing Atropine Possibly permanent demand pacemaker
Third-degree AV block	Anterior wall myocardial infarction Inferior wall myocardial infarction	Atropine if inferior wall MI Temporary transcutaneous or transvenous pacing Permanent demand pacemaker
Ventricular tachycardia (VT)	Monomorphic VT most likely caused by myocardial scar Polymorphic VT most likely caused by ischemia Electrolyte abnormalities Hypoxia Acid–base disturbances	If unstable, unsynchronized cardioversion If stable, administer amiodarone Maintain K^+ > 4 mEq/L and Mg^+ > 2.0 mEq/L
Ventricular tachycardia (VF)	MI Cardiogenic shock	Unsynchronized electrical countershock

HEART FAILURE

■ *During admission history, a patient with HF tells you that he is comfortable at rest but becomes short of breath during activities of daily living. In which New York Heart Association (NYHA) class is this patient?*

■ **NYHA Class II**

NYHA Class II is described as a person that is asymptomatic at rest but becomes dyspneic during normal activities of daily living.

The NYHA classification system was devised to classify the extent of HF based on functional capacity. It lists four categories of cardiac disease (Classes I-IV) ranging from mild to severe with progressively increasing symptoms of physical limitation associated with each class. For more information, please see www.my.americanheart.org.

■ *At which stage is a patient with normal EF, but a history of mitral regurgitation, according to the ACC/AHA stages?*

■ **Stage B**

The ACC/AHA stages of HF were developed for early identification of at-risk patients for HF (Table 1.1). The stages are not meant to replace the NYHA classification system. Patients in stages A and B are at risk for HF but are currently not symptomatic. The staging system includes therapy recommendations for each stage (Table 1.2).

Table 1.1 ACC/AHA Stages in Development of HF

Stage	Definition	Patients at risk
Stage A	At high risk for HF but without structural heart disease or symptoms of HF	Hypertension Atherosclerotic disease Diabetes Obesity Metabolic syndrome Using cardiotoxins Family history of cardiomyopathy
Stage B	Structural heart disease but without signs or symptoms of HF	Previous MI LV remodeling including LVH and low EF Asymptomatic valvular disease
Stage C	Structural heart disease with prior or current symptoms of HF	Known structural heart disease Shortness of breath Fatigue, reduced exercise tolerance
Stage D	Refractory HF requiring specialized interventions	Marked symptoms at rest despite maximal medical therapy

Adapted from the ACC/AHA practice guidelines.

Table 1.2 ACC/AHA-Recommended Therapy by Stage

Stage	Goals	Drugs	Devices/Options
Stage A	Treat hypertension Encourage smoking cessation Treat lipid disorders Encourage regular exercise Discourage alcohol intake, illicit drug use Control metabolic syndrome	ACE inhibitor or angiotensin receptor blocker (ARB) in appropriate patients for vascular disease or diabetes	
Stage B	Same as Stage A	ACE inhibitor or ARB in appropriate patients β-blockers in appropriate patients	
Stage C	All measures under Stages A and B Dietary salt restriction	Diuretics for fluid retention ACEI β-blockers Selected patients Aldosterone antagonist ARBs Digitalis Hydralazine/nitrates	Biventricular pacing Implantable defibrillators
Stage D	Appropriate measures under Stages A, B, and C. Decision regarding appropriate level of care		Compassionate end-of-life care/hospice Extraordinary measures Heart transplant Chronic inotropes Permanent mechanical support Experimental surgery or drugs

Adapted from the ACC/AHA practice guidelines.

PATHOPHYSIOLOGY

■ *Which type of HF causes a difficulty in filling the ventricles?*
■ **Diastolic dysfunction**

HF caused by diastolic dysfunction is a result of a difficulty with the filling of the ventricles. The difficulty with the ventricular filling may be caused by an incomplete ventricular relaxation, increased stiffness, pericardial restraint, or high intrathoracic pressure. The most common cause is hypertrophy of cardiac muscle.

■ *What is the most common underlying etiology of a diastolic dysfunction HF?*
■ **Hypertrophic cardiomyopathy**

Hypertrophic cardiomyopathy is the most common cause of diastolic dysfunction HF. It may be congenital or caused by chronic hypertension or aortic stenosis.

■ *Which commonly used drug classification in HF is contraindicated if the underlying abnormality is a diastolic dysfunction?*
■ **Inotropic agents**

The problem is not with the contractility of the pump (most patients with diastolic dysfunction actually have normal EF), but with a small ventricular chamber. An inotropic agent will constrict the chamber, limiting the filling even more. Calcium channel blockers are typically used to manage diastolic dysfunction. The goal is afterload reduction and relaxation of the ventricles.

> ❭ HINT
> Diastolic dysfunction HF frequently exhibits symptoms of failure but has a high EF.

■ *What type of HF has a decreased EF?*
■ **Systolic dysfunction**

Systolic dysfunction is caused by poor contractility or reduction in CO. It is commonly defined as an EF less than 35% to 40%. It is the most common cause of HF (Box 1.13).

Box 1.13 Etiology of Systolic Dysfunction HF

Myocardial ischemia	Obstructive cardiomyopathy
Myocardial infarction	Infection
Valvular heart disease	Toxin exposure
Chronic volume overload	Congenital heart defects
Dilated cardiomyopathy	

The goal is to decrease preload and afterload.

> ❭ HINT
> Remember:
> Preload = Volume
> Afterload = Resistance

■ *Drugs used to manage HF typically inhibit which neurohormonal compensatory mechanism?*
■ **Renin-angiotensin system (RAS)**

Aldosterone blockers, ACE inhibitors, and angiotensin receptor blockers (ARBs) all work on the RAS (Figure 1.1).

■ *What compensatory mechanism increases blood flow to the kidneys, thus decreasing the release of renin?*
■ **Brain natriuretic peptide (BNP)**

BNP is a peptide released by stretched myocytes during HF. The BNP will increase glomerular filtration rates, increase renal blood flow, decrease the release of renin, and decrease Na^+ reabsorption by the kidneys.

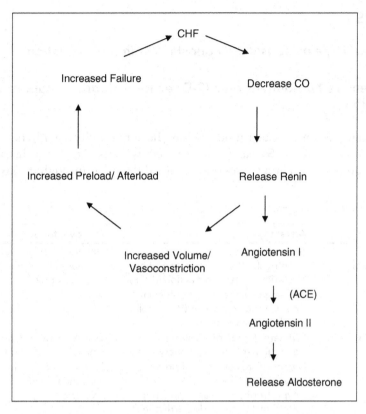

FIGURE 1.1 Renin–angiotensin system (RAS).

SYMPTOMS/ASSESSMENT

■ *Which abnormal heart sound is commonly associated with HF?*

■ **S_3**

S_3 is a gallop that occurs during early diastole and is frequently caused by ventricular over-load (Box 1.14).

> ❯ HINT
> A patient scenario with an S_3 is typically HF, whereas an S_4 is angina.

Box 1.14 Symptoms of HF

Left-Sided Failure	Right-Sided Failure	Other Symptoms
Crackles	Jugular venous distention	Fatigue
Tachypnea	Hepatomegaly	Weakness
Dyspnea	Splenomegaly	Decreased exercise tolerance
Hypoxemia	Elevated central venous pressure (CVP)	Unexplained confusion
Cough	Peripheral edema	
Pink, frothy sputum	Decreased CO	
Decreased CO	Tachycardia	
Orthopnea		
Tachycardia		

DIAGNOSIS

■ *What is the single most useful diagnostic test in the evaluation of a patient with HF?*

■ **Comprehensive two-dimensional (2-D) echocardiogram coupled with Doppler flow**

The 2-D echocardiogram can determine whether the abnormality is with the myocardium, heart valves, or pericardium. SV can be determined with use of echocardiogram by measuring the LV outflow tract and the amount of blood that goes through it (Box 1.15).

Box 1.15 Other Diagnostic Tests

Test	Advantage	Disadvantage
Radionuclide ventriculography	Accurate measurements of left ventricular (LV) function and right ventricular ejection fraction (RVEF)	Unable to assess valve abnormalities or cardiac hypertrophy
MRI	Evaluate chamber size, ventricular mass, right ventricular (RV) dysplasia, and pericardial disease	
Chest x-ray (CXR)	Estimate degree of cardiac enlargement and pulmonary edema	Unable to determine LV function or valvular abnormalities
12-lead ECG	Demonstrate evidence of prior myocardial infarction, LV hypertrophy, cardiac conduction abnormality, or cardiac arrhythmia	Unable to determine the mechanical function of the ventricles

■ *Which laboratory test may be used to determine the severity of HF?*

■ **BNP levels**

BNP levels may also be used to differentiate between HF and pulmonary disease. Elevated BNP levels accurately detect CHF in 95% to 97% of patients (100 pg/mL). The diagnostic "gray area" is between 100 and 500 pg/mL and anything greater than 500 pg/mL is positive.

■ *Are there false positives with elevated BNP levels?*

■ **Yes**

There are disease processes that can falsely elevate BNP levels, such as hypertension, LV hypertrophy, renal failure, and brain injury.

■ *What is the primary difference between BNP and NT-ProBNP levels?*

■ **Half-life of NT-ProBNP is longer than BNP**

The half-life of NT-ProBNP is 1 to 2 hours versus 20 minutes with BNP. The NT-ProBNP levels correlate to the NYHA classifications:

>
NYHA I = mean 1015
NYHA II = mean 1666
NYHA III = mean 3029
NYHA IV = mean 3465

MANAGEMENT

- *A patient on an ACE inhibitor is noncompliant. Which side effect of the ACE inhibitor is the most likely cause?*
- **Dry, nonproductive cough**

Some patients who cough while taking ACE inhibitors have this symptom because of CHF rather than ACE inhibitor intolerance and might improve with further diuresis. Others, develop a dry, hacking cough that can interfere with activities of daily living (i.e., eating, talking, sleeping) and may require changing to an ARB.

> **HINT**
> Recognize the drug is an ACE inhibitor when it ends in "-pril."

- *What electrolyte abnormality is common with an ACE inhibitor?*
- **Hyperkalemia**

ACE inhibitors promotes the excretion of Na^+ and water, thus increasing the reabsorption of K^+. Hyperkalemia may occur when patients are on ACE inhibitors, ARBs, and aldosterone antagonists. Serum potassium levels should be monitored closely in HF patients. Diuretics are commonly used in HF and can lead to hypokalemia. Hypokalemia may adversely affect cardiac conduction and lead to arrhythmias and sudden death.

> **HINT**
> Remember hypokalemia may increase the risk of digitalis toxicity.

- *Which class of drugs is used if a patient is ACE-inhibitor intolerant?*
- **ARB**

ARBs allow the conversion of angiotensin I to angiotensin II but block the receptor sites of angiotensin II. These drugs have side effects similar to an ACE inhibitor but do not exhibit the cough or angioedema. Following an episode of angioedema, the patient should have the ACE inhibitor changed to an ARB. ARBs may be used as a first-line treatment with mild to moderate HF and reduced LVEF.

- *A person with symptomatic HF on an ACE inhibitor and β-blocker has persistent symptoms. Which combinations of medications are recommended at this time?*
- **Hydralazine and nitrate**

The addition of a combination of hydralazine and nitrate is reasonable for patients with reduced LVEF, who are already taking an ACE inhibitor and β-blocker, but have persistent symptoms.

> **❯ HINT**
> The combination of hydralazine and nitrate is also recommended to
> improve outcomes for African Americans with moderate to severe
> symptoms.

■ *Which ECG finding indicates the need for cardiac resynchronization therapy?*
■ **QRS duration 0.12 seconds or longer**

Other indications include patients with LVEF 35% or less, sinus rhythm, and NYHA functional Class III or ambulatory IV.

DISSECTING THORACIC AND ABDOMINAL AORTA ANEURYSMS

■ *What is an aortic dissection?*
■ **Lengthwise separation of the medial layer of the aorta**

An aortic dissection involves the medial layer of the aorta. There is a lengthwise separation of the medial layer due to a tear in the intima with intramedial extravasation. Blood flows between the intimal and medial layers creating a double lumen, called a false lumen and a true lumen. Dissection can be acute, present within the first 14 days of initial injury, or chronic, with presentation longer than 14 days.

> **❯ HINT**
> A traumatic aortic aneurysm is a disruption of the intimal, medial, and
> adventitial layers. This is called a transection.

■ *What happens if blood flows into the false lumen, forming a large hematoma?*
■ **Partial to complete obstruction of the true lumen**

Following the intimal tear, blood enters the medial layer and can form a large hematoma, obstructing the true lumen and affecting distal perfusion. Shearing forces can also cause further tears, producing exit sites and flow back into the true lumen (Box 1.16).

> **❯ HINT**
> Thoracic aortic aneurysm occurs above the diaphragm and abdominal
> aortic aneurysm occurs below.

Box 1.16 Sites of Aortic Dissections

Ascending aorta	Descending aorta
Aortic arch	Thoracoabdominal aorta

■ *What genetic disorder of connective tissue resulting in above-average height*
  causes risk for an aortic dissection?
■ **Marfan's syndrome**

Marfan's syndrome is inherited as a dominant trait and symptoms vary from mild to severe. People with Marfan's syndrome tend to be very tall, with long limbs and fingers. They are at risk for aortic aneurysms and dissections (Box 1.17).

> **〉 HINT**
> Other connective tissue diseases that may be used in the scenario include Ehlers–Danlos or Loeys–Dietz

Box 1.17 Causes/Risk Factors of Aortic Dissention

Hypertension, especially uncontrolled	Chronic corticosteroid or immunosuppressive use
Pheochromocytoma	Congenital factors (bicuspid valve)
Cocaine or other stimulant use	Inflammatory vasculitis
Weight lifting or other Valsalva maneuvers	Atherosclerosis (e.g., peripheral vascular disease [PVD], coronary artery disease)
Pregnancy	Infections of the vascular wall
Genetic	Iatrogenic (e.g., aortic valve manipulation)
Polycystic kidney disease	

PATHOPHYSIOLOGY

- **What leads to the complication of organ ischemia with an aortic dissection?**
- **Obstruction of arterial branches off the aorta**

The dissection can propagate through the arteries that branch off of the aorta, leading to stenosis or obstruction. The obstruction of flow leads to end-organ ischemia and failure. Dissections can extend retrograde and antegrade (Box 1.18).

Box 1.18 Branch Arteries of the Aorta

Coronary	Renal
Brachiocephalic (e.g., subclavian, carotid)	Visceral (e.g., superior and inferior mesenteric arteries)
Intercostal	

> **〉 HINT**
> May present with symptoms of end-organ ischemia from loss of blood flow through these arteries.

- **What part of the aorta is involved in a DeBakey Type II dissection?**
- **Ascending aorta**

There are two major classification systems used in aortic dissections: DeBakey and Stanford systems. The DeBakey system uses Type I to Type III, whereas the Stanford system uses Type A and B (Box 1.19).

Box 1.19 Classifications of Aortic Dissections

DeBakey System	Type I	Type II	Type III
	Ascending and also involvement of descending aorta	Ascending aorta only	Only the descending is involved: IIIA: distal to the left subclavian artery to the diaphragm IIIB: descending aorta below the diaphragm
Stanford System	Type A	Type B	
	Ascending involved	Descending involved	

SYMPTOMS/ASSESSMENT

- *How is the pain of an aortic dissection frequently described?*
- **Ripping or tearing sensation**

The quality and severity of pain is frequently used to assist with the diagnosis of a dissection. The pain is initially described as a "ripping or tearing" sensation. It is of abrupt onset and severe in intensity. There is sometimes a "latency" period during which the pain will get better after the initial onset, but then it returns as a "knife-like" severe pain.

> ❯ HINT
> These patients typically report 10/10 pain despite pain management and will typically be agitated.

- *What specific physical examination should be performed in a suspected thoracic aortic dissection?*
- **Obtain BP in both arms**

Compare BPs obtained in each arm. A high-risk feature would be a discrepancy of systolic BP greater than 20 mmHg. Another assessment includes assessing pulses in the upper limbs compared to the lower limbs. A significant pulse deficit in the lower extremity should also increase level of suspicion (Box 1.20).

> ❯ HINT
> An associated new-onset diastolic murmur (aortic regurgitation) may indicate dissection of the ascending aorta.

Box 1.20 Signs of Aortic Dissection

Chest or abdominal pain (refers to the back)	Bruit (carotid, brachial, femoral)
Tracheal compression	Focal neurological deficits
Laryngeal hoarseness (pressure on recurrent laryngeal nerve)	Hemothorax
Dysphagia	Anxiety and premonition of death
Abdominal mass (pulsating)	Fever
Diastolic murmur (high-pitched blowing)	Hypertension
Pulse deficit	Manifestations of pericardial tamponade
Syncope	

■ *What are the three signs of Horner's syndrome?*

■ **Ptosis, miosis, and anhidrosis**

Horner's syndrome is caused by an interruption in the cervical sympathetic ganglia and manifests as ptosis, miosis, and anhidrosis. This can occur with a dissection of the aortic arch.

> ❯ **HINT**
> Horner's syndrome is the loss of sympathetic nervous system innervation.

DIAGNOSIS

■ *What diagnostic test is best used in an unstable patient with suspected aortic dissection?*

■ **Echocardiogram**

A chest x-ray (CXR) is frequently the initial evaluation but may not reveal any significant findings. A computed tomography (CT) scan is used in hemodynamically stable patients, whereas an echocardiogram is preferred if unstable. It is performed at the bedside, is rapid and noninvasive (unless a transesophageal echocardiogram [TEE] is used, which is minimally invasive). An emergency CT angiography with 3-D reconstruction is being used to obtain a view of the aorta without the potential complications of the more invasive aortogram.

> ❯ **HINT**
> The gold standard is still considered to be the aortogram for diagnosis of aortic dissection.

The aortogram can pinpoint the site of intimal tear, the true and false lumen entry site, appearance of dye outside of the aorta, and bulging of aorta.

■ *What is the disadvantage of a TEE in diagnosing aortic dissection?*

■ **Limited ability to visualize the distal ascending aorta**

TEE has limited ability to visualize the distal ascending aorta and proximal arch because of the air-filled trachea and main stem bronchus.

MEDICAL MANAGEMENT

■ *What class of drugs is recommended for the initial management of a thoracic aortic dissection?*

■ **β-blocker**

The initial treatment goal is to decrease the aorta wall stress by slowing the heart rate and lowering the BP. Esmolol (Brevibloc) is frequently used in acute management. If contraindicated to use a β-blocker, the second choice of drugs is nondihydropyridine calcium channel-blocking agents, which should be utilized as an alternative for rate control. β-blockers should be used cautiously in acute aortic regurgitation due to the block on compensatory tachycardia.

> **HINT**
>
> Vasodilator therapy, such as Nipride, should not be used until after heart rate control has been achieved to avoid reflex tachycardia.

■ *What is the target BP and heart rate in an acute aortic dissection?*

■ **Systolic rate between 110 and 120 mmHg and heart rate between 60 and 80 bpm**

During an acute aortic dissection, aggressive management of BP and heart rate should be initiated to lower the intraluminal pressure to limit extension of dissection. The end-organ perfusion also needs to be evaluated when managing BP to prevent hypoperfusion.

> **HINT**
>
> Most patients will be hypertensive; a hypotensive presentation may indicate pericardial tamponade or hemorrhage into the pleural or retroperitoneal space.

SURGICAL MANAGEMENT

■ *When is surgical repair recommended in an asymptomatic patient with a descending aortic aneurysm?*

■ **Aneurysm greater than 5.5 cm**

A patient with a stable chronic dissection may be observed for signs of progressive enlargement of the aorta. Surgical intervention is recommended with an aneurysm in the descending aorta greater than 5.5 cm. It is reasonable to follow up with CT scans or ultrasonography every 12 months to evaluate the size of the aneurysm, if less than 5.5 cm. Other indications for surgery include a saccular aneurysm or postsurgical pseudoaneurysm.

> **HINT**
>
> If the patient is symptomatic with acute dissection of any size, surgical intervention may be recommended.

■ *What technique is used in the operating room to protect organs from ischemia during repair of the aorta?*

■ **Cardiopulmonary bypass (CPB)**

Other correct answers include partial left heart bypass, deep hypothermic circulatory arrest, and retrograde perfusion. Goals of surgery include repair of aorta as well as prevention of ischemic insult to distal organs. Surgical procedures on aorta can include intimal flap repair, removal of thrombosis and false lumen, replacement of dilated aorta with a graft, repair of aortic root, and replacement of aortic valve. Endovascular repair may also be used in descending aortic dissections through femoral access.

> **HINT**
CPB requires heparinization. Postoperative management includes assessing for signs of coagulopathy and continued reversing of heparin.

■ *What technique may be used to protect the spinal cord during surgical or endovascular repair of descending aorta?*

■ **Cerebrospinal fluid (CSF) drainage**

CSF drainage is recommended in patients with high risk for spinal cord ischemia during surgical repair of the descending aorta. They may also use other spinal cord perfusion techniques such as proximal aortic pressure maintenance and distal aortic perfusion to optimize spinal cord perfusion (Box 1.21).

Box 1.21 Other Treatments Used in the Prevention of
Spinal Cord Ischemia

Intraoperative systemic hypothermia	Intrathecal papaverine
Epidural irrigation with hypothermic solution	Metabolic suppression with anesthetic agents
High-dose glucocorticosteroids	Reimplantation of intercostal arteries
Osmotic diuretic (i.e., Mannitol)	Distal perfusion

> **HINT**
A postoperative patient should be assessed for any motor or sensory abnormalities.

■ *What is the priority in the postoperative care of an aortic repair with graft placement?*

■ **BP management**

BP management is important in postoperative (as well as preoperative) care to prevent disruption of the graft, dissection, and hemorrhage. Antihypertensive agents used preoperatively may be continued in the postoperative period. Hemodynamic monitoring, prevention of fluid overload, correct coagulopathy, and administration of antibiotics to prevent graft infections are components of postoperative management.

■ *Where does an embolism from catheter manipulation during interventional graft placement typically travel?*

■ **Legs and viscera**

The internal surface of the aorta can be covered by atheromas. Manipulation of the catheter during interventional stent placement can break loose debris and become a distal embolism. This may involve the lower extremities or the abdominal viscera. Another complication can be migration of the graft.

> **HINT**
> May involve the renal, mesenteric, or iliac arteries. Assess for signs of organ hypoperfusion postprocedure.

COMPLICATIONS

■ *What part of the aorta is at the highest risk for aortic rupture?*

■ **Ascending aorta**

A high-risk aortic injury for rupture involves the ascending portion of the aorta and should be referred for emergent surgery to prevent life-threatening complications.

> **HINT**
> Ascending aortic dissections can dissect through the aortic valve resulting in acute aortic regurgitation and HF.

■ *Three days after the repair of a descending aortic dissection (Type B) with a graft placement, a patient develops severe abdominal pain and shows occult blood in stool. What is the most likely cause for the abdominal pain?*

■ **Bowel ischemia/infarction**

Dissection of the aorta can involve the branch arteries. The superior and inferior mesenteric arteries may be involved in a descending aortic dissection. Signs of malperfusion of the bowel with ischemia and infarction include new-onset severe abdominal pain, elevated lactate and CPK levels, and sometimes the presence of occult blood in stool. The diagnostic procedure is typically abdominal CT.

> **HINT**
> Most postoperative complications will involve the malperfusion of organs from branch artery occlusion (Box 1.22).

Box 1.22 Complications

Perioperative MI	Graft occlusion
Stroke	Arterial embolism to extremities
Hypertension	Aortic thrombosis/stenosis
Low cardiac output syndrome	Wound infection
Renal failure	Bowel ischemia
Dysrhythmias	Paraplegia
Coagulopathies/disseminated intra-vasular coagulopathy (DIC)	Hemorrhage (retroperitoneal, intraperitoneal)
Graft infections	

CARDIAC TRAUMA

PERICARDIAL TAMPONADE

■ *What is the most common mechanism for a traumatic pericardial tamponade?*
■ **Penetrating injury**

Pericardial tamponade is caused by bleeding into the pericardial sac due to a ruptured coronary artery, lacerated pericardium, or an injury to the myocardium.

Pathophysiology

■ *Is pericardial tamponade considered a diastolic or systolic dysfunction?*
■ **Diastolic dysfunction**

The pericardial sac usually contains 25 to 50 mL of fluid. Following an injury, blood accumulates within the pericardial sac, causing a constriction on the heart. The pericardial pressure becomes higher than the ventricular filling pressures, interfering with the ability of the ventricles to fill with blood (diastolic phase). The amount of blood required to impair filling depends upon the rate of the accumulation of blood and the compliance of the pericardial sac.

> ❯ HINT
> Pericardial tamponade is a constrictive cardiomyopathy.

Symptoms/Assessment

■ *What is the first sign of a traumatic pericardial tamponade?*
■ **Tachycardia**

A significant decrease in ventricular filling results in a decrease in SV. Tachycardia is a compensatory mechanism, an attempt to maintain a normal CO.

> ❯ HINT
> Suspect a pericardial tamponade in chest trauma if shock symptoms are unresponsive to fluid administration.

■ *What is the Beck's triad?*
■ **Increased jugular venous distention, hypotension, and muffled heart sounds**

The pressure caused by the blood in the pericardial sac limits the filling of the heart, backing the blood up into the venous circulation. This produces jugular venous distention. The decreased filling results in a decrease in SV leading to hypotension. The accumulation of blood in the pericardial sac muffles the heart sounds. The presentation of a classical Beck's triad occurs with an acute cardiac tamponade.

> ❯ HINT
> Look for distended jugular veins as a clue of the elevated central venous pressure. Trauma patients typically have flat neck veins due to hypovolemia (Box 1.23).

Box 1.23 Other Symptoms of
Pericardial Tamponade

Dyspnea
Cyanosis
Diaphoresis
Cold, clammy skin
Pulsus paradoxus
Pericardial friction rub
Agitation
Feelings of impending doom

> ❯ **HINT**
>
> Scenario of a penetrating chest wound in which the patient insists on sitting bolt upright, is agitated and confused, or has air hunger is more likely to be a condition of pericardial tamponade.

■ *What is the most common type of cardiac arrest?*

■ **PEA**

Pulseless electrical activity (PEA) occurs in cardiac tamponade due to the constriction interfering with the mechanical activity of the heart but the electrical activity continues.

> ❯ **HINT**
>
> Cardiac tamponade would be one of the differential diagnoses of PEA in a trauma patient.

Diagnosis

■ *What CXR changes would you expect to find in a pericardial tamponade?*

■ **Widened mediastinum (enlarged cardiac silhouette)**

The heart may also have the appearance of a water-bottle shape. Not all patients with a traumatic pericardial tamponade will demonstrate CXR findings and therefore it should not be used alone to rule out the injury. A CT scan may also be used to identify pericardial fluid but only on a stable patient.

■ *Which diagnostic test is frequently used in the emergency room to screen for a pericardial tamponade?*

■ **Ultrasonography**

Focused assessment sonography for trauma (FAST) is used to assess the abdomen and may frequently be used to assess the chest for pericardial tamponade. Ultrasonography is one of the most important tools for recognizing a tamponade. The classical pattern is a "swinging" heart. The heart oscillates within the pericardium side to side (this produces the pulsus alternans seen on the ECG). It may also detect pericardial fluid, thrombus, and collapsing of the ventricular wall during diastole.

Medical Management

■ *A patient is found to have a pericardial tamponade following a stab wound to the anterior chest. He is hypotensive. What would be the immediate medical management of this patient?*

■ **Oxygen, fluid bolus, inotropic agent**

Remember the ABCs of trauma. Oxygen is administered and pulse oximetry should be monitored. The effects of hypovolemia are profound in a cardiac tamponade and fluid bolus may be used to increase SV and perfusion. Volume overload may worsen the ventricular contractility and should be avoided. Passive elevation of the legs may also be used to increase venous return and improve ventricular filling. Positive inotropic drugs (i.e., dobutamine) may improve contractility without increasing SVR.

> **❯ HINT**
> Avoid positive pressure ventilation, if possible. If intubated and ventilated, minimize positive end-expiratory pressure (PEEP) levels.

Surgical Management

■ *What is the definitive care for a pericardial tamponade?*

■ **Remove the blood/fluid from the pericardial space**

This can be done with an emergency subxiphoid percutaneous aspiration in an unstable patient in the emergency department. Pericardiocentesis can also be performed using landmarks or guided by echocardiogram and by placing a drain tube. Pericardotomy can also be performed using a balloon to create the pericardial window. Open thoracotomy may be required in some cases. A minimally invasive technique commonly used is the video-assisted thorascopic (VAT) procedure.

■ *What is a life-threatening complication of a pericardiocentesis?*

■ **Puncture and rupture of the myocardium or coronary arteries**

Other complications include arrhythmias, puncture of the lungs, liver, or stomach. Continuous ECG monitoring to detect ventricular arrhythmias is recommended.

MYOCARDIAL CONTUSION

Pathophysiology

Myocardial contusion (MC) is a hemorrhage within the myocardium, marked by cellular injury and extravasation of red blood cells (RBCs) into the muscle fibers. Contusion severity ranges from subepicardial to intramural hemorrhage into the intraventricular septum. The hemorrhage can extend up to varying depths into the myocardium. During recovery, the healing occurs with scar formation.

■ *Which ventricle is the most susceptible to injury following a blunt chest trauma?*

■ **RV**

The RV is the most vulnerable because of its location under the sternum. The mitral and aortic valves are more likely to be injured than the tricuspid and pulmonic because of higher pressures in the LV.

Symptoms/Assessment

■ *What is the most common patient complaint of an MC?*

■ **Chest pain**

The chest pain is precordial and is frequently unrelieved by analgesics. The symptoms and presentation vary following a myocardial contusion. Some patients may present without symptoms.

■ *What is the most common arrhythmia following an MC?*

■ **Sinus tachycardia**

Following a trauma, most patients will present with sinus tachycardia, which is a sympathetic nervous system response. The most lethal arrhythmias of a myocardial contusion are ventricular tachycardia and VF. Other arrhythmias include AF, heart blocks, right bundle branch block, and right bundle branch block with hemiblock. The severity of the arrhythmia does not correlate with the severity of the contusion (Box 1.24).

> **❯ HINT**
> Tachycardia beyond expectation for hypovolemia based upon calculated blood loss is a high suspicion for MC.

Box 1.24 Other Symptoms of MCs

Bruising on chest wall	Pericardial friction rub/murmurs
Crackles	Presence of associated injuries
S_3 gallop	Hypotension

■ *When does a patient require cardiac monitoring?*

■ **Abnormal echocardiogram or ECG**

Monitoring is not required if both echocardiogram and ECG are normal in a hemodynamically stable patient.

Diagnosis

■ *Which of the cardiac markers is most specific to injury caused by MC?*

■ **Troponin levels**

CPK-MB levels will elevate following skeletal muscle trauma and myocardial injury and are nonspecific for myocardium. Troponin levels are more specific to myocardial injury.

■ *An echocardiogram is used to identify which specific change found in an MC?*
■ **Abnormal wall motion**

Transthoracic and esophageal echocardiograms can be used to identify abnormalities in cardiac function that can be used in diagnosing myocardial contusions. It is also used to identify patients requiring cardiac monitoring and the presence of complications, such as pericardial effusion. The abnormal wall motion results in a decrease in SV, CO, and BP.

Management

■ *Within what time period following an MC would arrhythmias most commonly occur?*
■ **Within 24 to 48 hours**

A patient sustaining a blunt chest trauma with a high suspicion of MC should have cardiac monitoring for 24 to 48 hours. Other management issues include hemodynamic stabilization and treatment of associated injuries.

Complications

■ *Following a blunt chest trauma, a patient develops a new-onset systolic murmur. Which valve abnormality is most likely the cause?*
■ **Mitral regurgitation**

The two most common valves to be damaged following a blunt chest injury are the mitral and aortic valves. A rupture (regurgitation) of the mitral valve results in a systolic murmur, whereas a rupture of the aortic valve would cause a diastolic murmur (Box 1.25).

> ❯ HINT
> Valve regurgitation causes a murmur to be heard during the cardiac cycle when the valve should be closed. The mitral valve should be closed during systole (systolic murmur) and the aortic valve must close during diastole (diastolic murmur).

Box 1.25 Complications of MCs

Arrhythmias	Cardiac rupture
LV dysfunction with CHF	Ventricular thrombosis
Acute valvular regurgitation (valve rupture)	Chronic constrictive pericarditis
Ventricular aneurysm	
Pericardial effusion (with or without tamponade)	Coronary vasospasm, thrombosis, or rupture
Intracardiac structural damage	Atrial fistula

TRAUMATIC AORTIC ANEURYSM

Traumatic aortic aneurysm is a cause of death at the scene due to a completely transected aorta (intimal, medial, and adventitia layers). If the patient survives to the emergency department, he or she will usually have a small tear or a partial-thickness tear of the aorta forming an aneurysm.

Pathophysiology

■ *A traumatic aortic aneurysm is most likely to be caused by what mechanism of injury?*
■ **Sudden deceleration**

A sudden deceleration may be either horizontal (i.e., high-speed motor vechile crash [MVC]) or vertical (i.e., fall). The aorta is relatively mobile in the chest and will continue to travel after the sudden deceleration except where it is secured by a ligament.

> ❯ HINT
> The scenario given will usually be a high-speed MVC with a sudden deceleration on impact.

■ *What is the most common site of the aorta for a traumatic aortic aneurysm?*
■ **Level of the isthmus**

The level of the isthmus is distal to the great vessels, where the aorta begins to descend. The ligamentum of arteriosum secures the proximal descending thoracic aorta, just distal to the arch (at the level of the isthmus). During the sudden deceleration, this ligament holds the aorta back while the arch of the aorta continues to travel. This causes the aorta to transect at the level of the isthmus. Other sites of fixation include the ascending aorta, the aortic root, and the diaphragmatic hiatus.

Symptoms/Assessment

■ *What is the classic sign of a traumatic aortic aneurysm?*
■ **Widened mediastinum on CXR**

Patients may be relatively asymptomatic for a traumatic aortic aneurysm. The CXR is used as a screening device. The patient may also present as hemodynamically unstable if there is bleeding into the thoracic cavity or in the presence of associated injuries. The patient may present with a cyclic pattern of responding to a fluid bolus, then becoming hypotensive again (Box 1.26).

> ❯ HINT
> Hemodynamic stability needs to be determined to guide management of these patients.

Box 1.26 Other Symptoms of Aortic Aneurysm

Retrosternal or intracapsular chest pain	Swelling at base of neck
Hoarseness (tracheal compression)	Paraplegia
Dysphagia (esophageal compression)	Pseudocoarctation syndrome
Systolic murmur over base of neck	

■ *What are the signs of pseudocoarctation syndrome?*

■ **Hypertension in upper extremities and hypotension in lower extremities**

The patient may present with bounding pulses in the upper extremities and hypertension. The pulses are diminished in the lower extremities and hypotensive. This is due to the formation of a hematoma, narrowing the lumen of the aorta. The narrowing creates a high pressure above and low pressure below the site. This can occur following a traumatic transection but is not common.

> **❭ HINT**
> The question may also have the nurse check BP in both arms, assessing for a significant difference in BP between the two.

■ *A chest tube is placed for left-sided hemothorax in a trauma patient. What finding following chest tube placement is a sign of an aortic injury?*

■ **Large volume of bright-red blood from the chest tube**

A rupture of the aorta frequently results in bleeding into the left pleural space and a resulting hemothorax. The sign is a large-volume hemorrhage from the chest tube, typically bright-red blood.

Diagnosis

■ *What are three findings on a CXR that would lead to suspicion of a thoracic aortic aneurysm?*

■ **Widened mediastinum, loss of aortic knob, or left apical cap**

A widened mediastinum is the most classic sign found on a CXR. The loss of the aortic knob (also called superior widened mediastinum) and an apical cap may also be commonly seen in a thoracic aortic aneurysm. Other CXR signs include a deviated nasogastric (NG) tube to the right, an obvious double lumen contour of the aorta, or depression of the left-stem bronchus.

■ *Which radiographic procedure has the most definitive diagnosis for a thoracic aortic aneurysm?*

■ **Arteriogram**

The CXR is used as a screening device and is used in combination with the mechanism of injury to warrant further workup for an aneurysm. A CT scan is the best screening tool. The arteriogram has been the gold standard for diagnosing an aortic injury but is being replaced with a multidetector helical CT scan. An older CT scan using a single slice helical view is not adequate to plan surgery by itself. If the multidetector CT scan findings are equivocal or do not visualize branch vessels or surrounding structures, an angiogram is used as a follow-up prior to surgery.

> ### HINT
> If the question asks for the gold standard, "arteriogram" as the answer.

Medical Management

■ *At what level should the systolic blood pressure (SBP) be maintained in a patient with thoracic aortic aneurysm?*

■ **Between 90 and 120 mmHg**

Allowing an increase in SBP above 120 mmHg will increase the risk of free rupture of the aneurysm. Lowering the SBP below 90 mmHg will cause hypoperfusion and may contribute to organ dysfunction. Short-acting antihypertensives may be used in the acute period to maintain BP within the acceptable range.

> ### HINT
> Avoid aggressive fluid resuscitation even in hemodynamically unstable patients due to risk of rupture.

Surgical Management

■ *What is the definitive management of an aortic aneurysm?*

■ **Graft replacement of the aorta**

Open thoracotomy is the most commonly used route to repair an aortic injury from a trauma. The endovascular route has also been used. Surgery may involve placing the patient on CPB or partial left heart bypass to maintain perfusion distal to the area of injury (Box 1.27).

Box 1.27 Indications for Surgical Management

Hemodynamically unstable
Large-volume hemorrhage from chest tubes
Contrast extravasation on CT scan or rapidly expanding mediastinal hematoma
Penetrating aortic injury

CARDIOMYOPATHIES

■ *What type of cardiomyopathy has a high incidence of SCD due to lethal arrhythmias?*

■ **Hypertrophic cardiomyopathy**

The hypertrophied LV wall places the patient at risk for increased myocardial oxygen consumption and fatal arrhythmias. The thickening of the ventricular wall is called remodeling.

> **HINT**
>
> A hyperthropic cardiomyopathy is an indication for the placement of automatic internal cardiac defibrillator (AICD).

■ *What are the two classifications of hypertrophic cardiomyopathy?*
■ **Obstructive and nonobstructive**

The obstructive hypertrophic cardiomyopathy has an obstruction to outflow from the LV in combination with ventricular hypertrophy. The obstruction to outflow is due to the enlarged septal wall causing the mitral valve to interfere with outflow during mid-systole.

■ *Your patient has a history of chronic alcoholism. Which type of cardiomyopathy would you suspect due to his history?*
■ **Dilated cardiomyopathy**

Dilated cardiomyopathy is the most common non-ischemic cardiomyopathy. It is classified as a systolic dysfunction (Box 1.28).

Box 1.28 Causes of Dilated Cardiomyopathy

Peripartum	Volume overload
Viral infection	Chemotherapeutic agents
Alcohol-induced	Idiopathic/genetic
Cocaine-induced Ischemia/infarction (previous myocardial infarction)	

■ *Which cardiomyopathy demonstrates a reduced diastolic volume but near-normal wall thickness?*
■ **Restrictive cardiomyopathy**

A restrictive cardiomyopathy is characterized by restrictive filling and reduced diastolic volume of either or both ventricles with normal to near-normal systolic function and wall thickness. A restrictive cardiomyopathy needs to be differentiated from a constrictive cardiomyopathy, which may be curable with surgical intervention. A restrictive cardiomyopathy is the least common form of cardiomyopathy.

> **HINT**
>
> A constrictive cardiomyopathy is caused by constriction around the heart (e.g., pericardial tamponade), whereas a restrictive cardiomyopathy is caused by stiffness of the ventricles.

■ *What causes the ventricles to become noncompliant or stiff in a restrictive cardiomyopathy?*
■ **Interstitial fibrosis or amyloid deposits**

A restrictive cardiomyopathy is characterized by intracellular accumulation of amyloid material sufficient to impair myocardial function. Deposits of protein fibrils throughout the myocardium create a rubbery consistency of the ventricular wall. Amyloid deposits are the most common cause (Box 1.29).

> ❯ HINT
> On autopsy, in a restricted cardiomyopathy, the heart does not collapse when removed from the chest cavity.

Box 1.29 Causes of Restrictive Cardiomyopathy

Idiopathic	Eosinophilic fibrosis

Heart muscle disease
  Amyloidosis
  Hemochromatosis
  Malignancy
	Postirradiation fibrosis

PATHOPHYSIOLOGY

■ *In an obstructive hypertrophic cardiomyopathy, what causes the obstruction to outflow tract from the LV?*

■ **Leaflet of the mitral valve**

During systole, there is an anterior motion of the mitral valve toward the hypertrophied septal wall. This abnormal motion of the mitral valve results in further narrowing of the outflow tract of the aortic valve. The outflow tract may already be narrowed from the hypertrophied septal wall.

■ *Which cardiomyopathy is associated with a high EF?*

■ **Hypertrophic cardiomyopathy**

Hypertrophic cardiomyopathy is characterized by increased contractility due to increased ventricular muscle mass. This increase in contractility results in near emptying of the LV at the end of systole.

> ❯ HINT
> Hypertrophic cardiomyopathy is the only cardiomyopathy with a high EF, whereas the others have a low EF.

■ *Is hypertrophied cardiomyopathy a diastolic or systolic dysfunction?*

■ **Diastolic dysfunction**

The LV chamber is small, decreasing the preload capability, and limiting the filling of the ventricle during diastole. The hypertrophic LV has increased contractility without significant systolic dysfunction.

■ *What effect does a dilated cardiomyopathy have on the CO?*
■ **Decreases the CO**

Dilated cardiomyopathy has a decrease in CO and an increase in pulmonary pressures caused by abnormal contractility, volume overload, and HF. It is characterized by an increase in end-diastolic and end-systolic volumes with a low EF.

> **❯ HINT**
> Dilated cardiomyopathies are classified as a systolic dysfunction in HF.

■ *Progressive dilation of the LV can lead to which valve abnormalities?*
■ **Mitral or aortic regurgitation**

The dilation of the LV stretches the leaflets of the valve, resulting in loss of integrity of the aortic and mitral valves. The regurgitation across these valves contributes to volume overload and further dilation of the ventricle (Box 1.30).

Box 1.30 Comparison of LV Dysfunction Cardiomyopathies

Type of Dysfunction	Hypertrophy Cardiomyopathy	Dilated Cardiomyopathy	Restricted Cardiomyopathy
Systolic dysfunction		X	
Diastolic dysfunction	X		X

SYMPTOMS/ASSESSMENT

■ *What is the most common presenting symptom of a hypertrophied cardiomyopathy?*
■ **Dyspnea**

Dyspnea is caused by elevated diastolic pressures (impaired diastolic compliance) and may occur in about 90% of people with hypertrophied cardiomyopathy.

■ *What is the most common cause of SCD in hypertrophied cardiomyopathies?*
■ **VF**

VF accounts for about 80% of SCDs of hypertrophied cardiomyopathies. Atrial arrhythmias (i.e., AF, paroxysmal supraventricular tachycardia, Wolff–Parkinson–White [WPW] syndrome) may degenerate to VF as well.

■ *Which cardiomyopathy frequently produces an S4 gallop?*
■ **Hypertrophy cardiomyopathy**

An S_4 is produced during atrial contraction against a noncompliant hypertrophied ventricle. A dilated cardiomyopathy is more likely to produce an S_3 due to volume overload. Atrial contraction against a noncompliant ventricle can also produce a double apical impulse and a double carotid arterial pulse.

> **HINT**
Remember, an S_3 occurs during passive filling of the ventricle and an S_4 occurs during the atrial kick. An S_3 is commonly caused by volume overload and an S_4 occurs with ventricle noncompliance.

■ *What is a common 12-lead ECG finding in hypertrophied cardiomyopathy?*
■ **Left-axis deviation**

The left-axis deviation is caused by the thicker LV wall mass. Other ECG changes include ST-T-wave changes, prolonged PR interval, sinus bradycardia, and atrial enlargement.

> **HINT**
A LBBB with a right-axis deviation is suggestive of a dilated cardiomyopathy.

■ *What is the most common arrhythmia associated with a restrictive cardiomyopathy?*
■ **Complete heart blocks and AF**

The amyloid and fibrous deposits within the SA and AV node can result in a complete heart block. Amyloid deposits within the bundle branches are rare. Ventricular arrhythmias are not as common as atrial arrhythmias (Box 1.31).

> **HINT**
SCD with restrictive cardiomyopathy is usually caused by PEA.

Box 1.31 Comparative Chart: Symptoms of Cardiomyopathies

Hypertrophic Cardiomyopathy	Dilated Cardiomyopathy	Restrictive Cardiomyopathy
Clinical findings		
Sudden cardiac death	Atrial fibrillation	Fatigue
Dyspnea	Dyspnea	Shortness of breath
Presyncope/syncope	Chest pain	Peripheral edema (pitting)
Fatigue	Syncope (due to arrhythmia)	Abdominal ascites
Angina	Jugular venous distension	Chest pain
Palpitations	(JVD)	Syncope (due to low CO
Orthopnea and paroxysmal	Tachycardia (loss of	syndrome)
nocturnal dyspnea	parasympathetic control)	Pleural effusions
Congestive heart failure		Hepatomegaly (splenomegaly
Dizziness		rare)
Heart sounds		
Split S_2	S_3 gallop	Loud S_3
S_3 and S_4 gallop		Rare S_4
Systolic murmur		Systolic murmur
(mitral regurgitation)		(mitral and tricuspid regurgitation)
Diastolic decrescendo murmur		
(aortic regurgitation)		

■ *What abnormal lab value is a predictor of poor outcomes in dilated cardiomyopathy?*

■ **Hyponatremia**

Hyponatremia parallels severity of HF. It is due to release of antidiuretic hormone (ADH) and volume overload (dilutional hyponatremia).

DIAGNOSIS

■ *Which lab value is found elevated in a dilated cardiomyopathy?*

■ **BNP**

BNP levels are increased in dilated cardiomyopathy due to the overstretched ventricle. Restrictive cardiomyopathy will also significantly elevate BNP levels.

> ### ⟩ HINT
> BNP levels will be normal in constrictive cardiomyopathy but grossly elevated in a restrictive cardiomyopathy.

■ *In a restrictive cardiomyopathy, how would the atria appear on an echocardiogram?*

■ **Dilated bilateral atria**

The ventricles are noncompliant and restrictive to filling so blood backs up in the atria, causing dilation of both the right and left atria. The echocardiogram would also show bilateral ventricular thickening with restrictive filling patterns, normal systolic function and EF (until later in the disease), and abnormal myocardial texture (amyloid deposits).

■ *What is the confirmation diagnosis of a restrictive cardiomyopathy due to amyloid deposits?*

■ **Cardiac biopsy**

A cardiac biopsy is used to confirm the diagnosis. A fine-needle aspiration of abdominal fat may also be used and is easier and safer for the diagnosis of amyloidosis. A liver biopsy is performed to diagnosis hemochromatosis (another cause of restrictive cardiomypathy).

MEDICAL MANAGEMENT

■ *Which antiarrhythmic agent has been found to lower the incidence of arrhythmogenic SCD in hypertrophied cardiomyopathy?*

■ **Amiodarone (Cardarone)**

Amiodarone is the only agent proven to reduce the incidence and risk of SCD, with or without obstruction to LV outflow. It is very effective at converting AF and flutter to sinus rhythm and at suppressing the recurrence of these arrhythmias. Disopyramide (Norpace) may be used to raise the atrial and ventricular arrhythmia threshold but is not recommended without concomitant β-blockade.

> ### ❭ HINT
> If Norpace is used, monitor QTc interval.

■ *Is the goal in managing hypertrophic cardiomyopathy to increase or decrease the inotropic state of the LV?*

■ **Decrease the inotropic state**

Hypertrophied cardiomyopathy is a diastolic dysfunction with a small LV chamber. An increase in the inotropic state of the LV will further limit the size of the LV chamber and filling capabilities. Agents that decrease the inotropic state of the LV and result in relaxation of the LV chamber are indicated. First-line agents include β-blockers to titrate the heart rate to 60 to 65 bpm.

> ### ❭ HINT
> β-blockers have also been shown to reduce the gradient across the LV outflow tract.

■ *Which type of calcium channel blocker would be contraindicated in managing hypertrophied cardiomyopathy?*

■ **Dihydropyridine calcium channel blockers**

An example of a dihydropyridine calcium channel blocker is nifedipine (Procardia). Cardiac glycosides (Digoxin) and other positive inotropic agents should also be avoided in patients with hypertrophic cardiomyopathy. The positive inotropic effect will increase the contractility and make the LV chamber size even smaller. This will worsen the filling capability of the ventricles, thus worsening CO and HF.

> ### ❭ HINT
> Verapamil (Calan) is an L-type calcium channel blocker and is indicated if β-blockade is not effective.

■ *What is the indication for anticoagulation therapy in dilated cardiomyopathy?*

■ **Severe LV dysfunction or at risk of AF**

Dilated cardiomyopathy presents as LV systolic dysfunction. As the LV dysfunction becomes severe with a low EF, a thrombus can form in the LV. Anticoagulation therapy is recommended to prevent a cardioembolic stroke or pulmonary embolism (from the RV). Dilated cardiomyopathy patients are at risk for the development of AF and should also be anticoagulated (Box 1.32).

Box 1.32 Pharmacological Management of Cardiomyopathies

Hypertrophic Cardiomyopathy	Dilated Cardiomyopathy	Restricted Cardiomyopathy
Amiodarone (Cordarone)	ACE inhibitor	Diuretics
β-blocker	β-blocker	Nitrates
Ca$^+$ channel blocker (L-type only)	Angiotensin receptor blocker	Anticoagulation therapy (AF)
Anticoagulation therapy (AF)	Cardiac glycosides	Antiplasma cell therapy
	Diuretics	Corticosteroids
	Antiarrhythmic	Interferon
	Vasodilator	
	Aldosterone antagonist	
	Inotropic agents	
	Anticoagulation therapy (AF)	
	Nesiritide (Natrecor)	

SURGICAL MANAGEMENT

■ *What is the surgical option for a restrictive cardiomyopathy?*
■ **Cardiac transplant**

A cardiac transplant may be considered if symptoms are refractory to treatment in idiopathic, familial, and amyloidosis cases of restrictive cardiomyopathy.

■ *What is the surgical option for an obstructive hypertrophic cardiomyopathy?*
■ **LV myomectomy**

An LV myomectomy is a procedure to remove the septal muscle, thus managing the obstruction to outflow in a hypertrophic cardiomyopathy. LV myomectomy is indicated for patients with severe symptoms refractory to therapy and outflow gradient greater than 50 mmHg. It is usually successful in abolishing the outflow gradient and can provide symptomatic relief for at least 5 years. The gradient outflow may increase gradually over time and return to the same level as before, requiring a repeat procedure. Other options to manage the outflow obstruction include mitral valve replacement, transcatheter septal alcohol ablation, and a dual-chamber pacemaker.

> ❯ HINT
> A patient with hypertrophic cardiomyopathy will have an implanted cardioverter-defibrillator (ICD) to prevent SCD.

COMPLICATIONS

■ *What is the primary complication of all of cardiomyopathies?*
■ **HF**

Whether the cardiomyopathy is hypertrophied, dilated, restrictive, or constrictive, HF is the common complication. AF can also complicate all types of cardiomyopathies (Box 1.33).

Box 1.33   Other Complications of Cardiomyopathies

Hypertrophic Cardiomyopathy	Dilated Cardiomyopathy	Restrictive Cardiomyopathy
SCD (due to arrhythmias)	Hypertrophy (remodeling)	MI
	Mitral and tricuspid regurgitation	Low output syndrome
	Pulmonary embolism	

HYPERTENSIVE CRISIS

■ *What BP is considered to be a hypertensive crisis?*

■ **Systolic greater than 180 mmHg and diastolic greater than 110 mmHg**

This definition of hypertensive crisis is derived from the seventh report of the Joint National Committee (JNC) on prevention, detection, evaluation, and treatment of high blood pressure in 2003. About 1% of people with hypertension will experience a hypertensive crisis.

■ *What makes the hypertensive crisis a "hypertensive emergency" instead of "hypertensive urgency"?*

■ **Evidence of acute damage of organs**

Acute hypertension can cause acute end-organ damage. When there is evidence of acute or ongoing injury to target organs, rapid reduction of BP is recommended. Hypertensive urgency, without evidence of organ involvement, can be treated less aggressively. It is not defined by the absolute BP, but by the presentation (Box 1.34).

> ❭ HINT
> The risk of a hypertensive emergency may not be the absolute BP but how rapidly the BP increased.

Box 1.34   Clinical Presentation of Organ Damage for Hypertensive Emergencies

Hypertensive intracranial hemorrhage	Aortic dissection
Hypertensive encephalopathy	Acute kidney injury
Angina/myocardial ischemia	Eclampsia/pre-eclampsia
Left ventricular failure with pulmonary edema	

PATHOPHYSIOLOGY

■ *What is the most common cause of a hypertensive emergency?*

■ **Pre-existing hypertension**

The most common history following a hypertensive emergency is noncompliance with antihypertensive medications or uncontrolled hypertension.

> **HINT**
> The test question may focus on a complete medication history
> assessment by the nurse on admission.

■ *Which hemodynamic change initiates hypertensive crisis?*

■ **Increase in SVR**

An abrupt increase in SVR initiates a hypertensive crisis. There is a loss of autoregulation causing greater sympathetic nervous system involvement. The vasoconstriction may be a result of release of vasoactive substances from the endothelium.

> **HINT**
> Remember that the diastolic pressure is the resistance the heart is
> pumping against (afterload).

SYMPTOMS/ASSESSMENT

■ *What is a common presentation of hypertensive emergency?*

■ **Chest pain, dyspnea, and neurological deficits**

The three most common presentations of hypertensive emergencies include chest pain, dyspnea, and neurological deficits. Other symptoms may include fatigue, nasal congestion, or a new-onset cough. The cardiac evaluation includes signs of ACS. If the presentation is consistent with aortic dissection, immediate evaluation is required.

■ *What is the usual presentation of hypertensive encephalopathy?*

■ **Headache and altered level of consciousness**

A focused neurological examination is required to assess for any focal neurological changes such as motor involvement. If present, it indicates potential hemorrhagic stroke. A sudden onset, "worst headache of my life" presentation may indicate an aneurysm rupture and subarachnoid hemorrhage.

> **HINT**
> Ocular/fundal examination finding of advanced retinopathy,
> hemorrhages, or papilledema assist with the recognition of hypertensive
> encephalopathy.

DIAGNOSIS

■ *What type of hemodynamic monitoring is recommended during the
management of hypertension?*

■ **Arterial BP monitoring**

Arterial BP monitoring allows for continuous monitoring of BP during the management of hypertensive emergencies. It is recommended when titrating infusions for targeted BP.

MANAGEMENT

■ *What is the percentage of decrease of mean arterial pressure (MAP) typically used as a goal in managing hypertensive emergencies?*
■ **25% decrease in MAP**

Multiple organizations have developed guidelines for the management of hypertension. The typical recommendation is to decrease MAP by 25% within 2 to 6 hours or to decrease diastolic pressure by 10% to 15% or below 110 mmHg within 30 to 60 minutes.

■ *What is a commonly used goal for systolic pressure in a hypertensive emergency?*
■ **Less than 160 mmHg**

The goal in a hypertensive patient should be to control the lowering of BP but should not be to "normalize" the BP. Chronic hypertension resets the autoregulation range for organ perfusion. A normal BP can cause hypoperfusion to vital organs (i.e., brain, heart, kidneys) in a chronic hypertensive patient.

> ❯ HINT
> Continue to monitor for signs of organ hypoperfusion while managing the BP.

■ *What is the mechanism of action of Labetalol?*
■ **Nonselective β-blocker and α$_1$-blocker**

Labetalol is frequently used in hypertensive emergencies and can be administered as a bolus or continuous IV infusion. It is a nonselective β-blocker (blocks both β$_1$ and β$_2$ receptors) as well as a selective α$_1$-blocker. It is not a pure β-adrenergic blocker, so does not decrease CO like other β-blockers. Potential adverse effects are AV nodal dysfunction (heart block) and bronchospasm.

> ❯ HINT
> If the hypertensive scenario presents a patient with a significant history of asthma, avoid labetalol (or any β-blockers) as the answer for the appropriate antihypertensive therapy due to bronchodilation.

■ *Which antihypertensive, administered as a continuous infusion, has a rapid onset of 1 minute and a potential side effect of bradycardia?*
■ **Esmolol**

Esmolol is a cardioselective β-blocker. It has a very rapid onset of 1 minute with a duration of 10 to 20 minutes (ultra-short acting). It is administered as a continuous infusion, titrated to a goal BP. It is a β-blocker, thus it decreases rate and contractility of the heart. It is frequently used in acute aortic dissection patients as an antihypertensive agent. It is contraindicated in patients with decompensated HF and bradycardia.

> **HINT**
> Esmolol would be a good answer for a hypertensive patient with acute pulmonary edema and underlying diastolic dysfunction.

■ *How is esmolol metabolized?*
■ **By hydrolysis**

Esmolol is metabolized by hydrolysis of ester linkages by RBC esterases. This agent may be administered to patients in hepatic dysfunction and kidney failure. This accounts for esmolol's rapid metabolism and ultra-short half-life.

> **HINT**
> Esmolol is a good answer for antihypertensive agent in hepatic or renal failure patients.

■ *Which antihypertensive has a vasodilatory effect in both coronary and cerebral vasculature?*
■ **Nicardipine**

Nicardipine is a dihydropyridine-derivative calcium channel blocker. It produces antihypertensive effects by blocking the influx of calcium, thus resulting in relaxation of smooth muscle in the vasculature. It also a coronary and cerebral vasodilator and has been shown to increase coronary and cerebral blood flow. Nicardipine is used as a continuous infusion with onset of 5 to 15 minutes, half-life of 1 hour, and duration of action of 4 to 6 hours.

> **HINT**
> Nicardipine is frequently used as an antihypertensive agent in a hemorrhagic stroke or in patients with coronary artery disease (CAD).

■ *What is the advantage of using fenoldopam in hypertensive emergencies?*
■ **Produces naturesis**

Fenoldopam (Corlopam) is an IV antihypertensive used to manage hypertensive emergencies. It is a dopamine-1-receptor agonist producing vasodilation by acting on dopamine type 1 receptors in the peripheral. It also activates dopaminergic receptors in the renal tubules, resulting in sodium excretion (naturesis). This agent improves creatinine clearance, urine output, and sodium excretion in patients with and without normal renal function. The onset is within 5 minutes and has a duration of 30 to 60 minutes.

> **HINT**
> Fenoldopam is a good answer as an antihypertensive agent in patients with acute renal failure.

■ *What is the greatest risk of using fenoldopam in hypertensive emergencies?*
■ **Hypersensitivity reactions**

Fenoldopam's solution contains sodium metabisulfate. Patients with sulfite allergies may have an allergic reaction to fenoldopam. It is metabolized rapidly and extensively in the liver.

> ❯ **HINT**
> Look at the scenario. If the patient has an allergy to sulfite, avoid fenoldopam as an appropriate antihypertensive agent.

■ *Which drug may be used as an adjunctive agent in a hypertensive patient with MI?*
■ **Nitroglycerin**

Nitroglycerin, at high doses, is an arterial dilator. It is both a venodilator and an arterial dilator. It is not considered a first-line drug for a hypertensive emergency, but it can be used as an adjunctive agent in a myocardial ischemic patient experiencing a hypertensive emergency.

> ❯ **HINT**
> Remember that the mechanism of nitroglycerin is dose dependent. Lower doses affect preload and higher doses affect afterload.

■ *What is the toxin that can accumulate with Nipride at higher doses?*
■ **Cyanide**

Sodium nitroprusside (Nipride) can lead to cyanide poisoning. The potential amount of cyanide accumulation depends on the dose and duration of the Nipride infusion. Typically, infusions more than 4 mcg/kg/min for 2 to 3 hours have led to toxic levels of cyanide. If higher infusions of Nipride are required, thiosulfate may be administered to prevent accumulation of cyanide.

■ *Does Nipride affect preload, afterload, or both?*
■ **Both preload and afterload**

Sodium nitroprusside (Nipride) dilates both the arterial and venous circulation, thus producing an effect on both preload and afterload. It has a rapid onset of 1 to 2 minutes and a half-life of 3 to 4 minutes. Due to the quick onset and short duration, Nipride is easily titrated. It should be avoided in patients with renal and hepatic failure due to dependence on these organs for metabolism. Nipride can cause a reduction in coronary blood flow to areas of ischemia (steal phenomenon), an increase in intracranial pressure, and may worsen hypoxia in acute respiratory failure.

> ❯ **HINT**
> Avoid Nipride as an answer in patients with ACS, acute respiratory failure, and in neurological patients with increased intracranial pressure (ICP).

■ *Which of the IV dihydropyridine calcium channel blockers has the shortest half-life?*

■ **Clevidipine (Cleviprex)**

Clevidipine's half-life is 1 to 2 minutes with rapid onset within 2 to 4 minutes and a duration of 5 to 15 minutes. Nicardipine, in comparison, has a half-life of 1 hour and a duration of 4 to 6 hours. They are both administered as a continuous infusion and are titrated to target BP. Clevidipine is more titratable due to its shorter half-life. It is metabolized by esterases in the blood and accounts for the ultra-short half-life of the drug. Clearance of the drug should not be affected by renal or hepatic impairment but requires more research.

> **❯ HINT**
> When titrating a drug for a targeted BP, clevidipine may be used as the answer over nicardipine, due to the shorter half-life.

■ *Clevidipine is contraindicated in patients with what allergies?*

■ **Allergies to soy products and egg or egg products**

Clevidipine is a milky, white emulsion that is high in lipids. It is contraindicated in patients who are allergic to soy products, eggs, or egg products. The lipid solutions provide 2 kcal/mL of clevidipine, so it needs to be counted in caloric intake.

■ *What antihypertensives should be avoided in hypertensive emergencies?*

■ **Nifedipine and hydralazine**

Nifedipine used by oral or sublingual route can cause a sudden, uncontrolled, and severe drop in BP and should not be administered for hypertensive emergencies. Hydralazine is a direct-acting vasodilator. It has a half-life of 3 hours and a half-life of approximately 10 hours. Hydralazine should be avoided because of its prolonged, unpredictable effects and difficulty in titration to target BP.

COMPLICATIONS

■ *What is a potential complication of antihypertensive therapy?*

■ **Hypotension and hypoperfusion of organs**

The targeted BP is 160/110 to prevent hypoperfusion to vital organs due to the resetting of autoregulation in chronic hypertensive patients. A shorter acting antihypertensive is recommended to prevent long periods of hypotension and is more titratable to targeted BPs.

VALVULAR HEART DISEASE

■ *Would a rapid onset of symptoms with valvular structural defect be a stenosis or regurgitation?*

■ **Regurgitation**

The stenosis of a valve occurs over time and is a more gradual process. Regurgitation can present with a sudden onset of symptoms of HF. In acute regurgitation, the heart has not compensated for the added volume in the ventricles or atria, so atrial and ventricular pressures can rise drastically in a short period of time. This results in HF.

> ❯ HINT
> If the scenario provides a "sudden onset" of HF, look for valvular abnormality of regurgitation. The most common is acute mitral regurgitation.

PATHOPHYSIOLOGY

- **What is the most common cause of aortic stenosis?**
- **Calcification of the aortic valve**

The most common cause of an aortic valve stenosis in adults is calcification of the valve, eventually causing reduction in leaflet motion.

- **Which cardiomyopathy can be caused by an aortic stenosis?**
- **Hypertrophied cardiomyopathy**

Over time, the LV has been contracting against greater resistance as the aortic valve area decreases and there is a reduction in leaflet motion. The heart compensates by increasing the wall thickness.

- **What are the complications that a patient with acute aortic regurgitation can typically develop?**
- **Pulmonary edema and cardiogenic shock**

There is a sudden large increase in blood volume in the LV due to the incompetence of the aortic valve. This results in a rapid increase in LV pressure with blood backing up into the LA. The elevated LA pressures cause congestion in pulmonary arteries. The LV is unable to compensate with the rapid volume overload and will decrease the CO. So, a patient with acute aortic regurgitation typically presents with either pulmonary edema or cardiogenic shock.

> ❯ HINT
> A dissection of the ascending thoracic aorta can damage the aortic valve, causing sudden onset of pulmonary edema.

- **What is the compensatory mechanism of the LV during chronic aortic regurgitation?**
- **Dilated followed by hypertrophy of LV**

The initial response of the ventricles is to dilate to hold the increase in end-diastolic volume following the onset of aortic regurgitation. The LV then begins to hypertrophy to maintain the high EF (due to the large volume or preload). There is an increase in systolic wall stress causing an increase in afterload, thus causing further hypertrophy. Initially, the

EF is maintained. Eventually, the hypertrophic response may become inadequate and the preload reserve fails, resulting in a low EF and signs of dyspnea.

> **HINT**
> Chronic aortic regurgitation occurs over time so the heart compensates and patients may remain asymptomatic for a time period.

■ *What is the most common cause of mitral stenosis?*
■ **Rheumatic carditis**

Rheumatic heart disease and a history of rheumatic fever may be found in 40% to 60% of the patients diagnosed with mitral stenosis. Rheumatic disease causes thickening and calcification of the mitral valve leaflets, resulting in a funnel-shaped mitral apparatus that narrows the orifice.

■ *Does mitral valve prolapse (MVP) always result in mitral regurgitation?*
■ **No**

MVP is the billowing of one or both the mitral valve leaflets back up in the LA. It may or may not be associated with mitral regurgitation. An echocardiogram is used to identify the MVP and determine the presence of mitral regurgitation. Other causes of mitral regurgitation include rheumatic heart disease, CAD, infective endocarditis, and ruptured chordae tendineae or papillary muscle.

> **HINT**
> The tricuspid valve may also have prolapse in 40% of patients with MVP.

■ *What is the most common arrhythmia induced by mitral regurgitation?*
■ **AF**

During mitral regurgitation, blood is pushed back up into the LA during systole. This causes LA overload and LA dilation. The dilating of the LA triggers the onset of AF. Pulmonary hypertension may also occur with CHF in later signs of mitral regurgitation.

DIAGNOSIS

■ *What is the most widely used screening for valvular heart disease (VHD)?*
■ **Auscultation for murmurs**

Murmurs are produced by three mechanisms:

1. High flow through normal or abnormal valve
2. Forward flow though a narrowed orifice (stenosis)
3. Backward flow through incompetent valve (regurgitation)

> **HINT**

Know the physiology of which valves are opened and closed during systole and diastole. This will help you determine whether a valve abnormality causes a systolic or diastolic murmur (Box 1.35).

Box 1.35 Valvular Murmurs

Questions to Ask Yourself	Answer	Potential Valve Abnormalities
Which two valves open during *diastole*?	Mitral and tricuspid	Mitral or tricuspid stenosis
Which two valves close during *diastole*?	Aortic and pulmonic	Aortic or pulmonic regurgitation
Which two valves are open during *systole*?	Aortic and pulmonic	Aortic or pulmonic stenosis
Which two valves close during *systole*?	Mitral and tricuspid	Mitral or tricuspid regurgitation

■ *What are the characteristics that describe a cardiac murmur?*

■ **Timing, quality, loudness, location, and radiation**

The timing is in relation to the cardiac cycle and may use exact descriptions (i.e., holosystolic or throughout systole). It is also described on the configuration of the murmur (i.e., crescendo, decrescendo, and crescendo–decrescendo). The loudness is written with the bottom number being the scale used and the top number being the loudness of the murmur itself (i.e., 3/6 murmur—murmur is rated a 3 out of 6 for loudness). The location of the chest sounds heard best assists with determining the valve producing the murmur (Box 1.36).

Box 1.36 Location of Auscultation

Chest Wall Landmarks	Referred Valve Sounds
Second intercostal space (ICS) right sternal border	Aortic valve
Second ICS left sternal border	Pulmonic valve
Fifth ICS midclavicular left side	Mitral valve
Fourth ICS left of sternal border	Tricuspid valve

> **HINT**

Use the location and timing of the murmur to determine the cause of the murmur. For example, a systolic murmur heard best at the second ICS right of the sternal border is most likely caused by aortic stenosis. Typically, the loudness of the murmur indicates the severity of the structural defect (Box 1.37).

Box 1.37 Abnormal Valve Characteristics

Valve Abnormalities	Murmur Characteristics	Other Associated Abnormal Heart Sounds	Hemodynamic Changes
Aortic stenosis	Crescendo-decrescendo systolic murmur	Paradoxical splitting of the S_2	Decreased CO
Aortic regurgitation	Short and/or soft diastolic murmur	S_3 due to increased volume	Tachycardia Decreased CO Widened pulse pressure Exaggerated "A" wave in pulmonary artery occlusive pressure (PAOP) tracing
Mitral stenosis	Mid-diastolic murmur		Large "V" wave in PAOP tracing
Mitral regurgitation	Late systolic or holosystolic murmur	S_3 systolic clicks	Exaggerated "A" waves

■ **Which diagnostic test is recommended for patients with cardiac murmurs and signs of HF?**

■ **Echocardiogram**

The presence of murmurs in symptomatic patients requires further evaluation of the cardiac structures. This includes patients with signs of HF, ACS, syncope, infectious endocarditis, and other evidence of structural heart disease. Other diagnostics include cardiac catheterization and exercise testing.

> ❯ **HINT**
>
> A suspected aortic root dissection with aortic valve involvement may require a thoracic CT scan for more rapid diagnosis.

■ **Which arrhythmia can trigger the onset of symptoms in a patient with mitral stenosis?**

■ **AF**

In mitral stenosis, the narrowed orifice decreases the speed of filling the LV during diastole. The LV diastolic volume is dependent on the gradient pressure caused by the atrial contraction. AF causes a significant decrease in LV end-diastolic volume due to loss of the atrial kick and onset of dyspnea. Exercise-induced dyspnea may also be found in patients with mitral stenosis due to the tachycardia and decreased ventricular filling time that occurs with exercise.

Aortic stenosis can also become symptomatic with new-onset AF. The hypertrophied ventricle has a greater resistance to filling and requires a strong atrial contraction to fill the chamber. A person may be asymptomatic until the onset of AF. The atrial contraction is lost in AF, resulting in less filling of the LV during diastole and a decrease in CO and clinical deterioration in symptoms.

> **❯ HINT**
> Symptoms of HF with exercise or new-onset AF should be red flags
> for the diagnosis of mitral stenosis but aortic stenosis may also be a
> differential diagnosis.

■ *While obtaining BP, you notice that Korotkoff sounds continue down to zero.*
Which valve abnormality would be the cause of loss of diastolic pressure?

■ **Aortic regurgitation**

The aortic valve does not close completely during diastole, allowing for the equilibration
of pressures in the aorta and LV during diastole. This frequently presents with a loss of
diastolic pressure being obtained when auscultating BP. Arterial BP may demonstrate a
widened pulse pressure (very low diastolic pressure).

■ *Which ECG change may contribute to SCD in patients with MVP?*

■ **Prolongation of QT interval**

SCD is not common in mitral regurgitation but is more likely in familial versus nonfamilial
forms of MVP. They have been frequently found to have prolongation of the QT interval,
which may result in ventricular tachycardia (VT) and SCD.

MEDICAL MANAGEMENT

■ *What is the drug therapy of choice in severe acute aortic regurgitation?*

■ **Vasodilator and positive inotropic support**

Treatment of severe acute aortic regurgitation is surgery. The goal for medical management
temporarily before surgery is to augment the forward flow by increasing contractility and
decreasing LV end-diastolic pressures. Nipride with dobutamine may be used in combination. Vasodilator therapy may also be used in severe chronic aortic regurgitation to lower
LV resistance (afterload).

> **❯ HINT**
> Remember, an intra-aortic balloon pump (IABP) is contraindicated in a
> patient with aortic valve incompetence.

■ *Which drug therapy should be avoided in severe acute regurgitation?*

■ **β-blockers**

β-blockers will block the compensatory tachycardia, which may benefit the patient by
increasing CO. β-blockers are typical drugs for managing an aortic dissection but should
be avoided if the dissection involves the aortic root and aortic valve.

> **❯ HINT**
> The scenario may use an ascending thoracic dissection with aortic valve
> involvement, giving esmolol as a potential answer. In this scenario,
> Nipride may be the better answer.

■ *What is the heart rate goal in managing mitral stenosis?*
■ **Slow the heart rate**

Medical management involves the use of drugs, which may slow the heart rate, allowing for greater time for the LV to fill during diastole. Agents with negative chronotropic effects, including β-blockers and heart rate regulating calcium channel blockers, are recommended.

> **❯ HINT**
> Avoid any medication that will increase the heart rate and worsen diastolic filling.

■ *What are the treatment recommendations in patients with mitral stenosis and acute-onset AF or atrial flutter?*
■ **Anticoagulation and control of heart rate response**

Anticoagulation is to prevent systemic or pulmonary embolism during AF. Control of rapid ventricular response to AF includes the use of IV digoxin, heart rate-regulating calcium channel blockers, and β-blockers. If unable to use these previous agents, the second-line drug is an IV or oral amiodarone. If hemodynamically unstable, urgent electrical cardioversion is recommended.

> **❯ HINT**
> If the scenario indicates a need for electrical cardioversion, IV heparin is recommended before, during, and after the procedure.

■ *What is the drug of choice to stabilize acute mitral regurgitation in preparation for surgery?*
■ **Nitroprusside (Nipride)**

Medical management of acute mitral regurgitation is limited and is typically used to stabilize and prepare the patient for surgery. Nitroprusside increases forward flow and reduces pulmonary congestion.

> **❯ HINT**
> Nipride should not be used alone if the patient is hypotensive. May combine with positive inotropic agent.

SURGICAL MANAGEMENT

■ *What would be the indication for aortic valve replacement in aortic stenosis?*
■ **Presence of symptoms**

The decision to replace the aortic valve in aortic stenosis depends upon the severity of symptoms more than on the actual aortic valve area (size of the orifice). Some people have very severe stenosis but are asymptomatic. Others have mild stenosis but are symptomatic.

■ *What symptoms would indicate the need to evaluate a patient with chronic aortic regurgitation for surgery?*

■ **Dyspnea, angina, or syncope**

It is recommended that symptomatic patients with severe aortic regurgitation undergo aortic valve replacement instead of long-term medical management.

■ *What echocardiogram finding would be a contraindication for percutaneous mitral balloon valvotomy?*

■ **LA thrombus**

An echocardiogram is recommended before percutaneous mitral balloon valvotomy to assess for the presence of an LA thrombus. If an LA thrombus is found, the patient should be anticoagulated with warfarin for 3 months for the resolution of the thrombi.

■ *What can be used as a "bridge" for a hypotensive patient with acute mitral regurgitation caused by papillary muscle rupture?*

■ **IABP counterpulsation**

An acute mitral regurgitation may be treated with Nipride, but if hypotensive, an IABP may be beneficial. The IABP will increase forward flow and MAP while decreasing regurgitant volume and LV filling pressures.

COMPLICATIONS

■ *What is the primary complication of acute valvular dysfunction in left-sided valves?*

■ **CHF**

Acute aortic and mitral valve dysfunction result in higher pressures within the LV and/or LA. The high pressures result in congestion and pulmonary edema. Other complications include cardiomyopathy, low CO syndrome, and thrombus formation.

PERIPHERAL ARTERY DISEASE

PATHOPHYSIOLOGY

■ *What is the primary cause of peripheral arterial disease (PAD)?*

■ **Atherosclerosis**

PAD is atherosclerosis of the extremities causing ischemia. The risk factors are the same as for CAD (Box 1.38).

Box 1.38 Risk Factors of PAD

Hypertension	Male
Diabetes	Obesity
Dyslipidemia	High homocysteine levels
Cigarette smoking	

■ *What is the most common location of a thrombus in the peripheral vascular system of the lower extremities?*

■ **Popliteal bifurcation**

Obstruction of the thrombus occurs at arterial bifurcations just distal to the common femoral bifurcation and at the popliteal bifurcation.

SYMPTOMS/ASSESSMENT

■ *What is the most classic symptom of PAD in the lower extremities?*

■ **Intermittent claudication**

Intermittent claudication is painful cramping or ache in the legs with exercise that is alleviated by rest. The most common site of claudication is the calves but it can also occur in thighs, hips, buttocks, or feet. Claudication is exercise-induced reversible ischemia, similar to a stable angina. Some have atypical pain, including exercise intolerance, hip pain, and other joint pain.

> ❭ **HINT**
> Pain at rest may indicate irreversible muscle ischemic injury and requires immediate intervention.

■ *What aggravates the pain at rest?*

■ **Elevating the leg**

Pain worsens when the leg is elevated and improves when lowered (below the level of the heart). The pain may be described as cramping, burning, aching, or tightening (Box 1.39).

Box 1.39 Other signs of PAD in the Lower Extremities

Diminished or absence of peripheral pulses	Cyanotic
Dependent rubor	Increased sweating in extremities
Prolonged capillary refill (dependent)	Extremity cool to touch
Edema (if immobile)	Leg ulcers
Thin, pale (atrophic) skin	Erectile dysfunction (Leriche's syndrome)

DIAGNOSIS

■ *What is the noninvasive test used to recognize PAD?*

■ **Ankle–brachial index (ABI)**

A low ABI indicates the presence of PAD. A normal index is between 1.00 and 1.40. ABI values of 0.91 to 0.99 are considered "borderline" and values greater than 1.40 indicate noncompressible arteries (Boxes 1.40 and 1.41). Ultrasonography is also used to evaluate noninvasively by determining pressure gradients and pulse–volume waveforms.

> ❯ HINT
> The lower the index, the more severe the PAD.

Box 1.40 How to Measure ABI

Obtain SBP in bilateral arms
Obtain SBP in bilateral ankles (may use a Doppler probe)
Calculate ankle-to-arm ratio (divide SBP of ankle by SBP of brachial)

Box 1.41 ABI Severity

Mild	Moderate	Severe
0.71–0.90	0.41–0.70	< 0.40

■ *What is the diagnostic test obtained prior to surgery for PAD?*

■ **Arteriogram**

An arteriogram provides details of the location and extent of arterial occlusion. It is typically performed before surgery or percutaneous transluminal angioplasty (PTA). It does not provide information about the functional significance of the abnormal findings.

■ *When measuring transcutaneous oximetry (TcO$_2$), what level is predictive of poor wound healing?*

■ **Less than 40 mmHg**

TcO$_2$ may also be used to evaluate peripheral arterial insufficiency. A value less than 40 mmHg is predictive of poor wound healing and less than 20 mmHg indicates critical limb ischemia.

MEDICAL MANAGEMENT

■ *What is the primary pharmacological management of PAD?*

■ **Antiplatelet therapy**

Antiplatelet therapy is used to modify atherogenesis and reduce the risk of CAD, stroke, and vascular death. In lower extremity PAD, it may also lessen the symptoms and improve the walking distance. Antiplatelet therapy is also used after lower extremity revascularization (endovascular or surgical bypass). Aspirin is the recommended antiplatelet therapy and clopidogrel (Plavix) is an effective alternative. The combination of aspirin and clopidogrel may be considered in a high-risk patient for CAD or loss of a limb who is not at increased risk of bleeding.

> **HINT**
> ACE inhibitor may also be used to relieve symptoms of claudication by
> improving blood flow.

SURGICAL/INTERVENTIONAL MANAGEMENT

■ *What is the nonsurgical intervention for the treatment of PAD?*

■ **PTA**

Angioplasty, with and without stent placement, is recommended in patients with severe
PAD that is amendable by the nonsurgical route. Stents may keep the arteries open with a
lower restenosis rate over angioplasty alone.

> **HINT**
> Stents work best in larger arteries with a higher flow, such as iliac and
> renal arteries (Box 1.42). PTA is not as useful in diffuse disease or long
> occlusions (typically > 3–5 cm).

Box 1.42 Indications for PTA

Indications	Suitable Lesions
Claudication inhibiting daily activities	Short iliac stenosis (< 3 cm)
Rest pain	Short, single, or multiple lesions that are superficial on the femoropopliteal segment
Gangrene	Complete occlusions superficial on the femoral artery
	Iliac stenosis proximal to bypass femoropopliteal artery

■ *What is a complication of PTA?*

■ **Loss of blood flow distal to the extremity**

Complication following a PTA is loss of blood flow distal to the site of angioplasty and
stent placement. Postprocedural assessment includes frequent neurovascular checks on the
involved extremity. The loss of blood flow may be due to a thrombosis at the site of dilation,
distal embolization, or the dissection of intimal lining causing an obstruction to flow.

> **HINT**
> Sudden arterial occlusion may require immediate revascularization
> surgery or thrombolytic therapy.

■ *What is the recommended conduit in surgical bypass procedures of the
lower extremities?*

■ **Autogenous vein**

Surgical bypass procedures with an autogenous vein conduit are recommended in severe
PAD with critical limb ischemia in patients with life expectancies longer than 2 years.
Outcomes using a prosthetic bypass are poor and balloon angioplasty with stent place-
ment may be recommended over the use of a prosthetic conduit.

COMPLICATIONS

■ *What is a common complication of PAD?*

■ **Foot or heal ulcers**

Lower extremity ulcers that are not healing can indicate PAD. Skin ulcerations and presence of gangrene in the extremities meet the criteria for critical limb ischemia. Amputation of the extremity is also a resulting complication of severe PAD and critical limb ischemia.

HYPOVOLEMIC SHOCK

■ *What is the major component in defining shock?*

■ **Hypoperfusion**

Shock is the pathophysiological state in which there is defective vascular perfusion of tissues and organs. It is a state of inadequacies between delivery of oxygen and the removal of end products of metabolism from peripheral tissues. This results in widespread reduction in tissue perfusion, hypoxia, and conversion of cellular respiration to an anaerobic form of metabolism, which produces lactate as a by-product. Rapid restoration of oxygen delivery can be a major factor in preventing the development of multiple organ dysfunction syndrome.

> ❯ **HINT**
> Remember, shock is defined by hypoperfusion not hypotension.

PATHOPHYSIOLOGY

■ *During hypovolemic shock, which compensatory mechanism decreases urine output in an attempt to restore circulating blood volume?*

■ **RAS**

During periods of hypovolemia and hypoperfusion, the kidneys release renin, which converts angiotensin I to angiotensin II. Angiotensin II is a potent vasoconstrictor, shunting blood away from nonvital organs. Angiotensin II stimulates the release of aldosterone, which results in reabsorption of sodium and water. This decreases the urine output while increasing vascular volume. The sympathetic nervous system is another compensatory system activated during hypovolemic shock. It results in tachycardia, increased myocardial contractility, and vasoconstriction.

> ❯ **HINT**
> Vasoconstriction may maintain a BP during hypovolemic shock. Vital signs may not reflect the presence or severity of shock.

■ *What are the hemodynamic findings of hypovolemic shock that differentiate it from other types of shock?*

■ **Low filling pressures and high SVR**

Hypovolemic shock is due to a decrease in circulating blood volume causing a low SV/CO ratio. Hypovolemia can be caused by blood loss, poor intake, increased fluid losses, or redistribution of fluid (third spacing).

> ❯ HINT
> Both the central venous pressure (CVP) and pulmonary artery occlusive pressure (PAOP) are low.

■ *What compartmental fluid shift occurs with hemorrhagic shock?*
■ **Extravascular to intravascular**

In hemorrhagic shock, fluid shifts from the extravascular space into the intravascular space in an attempt to replace volume due to acute blood loss. In disease states in which plasma volume is lost, the fluid shifts from intravascular to the interstitial space. This is frequently called third spacing and can result in hypovolemic shock. Examples include peritonitis, burns, and crush injuries.

SYMPTOMS/ASSESSMENT

■ *Following a trauma, a patient presents with the following vitals signs on admission: HR 124, RR 32, BP 94/60, and UO 15 cc/hr. Based on these vital signs, what is the class of hemorrhagic shock?*
■ **Class III hemorrhagic shock**

The American College of Surgeons has developed a classification of hemorrhagic shock based on vital signs to indicate the severity of blood loss. This is not exact and patient presentation can vary.

■ *A Class III hemorrhagic shock would indicate what percentage of blood loss?*
■ **30% to 40%**

The classification is based on the percentage of total blood loss (TBV). The estimated amount of blood volume loss is based on a 70-kg male (TBV approximately 5 L). A 30% to 40% TBV loss (Class III) would be approximately 1,500 to 2,000 mL (Box 1.43).

Box 1.43 American College of Surgeons Classification of Hemorrhage

	Class I	Class II	Class III	Class IV
Blood loss (mL)	<750	750–1,500	1,500–2,000	>2,000
Blood loss (%)	<15	15–30	30–40	>40
Systolic blood pressure	Normal	Normal	Decreased	Decreased
Heart rate (bpm)	<100	>100	>120	>140
Respiratory rate (breaths/min)	14–20	20–30	30–40	>35
Mental status	Anxious	Agitated	Confused	Lethargic

Source: Adapted from the American College of Surgeons on Trauma. (1993). *Advanced Trauma Life Support for Physicians,* Students and Instructor Manual, Chicago, American College of Surgeons.

> ❭ HINT
> Young patients may have normal BP/HR in the presence of significant blood loss due to the effectiveness of their compensatory mechanisms. Elderly patients may be hypotensive with minimal blood loss.

■ **What classification of drugs limits tachycardic response that occurs during hemorrhagic shock?**

■ **β-blockers**

Blocking β-receptors of the heart results in limited ability to respond to the sympathetic nervous system with tachycardia. The lack of tachycardia does not rule out hemorrhagic shock in patients taking β-blockers.

Other signs of hypovolemic shock include pale, cool, clammy skin. The urine output will progressively decrease as the shock worsens.

> ❭ HINT
> Hypovolemic/hemorrhagic shock patient may narrow the pulse pressure before decreasing systolic BP.

DIAGNOSIS

■ **Which laboratory studies may be used to identify the presence of shock in a normotensive patient?**

■ **Lactate and base deficit**

Vital signs are not reliable in identifying all patients in shock. Cellular metabolism is limited by inadequate tissue hypoperfusion and results in mandatory changes from an aerobic to an anaerobic metabolism. In anaerobic metabolism, the production of lactic acid is an end product that creates lactic acidosis. Elevated lactate levels and the presence of a base deficit are used to identify anaerobic metabolism.

■ **What is a base deficit?**

■ **Amount of base needed to titrate 1 L of whole blood to pH 7.40**

The base deficit reflects the extent of anaerobic metabolism and the severity of the metabolic acidosis. This value is obtained from an arterial blood gas. The normal base is +2 to –2 mEq/L with positive numbers indicating a base excess and negative numbers indicating a base deficit.

> ❭ HINT
> Base deficit is used as an end point of resuscitation.

■ **Why does the hgb/hct not accurately reflect the RBC mass during an acute hemorrhage?**

■ **Equal loss of all blood components**

Hematocrit and hemoglobin concentration are indices of balance between loss of blood and movement of extravascular fluid to intravascular space. During an acute hemorrhage, there is loss of whole blood with a decrease in all blood components in a similar ratio. If the initial hgb is low, it is caused by fluid administration and hemodilution. The rate of change in hgb over time is more predictive of the severity of bleeding.

> **HINT**
A normal hgb/hct does not rule out active bleeding in acute situations.

MANAGEMENT

■ *What is the primary treatment for hypovolemic/hemorrhagic shock?*
■ **IV fluids**

IV fluids are the mainstay treatment for hypovolemia. In the case of trauma or acute bleeding, finding the source of blood loss and stopping the bleeding surgically may be required. If the patient is hypothermic, the resuscitation fluids should be warmed prior to or during infusion.

> **HINT**
Remember airway and breathing are still priority of care in all hemorrhagic shock patients.

■ *What is the greatest disadvantage of resuscitating with crystalloids?*
■ **Fluid shifts from intravascular to interstitial space**

Crystalloids are electrolyte solutions with small molecules, which can shift across the spaces. A large amount of infused crystalloids will shift from the intravascular to the interstitial space within minutes of administration. This requires larger volumes of fluids to be administered to replace vascular losses. Frequently used crystalloids for resuscitation include lactated Ringer's (LR) and normal saline (NS). These fluids are both isotonic solutions.

> **HINT**
A 3:1 replacement rule has been used to determine the amount required for crystalloid resuscitation (3 L of crystalloids for every 1 L of blood loss).

■ *Which acid–base imbalance is caused by large-volume infusions of NS?*
■ **Metabolic acidosis**

A 1-L bag of NS contains 154 mEq/L of sodium and chloride. Large amounts of NS administered during resuscitation can cause hyperchloremic metabolic acidosis. An LR solution is a more balanced salt solution and may be used in large-volume resuscitations to prevent metabolic acidosis (Box 1.44).

> ❯ HINT
> The patient's respiratory rate may be rapid to compensate for metabolic acidosis.

Box 1.44 Crystalloids Versus Colloids

	Crystalloids	Colloids
Advantages	Replaces interstitial fluid losses that may have occurred Cheaper Easier to store	Uses less fluid to resuscitate May draw fluid into the vascular space from interstitial space Albumin may have anti-inflammatory effects
Disadvantages	Uses larger amounts of fluid to resuscitate	During periods of increased capillary permeability, albumin will third-space into the extravascular space. Synthetic colloids (i.e., Dextran) activate immune response May cause hypersensitivity reaction Synthetic colloids increase bleeding tendencies More expensive Difficult to store

■ *Which crystalloid is used to increase serum osmolality and rapidly expands the intravascular space?*

■ **Hypertonic saline**

Small amounts of hypertonic saline (4–5 mL/kg) can decrease the total amount of crystalloids used during resuscitation. Hypertonic saline increases serum osmolality and draws fluid from the extravascular space into the intravascular space. It may improve blood flow to organs and has been found to lower intracranial pressure.

> ❯ HINT
> Metabolic acidosis and hypernatremia are complications of a hypertonic saline because of large amounts of chloride, even greater than an NS.
>
> Na^+ in 3% NS is 513 with Cl^- of 513
> Na^+ in 7.5% NS is 1,283 with Cl^- of 1,283

■ *What is a benefit of "hypotensive resuscitation" in a bleeding patient?*

■ **Limited blood loss**

Avoiding aggressive fluid resuscitation to increase BP may limit the amount of blood volume loss in a bleeding patient prior to surgery. Hypotensive resuscitation aims to maintain the systolic BP between 80 and 90 mmHg with smaller boluses of fluid (200-mL bolus). Higher systolic BPs increase intravascular hydrostatic pressure, worsening blood loss in a bleeding patient. The risk of this strategy is hypoperfusion.

> ❯ HINT
> The exception is traumatic brain injured patients. They require a SBP greater than 90 mm Hg. Maintain the systolic BP more than 90 for those with traumatic brain injury.

■ *When giving multiple units of packed red blood cells (PRBCs), what other blood products need to be administered?*

■ **Fresh frozen plasma (FFP) and platelets**

Administering PRBCs and fluid causes a dilutional coagulopathy. PRBCs are void of clotting factors and platelets. Transfusion practice is changing by adding more FFP and platelet transfusions into the resuscitation. Some practitioners are using the 1:1 replacement rule. For every one unit of blood, one unit of FFP is administered.

■ *A patient without a history of cardiac problems was given PRBCs for acute blood loss. Within 4 hours of the transfusion, the patient became hypoxic, febrile, showing pulmonary edema on a chest x-ray, requiring intubation. What is the most likely cause of this change in clinical status?*

■ **Transfusion-related acute lung injury (TRALI)**

TRALI is the most common cause of transfusion-related deaths. The theory behind TRALI is a "two hit" insult. The first hit is a stressful situation (such as trauma, sepsis, massive transfusion, cardiopulmonary bypass [CPB] surgery), which causes the neutrophils to be "primed" and adhere to the pulmonary endothelial bed. The second hit is the actual transfusion of the blood. The transfused blood contains donor antibodies against neutrophil antigens and human leukocyte antigens. These antibodies activate the "primed" neutrophils and monocytes resulting in increased capillary permeability and noncardiogenic pulmonary edema.

> **❯ HINT**
> Think of TRALI if there is a sudden onset of hypoxia, fever, and cough within 1 to 6 hours after a blood transfusion.

■ *What is the laboratory value that can be used as an end point of resuscitation?*

■ **Base deficit**

The base deficit has been found to be a better prediction of metabolic dysfunction during hypovolemic shock and correlates with lactate levels and SVO_2 (guide to determine magnitude of volume deficit). Lactate levels are used to determine the presence of anaerobic metabolism but do demonstrate rapid adjustments to identify the return to aerobic metabolism.

> **❯ HINT**
> A base deficit of –3 to –5 may be seen on a postoperative patient and may indicate the need for further fluids (Box 1.45). A base deficit of more than –15 may indicate an ongoing blood loss.

Box 1.45 Base Deficit Determines Severity Hypovolemia

Mild	–3 to –5
Moderate	–6 to –14
Severe	> –15

COMPLICATIONS

- ■ *What is the "lethal triad" that can occur with hemorrhagic shock and resuscitation?*
- ■ **Coagulopathy, hypothermia, acidosis**

A worsening of one of these can lead to a cycle that results in rapid deterioration and ultimately death in a bleeding patient. All IV fluids should be warmed during the resuscitation, adequate replacement of clotting factors and platelets must be done to limit the coagulopathy, and maintaining perfusion of tissues and organs to help prevent these complications.

> ❯ **HINT**
> Remember hypothermia worsens coagulopathy, and tissue hypoxia (shifts oxyhemoglobin dissociation curve), and decreases CO (decreasing myocardial contractility).

- ■ *What are the electrolyte abnormalities commonly found after a massive resuscitation?*
- ■ **Hypocalcemia, hypomagnesium, hypo- or hyperkalemia**

Blood transfusions contain citrate to increase the shelf-life of stored blood. Citrate binds calcium and magnesium, lowering the ionized levels of both. Multiple transfusions of blood can also increase potassium levels due to cell lysis, but frequently potassium levels are low after resuscitation. The low potassium may be caused by the release of aldosterone. The kidneys hold on to sodium and excrete potassium.

> ❯ **HINT**
> Signs of low magnesium are similar to that of low calcium. Look for either answer if the scenario provides symptoms of muscle spasms, Chvostek's sign, or Trousseau's sign following blood transfusions.

- ■ *What is the abdominal complication associated with aggressive fluid resuscitation?*
- ■ **Abdominal compartment syndrome**

Excessive fluid administration increases the third spacing, resulting in compartment syndromes (cranium, thoracic, abdominal). The elevated pressure in the abdominal cavity results in pulmonary and renal complications, elevated intracranial pressure, and decreased venous return. Abdominal compartment syndrome affects almost all organ functions.

> ❯ **HINT**
> Bladder pressure measurements are used to monitor abdominal compartment syndrome.

CARDIAC SURGERIES

- ■ *What is an indication for a CABG surgery?*
- ■ **Left main coronary artery stenosis**

Other indications include severe triple vessel disease, recurrent HF due to ischemia, multiple coronary artery occlusions, and any contraindication to angioplasty/stent procedures (Box 1.46).

Box 1.46 Cardiac Surgeries

CABG	Repair or replacement of aorta root
Valve repair or replacement	Intracardiac tumors
Repair congenital or acquired defects (atrial septal defect [ASD] and ventricular septal defect [VSD])	LV aneurysmectomy

- ■ *What is the purpose of the use of cardioplegic hyperkalemic solution in open heart procedures?*
- ■ **Induce asystole**

The induction of asystole with cardioplegic hyperkalemic solutions on the heart during the surgery decreases myocardial metabolism and oxygen consumption. This potentially protects the heart during the period of ischemia.

PATHOPHYSIOLOGY

- ■ *What aspects of CPB stimulate the release of the inflammatory system?*
- ■ **Nonpulsatile flow and exposure to bypass circuit**

CPB can cause a systemic reaction with the release of inflammatory mediators similar to sepsis. This inflammatory response is responsible for many of the adverse effects that can occur with CPB, including multisystem organ failure.

- ■ *What are potential advantages of "off-pump" CABG?*
- ■ **Lowers risk of bleeding and multisystem organ failure**

The development of off-pump or "beating heart" CABG procedures lower the incidence of complications attributed to CPB. This technique does not require CPB to be used.

> ❯ HINT
> The greatest risk of off-pump CABG is requiring early revascularization procedures.

SYMPTOMS/ASSESSMENT

▪ *What is the major focus of hemodynamic monitoring on a postoperative cardiac patient?*

▪ **Ventricular function**

Ventricular function must be continuously assessed postoperatively in a cardiac surgery patient. Hemodynamic monitoring is used to determine ventricular function. Even after the heart abnormality is repaired, the ventricular function may continue to be affected for a period of time. Cardiac function has been found to be depressed postoperatively, peaking at 4 to 6 hours after surgery and typically improving within 24 hours.

> ❭ HINT
>
> Interventions will be aimed at improving ventricular function pharmacologically or mechanically.

DIAGNOSIS/POSTOPERATIVE MONITORING

▪ *Following a CABG procedure in which the left internal mammary artery (LIMA) was grafted to the left anterior descending (LAD) artery, what would ST elevation in all anterior leads indicate?*

▪ **LIMA spasm**

ST elevation in all anterior leads following the procedure of grafting the LIMA to the LAD indicates spasm of the LIMA. This 12-lead ECG finding should be reported to the physician immediately. It is important on a post-CABG patient to perform ST-segment monitoring. The lead frequently used for continuous monitoring is a lead in the territory of the graft.

> ❭ HINT
>
> ST elevation in two or more contiguous leads in a territory that was grafted indicates acute graft failure.

▪ *Which electrolytes are commonly monitored closely in a postcardiac surgery patient?*

▪ **Potassium and magnesium**

Hypokalemia and hypomagnesium are frequent electrolyte abnormalities encountered in a postcardiac surgical patient and require careful monitoring to treat. Hypokalemia and hypomagnesium can significantly increase the likelihood of postoperative arrhythmias.

> ❭ HINT
>
> Remember, to effectively treat the low potassium, the magnesium needs to be corrected first.

MANAGEMENT

■ *What is the hemodynamic complication that occurs during the rewarming of a postcardiac surgery patient?*

■ **Hypotension**

Hypothermia causes vasoconstriction and an increase in SVR. Most postcardiac patients have been cooled in the operating room (usually < 34°C). Vasodilation occurs during the rewarming process resulting in hypotension. Patients are rewarmed with the use of air convection that blows warm air over the patient.

> ❯ HINT
> Rewarming is important in the management of patients to prevent complications of hypothermia (Box 1.47).

Box 1.47 Complications of Hypothermia

Myocardial contractility depression	Causes shivering and increased oxygen consumption
Predisposes to ventricular arrhythmias	
Increases afterload and myocardial workload	Decreases CO_2 production
	Causes coagulopathy

■ *Which of the inotropic agents is a phosphodiesterase inhibitor?*

■ **Milrinone (Primacor)**

Inotropic agents are used in postcardiac surgery patients to increase the contractility of the ventricles. Milrinone, being a phosphodiesterase inhibitor, does not rely on either α or β stimulation for inotropic effects. Milrinone increases the levels of cyclic adenosine monophosphate (CMP) and intracardiac calcium, which promote increased contractility. The influx of calcium in the vascular beds leads to vasodilation and lowering of SVR.

> ❯ HINT
> If the patient develops tolerance due to catecholamine depletion, milrinone is the drug of choice (Box 1.48).

Box 1.48 Other Inotropic Agents

Dopamine	Epinephrine
Dobutamine	Norepinephrine

■ *What hemodynamic profile needs to be assessed before administering a vasopressor?*

■ **Fluid status**

Vascular fluid status needs to be assessed before administering a vasopressor. The vascular volume should be replaced before administering a vasoconstricting drug. The vasoconstriction and increased afterload can result in organ hypoperfusion in a hypovolemic patient. Adequate volume status during the administration of a vasoconstrictor will limit the hypoperfusion.

> ❯ HINT
>
> Do not attempt to squeeze an empty vessel. Replace fluid volume first,
> then vasoconstrict with pharmacological agents to increase MAP.

■ *Which vasoconstrictor is a pure α-agonist drug?*

■ **Phenylephrine**

Phenylephrine is a pure α-agonist that has no β-receptor effects. Norepinephrine is both an α- and β-receptor agonist. Vasopressin may also be used as a vasoconstrictor. It is an exogenous production of antidiuretic hormone (ADH).

COMPLICATIONS

■ *Why is bleeding a common postoperative complication of open heart surgery with the use of CPB?*

■ **Heparinization**

During the period of CPB, the patient must be heparinized and the activated clotting times (ACT) must be maintained at more than 400 seconds to prevent clotting in the bypass circuit. Longer CPB times result in greater incidence of bleeding complications, even with the reversal of heparin at the end of the surgery with protamine. If the ACT is elevated, administer protamine to further reverse the heparin. The patient may not have been completely reversed (inadequate dose) or received additional heparin at the time of discontinuation from the pump (Box 1.49).

> ❯ HINT
>
> An ACT test should be performed on admission to the intensive
> care unit (ICU) to assure adequate reversal of heparin (normal values
> between 100 and 120 seconds). Always consider a surgical source of
> bleeding with sudden onset of fresh, rapid bleeding from mediastinal
> chest tubes.

Box 1.49 Other Causes of Postoperative Bleeding

Thrombocytopenia and abnormal function of platelets	Bleeding from small arteries or veins
Hypothermia	Leaks at vascular anastomosis
Preoperative anticoagulation or antiplatelet drugs	

■ *What are the signs of a protamine reaction?*

■ **Hypoxia and hypotension**

A protamine reaction can occur with any administration of protamine, even if the patient had tolerated the drug previously. Pulmonary hypertension with resulting hypoxia and systemic hypotension are the signs of a protamine reaction. Monitor for this adverse reaction when administering protamine.

> **HINT**
> Excessive use of protamine can also cause coagulopathy.

■ *Administration of five units of platelets should increase the platelet count by how much?*

■ **25,000 to 50,000**

Correction of the bleeding complication includes administration of platelets, FFP, cryoprecipitate, and PRBCs. Monitoring PT/PTT will guide the replacement of FFP. Cryoprecipitate contains fibrinogen and factor VIII. Other methods to control small venous bleeding in the thoracic cavity include raising the head of the bed and adding PEEP on the ventilator to increase pleural and mediastinal pressures. There are no definitive studies on these methods.

> **HINT**
> The main purpose of giving PRBC in a postcardiac bleeding patient is to improve oxygen delivery. Otherwise, a stable patient may tolerate hgb of 7.0 g/dL.

■ *When would aminocaproic (Amicar) be indicated in a postoperative cardiac patient?*

■ **Actively bleeding**

Rescue Amicar may be used in a postoperative cardiac patient who is actively bleeding when all other causes of bleeding have been addressed. Amicar and tranexamic acid (TXA) are frequently administered to cardiac surgical patients in the operating room to reduce the amount of blood loss and limit the amount of required blood transfusions. They are antifibrinolytic agents that inhibit conversion of plasminogen to plasmin thus preventing activation of fibrinolysis. The major risk of both drugs is thrombosis, including complete occlusion of the new graft.

> **HINT**
> Amicar may cause renal failure and tranexamic acid may increase the risk of seizures.

■ *How does desmopressin acetate potentially work to prevent bleeding complications?*

■ **Improves platelet function**

Desmopressin acetate elevates the levels of factor VII and von Willebrand's factor. This may improve the platelet function following cardiac surgery.

■ *Following an aortic valve replacement, a patient suddenly becomes hypotensive and decreases output from the mediastinal chest tubes. What complication would you suspect?*

■ **Cardiac tamponade**

Cardiac tamponade can be a complication of cardiac surgeries. It is more common in open heart procedures such as valvular surgeries. The classic signs of pericardial tamponade may not be present but the presence of hypotension needs to be evaluated for potential cardiac tamponade. Decreasing or abrupt cessation of output from the mediastinal chest tubes should increase the suspicion of a cardiac tamponade. TEE may be used to diagnose the cardiac tamponade. Volume resuscitation, inotropes, and vasopressors may be temporary measures until surgery.

> **HINT**
> Cardiac tamponade can have a regional effect such as compression of RV with the onset of symptoms of RV failure.

▨ *Which arrhythmia commonly presents in elderly patients 2 to 3 days post–cardiac surgery?*
▨ **AF**

AF is common following cardiac surgeries, in particular, valve surgeries. It may be seen in patients of all ages but occurs most frequently in the older population. Other common arrhythmias that occur after cardiac surgery are heart blocks and ventricular arrhythmias.

> **HINT**
> New onset AF should be immediately converted to prevent the formation of intracardiac thrombi.

▨ *What type of stroke is more common following CPB surgeries?*
▨ **Watershed stroke**

Watershed strokes are ischemic strokes, which occur between major cerebral vascular territories. Periods of hypotension or hypoperfusion during the nonpulsatile flow state of CPB leads to the ischemia. Other causes of stroke following CPB include showing of atherosclerotic emboli mobilized by surgical manipulation of the aorta and embolic strokes with the development of AF.

▨ *What is the primary symptom of an air embolus following CPB surgeries?*
▨ **Seizures**

An air embolus is a risk when the surgery requires aortotomy or when an open heart procedure is performed. The symptoms include seizures, delayed emergence from anesthesia, and focal neurological deficits. In contrast to strokes, an air embolus rarely shows changes on CT or magnetic resonance imaging (MRI) (Box 1.50).

> **HINT**
> A scenario with valve replacement in a postop patient who is not waking up, but shows nothing on CT/MRI, would most likely be caused by an air embolus.

Box 1.50 Neurological Complications of CPB

Stroke	Seizures
Coma	Memory deficits
Paralysis	

■ *Following a mitral valve replacement, what signs would indicate an acute dehiscence of the valve repair?*

■ **New systolic murmur and new "V" wave**

Acute dehiscence of a valve repair is rare. The signs would be a new regurgitant murmur. A mitral regurgitation produces a systolic murmur whereas an aortic valve regurgitation produces a diastolic murmur. A new "V" wave develops in the PAOP waveform due to high pressures in the LA during ventricular systole due to the backflow of blood into the LA.

TESTABLE NURSING ACTIONS

HEMODYNAMIC MONITORING

See Table 1.3.

■ *A patient develops hypotension. The CVP is 14 and PAOP is 7. What is the most likely cause of these hemodynamic findings?*

■ **RV failure**

RV failure will result in an elevation of CVP due to backward flow and a lower PAOP due to less blood flow to the left side of the heart. This may be caused by RV infarct, pulmonary hypertension, or pulmonary embolism.

Table 1.3 Hemodynamic Profiles

Parameter	Method Calculation	Normal
MAP	(Systolic BP – diastolic BP/3) + Diastolic	70–105 mmHg
CO	Liters per minute	4–8 L
Cardiac index	CO/body surface area	2.5–4.0 L/min/m²
Stroke volume (SV)	CO/Heart rate (HR)	50–100 mL/beat
Stroke index (SI)	SV ÷ BSA	25–45 mL/m²/beat
Systemic vascular resistance (SVR)	(MAP – CVP) × 80 ÷ CO	800–1200
Pulmonary vascular resistance (PVR)	(Mean PA – PAOP) × 80 ÷ CO	50–250
Left Ventricular Stroke Work Index (LVSWI)	SI × (MAP – PAOP) × 0.0136	40–65 g·m/m²
Right Ventricular Stroke Work Index (RVSWI)	SI × (Pam – CVP) × 0.0136	5–12 g·m/m²
Pulmonary artery pressure (PA)	(MPAP = 9–18)	25/10
Pulmonary artery occlusion pressure (PAOP)		4–12
CVP		2–6

> **HINT**
> If both the CVP and PAOP are elevated, it could be because of LV
> failure or volume overload (see Figure 1.2).

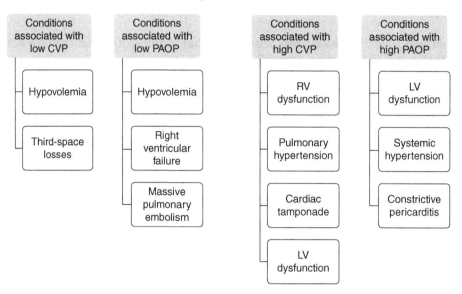

FIGURE 1.2 Hemodynamic interpretation.

■ *Which valve abnormality interferes with the ability to obtain an accurate pulmonary artery occlusive pressure?*

■ **Mitral stenosis**

For the LA pressure to be equal to the LV end-diastolic pressure (LVEDP), the mitral valve must be open for the pressures to equalize. In mitral stenosis, the valve does not open completely, thus limiting the ability of the LA pressure to accurately reflect LV pressure. After obtaining a CVP reading that is the same on the right side of the heart, the tricuspid valve must be open completely to obtain an accurate reading of the RV end-diastolic pressure (RVEDP).

> **HINT**
> An accurate pressure reading can be obtained in mitral regurgitation if
> read during the A wave only (when the mitral valve is open).

■ *PAOP and CVP readings in patients with hypertrophied cardiomyopathy are falsely high or low?*

■ **High**

PAOP and CVP are readings of pressures in the heart chambers. Pressure is not always equal to volume and can cause an erroneous reading. Hypertrophied cardiomyopathies will read the pressures higher than the actual volume. This is due to the high pressure of the thickened myocardial muscle placed on the heart chambers. Dilated cardiomyopathies exert little pressure but are dilated chambers that hold large volumes of blood. In dilated cardiomyopathy, CVP and PAOP readings are lower than the actual volume.

> **HINT**
> Pressure is not always equal to volume. Read the scenario and interpret findings based on the patient case study presented in the question.

■ *What is SV variance (SVV) an indicator of?*
■ **Preload responsiveness**

SVV is frequently used to determine the need for fluid. SVV is not an indicator of actual preload but of relative preload responsiveness. The goal is to maintain SVV less than 13%.

> **HINT**
> The patient must be intubated for accuracy of measurement (Box 1.51).

Box 1.51 Limitations of SVV

Requires mechanical ventilation (improves accuracy)
Arrhythmias (affect accuracy)
Positive end-expiratory pressure (PEEP; SVV)
Vascular tone (vasodilation may increase SVV)

■ *What maneuver could be used instead of SVV to determine fluid responsiveness in a spontaneous breathing patient?*
■ **Passive leg raising**

Without the availability of SVV, raising the legs has proven clinically to act like a "self volume challenge" to indicate the patient's status on the Fran–Starling curve. This provides a physiologic fluid bolus and may be performed if the patient has arrhythmias or spontaneous breathing.

■ *What are the three components of oxygen delivery (DO$_2$)?*
■ **Oxygen saturation, hemoglobin (hgb), and CO**

DO$_2$ is the amount of oxygen leaving the heart per minute and delivered to the tissue level. The components of DO$_2$ include oxygen saturation, hgb, and CO. If DO$_2$ decreases, the body compensates by offloading more oxygen from the hgb to the tissues. CO is the most important component of this equation.

> **HINT**
> If the tissues take more oxygen from the hgb, then less oxygen is returned to the right side of the heart.

■ *What is oxygen consumption (VO$_2$) equal to in a normal situation?*
■ **Oxygen demand**

In a normal situation with adequate oxygen delivery, an increase in oxygen demand will increase oxygen consumption. VO$_2$ will vary based on the metabolic needs of the tissues.

> **HINT**
Intervention may be to increase the delivery of oxygen or decrease the demand of oxygen (Box 1.52).

Box 1.52 Causes of Increased VO_2

Fever	Anxiety
Shivering	Hyperthermia
Increase in work of breathing	Response to major illness or surgeries
Pain	Seizures

■ *Are critically ill patients usually supply independent or supply dependent?*
■ **Supply dependent**

VO_2 is a good measurement of the overall aerobic metabolism but by itself is an unreliable indicator of adequacy of tissue perfusion. Adding DO_2 in relation to VO_2 tells more about oxygen use. Supply independency occurs when the VO_2 remains constant during a period of increased demand or decreased supply. This indicates that DO_2 is sufficient for the demand, indicating adequate tissue perfusion. In critically ill patients, it is difficult to achieve this supply independency. Supply dependency occurs as the tissue demand increases and requires an increase in blood flow. This indicates that the DO_2 was not sufficient for the tissue demands.

> **HINT**
An increase in VO_2 after increasing DO_2 indicates an oxygen debt (see figure below).

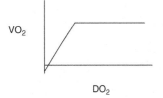

■ *What is a normal SvO_2 obtained from a PAC?*
■ **60% to 80%**

SvO_2 monitoring is used to allow for continuous monitoring of O_2 supply and demand. SvO_2 measures oxygen saturation of the venous blood from the right side of the heart (it is the amount of oxygen returning to the right side after tissue extraction). A change in SVO_2 may indicate a change in either DO_2 or VO_2 or both.

> **HINT**
If the question gives a change in the SvO_2, look at both the demand and delivery to determine the cause.

■ *What is the difference between SvO_2 and $ScvO_2$ monitoring?*
■ **SvO_2 is a true mixed venous gas**

$ScvO_2$ is obtained from a central line (central venous circulation), whereas SvO_2 is obtained from the PAC (pulmonary artery). $ScvO_2$ is not a true "mixed" venous gas but can be used to determine oxygen consumption. The goal is to maintain $ScvO_2$ at greater than 70%.

INTRA-AORTIC BALLOON PUMP COUNTERPULSATION

- *Where is the balloon positioned in the aorta?*
- **Descending thoracic aorta**

The tip of the catheter should be positioned just distal to the left subclavian artery and above the renal and mesenteric arteries.

> ❯ **HINT**
> Sudden cessation of urine may indicate migration of the balloon distally, obstructing the renal arteries.

- *When does inflation of the balloon occur?*
- **Beginning of diastole**

The inflation of the balloon just after the closure of the aortic valve, the beginning of diastole, increases the aortic pressure and augments perfusion. It elevates the diastolic pressure in the aorta, thus improving coronary perfusion.

> ❯ **HINT**
> Remember coronary perfusion pressure (CPP) is the difference between aortic diastolic pressure (ADP) and right atrial pressure (RAP):
>
> $$CPP = ADP - RAP$$

- *What is the purpose of balloon deflation immediately prior to systole?*
- **Decreased afterload**

The balloon should deflate just before the opening of the aortic valve, immediately prior to systole. This results in a sudden decrease in aortic pressure and decreases the afterload or resistance of the LV.

> ❯ **HINT**
> If the balloon deflates after the onset of systole, it will increase the workload of the heart. It is important that deflation occurs immediately prior to systole.

- *Which of the following provides the most support to the heart: the 1:1, 1:2, or 1:3 cycle?*
- **1:1**

A 1:1 cycle indicates that the balloon inflates and deflates with every heartbeat. It provides support with every contraction. A 1:2 cycle provides support with every second cardiac cycle, and the 1:3 cycle every third.

> **> HINT**
> Weaning the IABP is typically performed by decreasing the cycle frequency from 1:1 to 1:2, then to 1:3 before removing the balloon.

■ *Which valve abnormality would be a contraindication for the use of IABP?*
■ **Aortic insufficiency**

Inflates after closure of the aortic valve. An aortic insufficiency would cause the blood to flow back into the LV during balloon inflation, increasing the LV volume. This would increase the workload of the heart and worsen LV failure. Other contraindications include aortic dissection and severe peripheral vascular disease (due to placement of the catheter in femoral location).

> **> HINT**
> IABP is indicated for mitral valve insufficiency to lower the resistance of the LV (Box 1.53).

Box 1.53 Indications for an IABP

Cardiogenic shock: medically refractory	Acute ventricular septal rupture
AMI: medically refractory	Bridge to cardiac transplantation
Acute mitral regurgitation	

■ *A common complication of IABP is lower extremity ischemia. What should be performed routinely to assess for this potential complication?*
■ **Check distal pulses hourly**

The catheter is placed in the femoral artery and can diminish or occlude blood flow distally. It is recommended to assess distal pulses hourly for as long as the balloon is in place. Hematomas can occur at the insertion site contributing to a decrease in distal flow. Assessment of the insertion site hourly for the presence of hematoma is recommended (Box 1.54).

Box 1.54 Other Complications of Using an IABP

Occlusion of the renal, superior mesenteric, or subclavian artery	Thrombocytopenia
	Thromboembolism
Acute aortic dissection or perforation with retroperitoneal hemorrhage	
Wound infection	

PACEMAKERS

■ *According to the pacemaker code, where does a DVI pacemaker sense and pace?*
■ **Senses in ventricles, paces in both atrium and ventricles**

A DVI pacemaker paces in both the atrium and ventricles and senses in the ventricles only. The first letter in the code is chamber paced, and the second letter is chamber sensed (Box 1.55).

Box 1.55 Inter-Society Commission for Heart Disease (ICHD) Pacemaker Codes

I	II	III
Chamber Paced	**Chamber Sensed**	**Mode of Response (s)**
V = Ventricle	V = Ventricle	T = Triggered
A = Atrium	A = Atrium	I = Inhibited
D = Double	D = Double	D = Double
O = None	O = None	O =None

> **HINT**
> A fourth letter would indicate whether the pacemaker is rate responsive. For example, VVIR.

- *Following placement of a permanent pacemaker, the patient's BP decreased from 142/76 to 99/40 on admission to the ICU. What is the most likely cause of the hypotension?*
- **Cardiac tamponade**

During placement of lead, manipulation or fixation of the screw into the wire causes bleeding into the pericardial space. The most common symptom is hypotension. Emergency pericardiocentesis is required to manage pericardial tamponade (Box 1.56).

Box 1.56 Potential Complications of an Implanted Pacemaker

Rejection phenomena	Surgical complications (hematoma, infection, thrombosis)
Skin erosion	Lead problems (fractured, compressed, dislodgement)
Muscle or nerve simulation	Cardiac perforation, cardiac tamponade

- *Which pacemaker would be contraindicated in a patient with a complete AV heart block?*
- **Atrial pacemaker (AAI)**

An atrial pacemaker senses and paces in the atrium only. The impulse travels to the AV junction and requires an intact pathway to travel down to the ventricles. A patient with an AV block requires either a ventricular (VVI) or dual chamber pacemaker (DDD) to pace below the level of the block.

> **HINT**
> Ventricular pacemakers (VVI) sense and pace only in the ventricles. Without any coordination with the atrium, the atrial kick is lost and can decrease the SV.

- *If the patient does not know what type of pacemaker he or she has, what test must be ordered?*
- **CXR**

A CXR can identify the types of leads, the number of leads, and their positions. This indicates what system the patient has implanted. The shape of the pacemaker and manufacturer can assist with further identifying the type of pacemaker.

> ❯ HINT
> Two wires would indicate a dual-chamber pacemaker.

■ *If CXR reveals three leads, what type of pacemaker does the patient have?*
■ **Biventricular pacemaker (three-chamber pacemaker)**

A biventricular pacemaker is also called cardiac resynchronization therapy (CRT). Single- and dual-chamber pacemakers pace in the right side of the heart. Depolarization of the LV occurs after the RV, resulting in dyssynchronization of the ventricles and can decrease CO. Pacing both LV and RV will resynchronize the ventricular contraction and improve CO. It is indicated for the reduction of the symptoms of moderate to severe HF (NYHA Functional Class III or IV) in those patients who remain symptomatic despite stable, optimal medical therapy and have an LVEF of 35% or less and a prolonged QRS duration.

> ❯ HINT
> The paced QRS complex on a triple-chamber pacemaker has a normal width compared to the wide QRS complex on a paced beat with ventricular or dual-chamber pacemaker.

■ *What pacemaker problem can lead to competition between the pacemaker and the heart?*
■ **Undersensing**

Failure of the heart to sense the underlying electrical activity (P wave or QRS complex) is called undersensing. The pacemaker sends electrical impulses when the heart does not need it. This results in competition.

> ❯ HINT
> Competition can cause an R-on-T phenomenon resulting in deadly arrhythmias, such as ventricular tachycardia (torsades de pointes).

■ *What is it called when the pacemaker detects other activities besides the intended P wave or QRS complex?*
■ **Oversensing**

Oversensing results in the chamber not being paced when indicated because the pacemaker sensed other activity. Unwanted signals commonly sensed can be T wave (sensed as a QRS), skeletal muscle myopotentials, and signals from the pacemaker (cross-talking) in which the pacemaker senses the pacemaker spike as intrinsic activity.

> **HINT**
>
> On an ECG strip, this can look like a failure to pace.

■ *What does a "failure to capture" look like on an ECG strip?*
■ **Pacer spike without electrical activity**

Capture is the depolarization of the paced chamber. This is influenced by the amplitude and duration of the stimulus.

> **HINT**
>
> To correct failure to capture, the milliamps (mA) are increased.

BIBLIOGRAPHY

ACCF/AHA. (2009). Practice guideline: Focused update for diagnosis and management of heart failure in adults. *Circulation, 119,* 1977–2016.

ACCF/AHA. (2010). Guidelines for the diagnosis and management of thoracic aortic disease. *Circulation, 121,* 1544–1579.

ACCF/AHA. (2011). Focused update of the guideline for the management of patients with peripheral artery disease. *Circulation, 58,* 19.

ACCF/AHA. (2013). Guidelines for the management of ST-elevation myocardial infarction: Executive summary. *Circulation, 127,* 529–555.

AHA. (2013). Guidelines for ST elevation myocardial ischemia. *Circulation, 127.*

American Association of Critical-Care Nurses (AACN). (2009). AACN practice alert: ST segment monitoring.

American College of Surgeons on Trauma (1993). Advanced Trauma life Support for *Physicians, Students and Instructor Manual,* Chicago, American College of Surgeons.

Bodson L., Bouferrache K., & Vieillard-Baron, A. (2011). Cardiac tamponade. *Current Opinion in Critical Care, 17,* 416–424.

Little W., & Freeman G. (2006). Pericardial disease. *Circulation, 113,* 1622–1632.

Smithburger, P., Kane-Gill, S., Nestro, B., & Seybert, A. (2010). Recent advances in the treatment of hypertensive emergencies. *Critical Care Nurse, 30*(5), 24–30.

Questions

1. Mr. M begins to complain of chest pain. A 12-lead ECG is obtained and shows new-onset ST-segment elevation in leads II, III, and aVF. Which of the following would be the most appropriate assessment following this finding?

   A. Measure the QTc interval
   B. Place the precordial leads on the back of the patient
   C. Perform an ECG with right precordial leads
   D. Extend the left precordial chest leads

2. A patient is admitted to the ICU for a syncopal episode and is being evaluated. A 12-lead ECG and cardiac enzymes are obtained. His troponin levels are elevated and myocardial ischemia is suspected. Which of the following disorders can also elevate troponin levels and would need to be ruled out?

   A. Acute cardiomyopathy
   B. Scleroderma
   C. Sepsis
   D. Glioblastoma

3. ECG findings of ST-segment elevation may be found in other disorders and mimic STEMI. Which of the following disorder may elevate the ST segment?

   A. Hypovolemic shock
   B. Brugada's syndrome
   C. Dilated cardiomyopathy
   D. Mitral regurgitation

4. A preoperative cardiology consult was obtained on a patient admitted for a hip repair. The cardiologist recommended a cardiac catheterization procedure for evaluation. Significant coronary artery narrowing was found in two vessels. Which of the following is the most likely intervention to be performed?

   A. BMS placement
   B. CABG surgery
   C. DES placement
   D. Thrombolytic therapy

5. You have received report of a patient with a stent placed for a STEMI. During the report, the nurse tells you that there has been a recent increase in ST elevation, which occurred after the patient was bathed. Which of the following would be the most appropriate response?

   A. Ask the patient whether he wishes to be resuscitated.
   B. Ask the nurse whether the ECG patches were replaced during the bath.
   C. Call the physician stat and prepare for cardiac catheterization.
   D. Tell the nurse that it is normal to have an increase in ST segment in the acute period after a stent is placed.

6. Which of the following medications has been found to lower the efficacy of clopi-dogrel (Plavix) by reducing the formation of the active metabolite?

   A. Proton-pump inhibitors (PPIs)
   B. Calcium channel blockers
   C. β-blocker
   D. Antihistamine

7. A patient presents to the hospital with ACS within a month of a previous STEMI and stent placement. On assessment, the patient's home medications were found to include aspirin, clopidogrel (Plavix), and a statin. Which of the following is the most accurate statement regarding the restenosis?

   A. This is very common following placement of a BMS.
   B. The patient may have a CYP2C19 deficiency, resulting in a lowering of the efficacy of clopidogrel.
   C. The early restenosis indicates that the patient is noncompliant with the medications.
   D. Following a restenosis, the patient will require a CABG procedure to reopen the stenosis.

8. A β-blocker is frequently ordered following an ACS. In which of the following situa-tions would you expect the β-blocker to be discontinued?

   A. Cardiogenic shock
   B. CHF
   C. An elderly patient with cardiovascular disease
   D. Chronic lung disease without active bronchospasm

9. A patient received eplerenone (Inspra) for LV failure following an AMI. Which of the following laboratory values should be followed closely?

   A. Calcium
   B. Sodium
   C. Potassium
   D. Magnesium

10. A patient presents with an acute inferior wall MI with hypotension, clear breath sounds, and elevated jugular distention. Which of the following diagnosis would be the most likely based on the findings?

    A. CHF
    B. Dilated cardiomyopathy
    C. Septal wall infarction
    D. RV infarction

11. Which of the following class of medications should be avoided in patients with HF?

    A. Antidepressants
    B. Anticonvulsants
    C. Opioids
    D. Nonsteroidal anti-inflamatory drugs (NSAIDs)

12. A cardiologist ordered eplerenone, an aldosterone antagonist, to be started on a patient with HF in the ICU. Which of the following lab values would be a contraindication to administering the aldosterone antagonist?

    A. Potassium < 3.4 mEq/L
    B. Serum creatinine > 2.5 mg/dL
    C. Sodium < 135
    D. pH > 7.45

13. Mr. M presents with symptoms of HF. An echocardiogram finds an EF of 30%. The ECG demonstrates an abnormally wide QRS complex measuring 0.16 seconds. Which of the following therapeutic interventions would be recommended?

    A. Cardiac resynchronization therapy
    B. Implantable cardioverter–defibrillator
    C. Atrial ventricular pacemaker
    D. IABP

14. A patient presents with STEMI and has a history of stroke. Which of the following drugs or drug combinations may be administered to this patient during the PCI?

    A. ASA and prasugrel
    B. Fondaparinux alone
    C. Prasugrel
    D. ASA and clopidogrel (Plavix)

15. A patient presents to the ICU with angioedema after being on captopril (Capoten) for 1 year. Which of the following drugs would you expect the physician to order for this patient instead of captopril?

    A. Lisinopril (Prinivil)
    B. Losartan (Cozaar)
    C. Eplerenone (Inspra)
    D. Nesiritide (Natrecor)

16. A patient with parasternal penetrating chest wounds is sitting bolt upright, agitated, confused, and demonstrating air hunger. What is the most likely cause?

    A. Pericardial tamponade
    B. Flail chest
    C. Bronchial tear
    D. Aortic dissection

17. A patient is suspected of having a pericardial tamponade following a trauma. Which of the following is the best diagnostic test to rapidly identify excess pericardial fluid?

    A. CXR
    B. CT scan
    C. MRI
    D. FAST

18. Which of the following is a symptom of the Beck's triad?

    A. Increased jugular distention
    B. Agitation
    C. Hypertension
    D. S$_3$ gallop

19. Which of the following findings on an ultrasonography is a classic sign of pericardial tamponade?

    A. Dilated RV
    B. New-onset mitral regurgitation
    C. Dyskinesia
    D. "Swinging" heart

20. A common finding in a pericardial tamponade includes which of the following?

    A. Water Hammer's sign
    B. Pulsus alternans
    C. Auscultatory gap
    D. Levine's sign

21. Following a traumatic pericardial tamponade, which of the following statements would be most accurate in managing the patient?

    A. The priority of care is to intubate and ventilate the patient with positive pressure
    B. Maintain ventilation with bilevel positive airway pressure (BiPAP)
    C. Use higher levels of PEEP to manage the hypoxia
    D. Apply oxygen and avoid intubation if possible

22. Following an MVC, a patient was found to have rib fractures, pneumothorax, and a tibial/fibula fracture. The following vital signs are obtained on admission to the ICU:

    BP 126/78
    HR 138
    RR 22

    Which of the following would you suspect based on the above findings?

    A. Pericardial tamponade
    B. Myocardial contusion
    C. Hypovolemic shock
    D. Septic shock

23. Mr. M was involved in a high-speed MVC. Upon presentation to the emergency department, his vital signs are:

    BP 90/40
    HR 98
    RR 32

Fluid bolus is administered with BP increasing to 120/82. A left hemothorax and widened mediastinum is noted on CXR. A CT is placed on the left to drain the hemothorax. BP begins to decrease within 30 minutes of the initial bolus. Which of the following is the most likely cause of this patient's hemodynamic instability?

A. Aortic aneurysm
B. Myocardial contusion
C. Pericardial tamponade
D. Tension pneumothorax

24. Which of the following would be the most appropriate intervention in managing a hemodynamically unstable traumatic aortic aneurysm?

A. Provide aggressive fluid resuscitation
B. Maintain systolic BP < 120 mmHg
C. Perform passive leg raise procedure
D. Administer dopamine

25. A patient is admitted to the ICU with acute pulmonary edema. He has no history of HF. He had received mediastinal irradiation treatments about 2 years ago. An echocardiogram is ordered. Which of the following forms of cardiomyopathy would be the most likely cause of his congestion?

A. Hypertrophic cardiomyopathy
B. Dilated cardiomyopathy
C. Restrictive cardiomyopathy
D. Constrictive cardiomyopathy

26. A patient presents with HF and dyspnea. He is diagnosed with a hypertrophied cardiomyopathy based on the echocardiogram. Which of the following medications will most likely be used as a first-line management for his HF?

A. Digoxin
B. Nifedipine
C. Verapamil
D. Metoprolol (Lopressor)

27. Mr. M is admitted from the emergency room to the ICU with a diagnosis of hypertensive emergency. His initial BP in the emergency room was 225/122. The following are his admitting vital signs in the ICU:

BP 195/104
HR 86
RR 22

Which of the following is the most correct statement?

A. Hypertensive urgency requiring rapid decrease in systolic BP.
B. Hypertensive emergency is defined as a BP greater than 220 systolic or 120 diastolic.
C. Hypertensive urgency and hypertensive emergency are most commonly caused by acute kidney injury.
D. Hypertensive emergency is defined as hypertension accompanied by organ dysfunction.

28. A patient presents in a hypertensive crisis with a BP of 220/125. Which of the following medications would be the most appropriate for this patient?

    A. Enaloprit IV
    B. Esmolol IV
    C. Nifedipine SL
    D. Clonidine orally

29. Which of the following statements is the most correct regarding esmolol (Brevibloc)?

    A. It should be avoided in renal-failure patients due to excretion through the kidneys.
    B. The metabolism is via rapid hydrolysis and can be used in hepatic dysfunction.
    C. The half-life is 4 to 6 hours and may result in accumulation of the drug.
    D. It should be avoided in tachycardic patients due to reflex tachycardia.

30. An antihypertensive is ordered for a patient experiencing acute pulmonary edema and hypertension. On review of the patient's chart, it is noted that the patient is allergic to sulfites. Which of the following antihypertensive agents should be avoided in this patient?

    A. Fenoldopam (Corlopam)
    B. Esmolol (Brevibloc)
    C. Nicardipine (Cardene)
    D. Hydralazine

31. A physician ordered an antihypertensive agent to maintain systolic BP between 130 and 150 mmHg in a patient with hemorrhagic stroke. Which of the following antihypertensive agents is the most likely choice by the physician for this patient?

    A. Nimodipine (Nimotop)
    B. Sodium nitroprusside (Nipride)
    C. Nitroglycerin
    D. Nicardipine (Cardene)

32. Which of the following medications is contraindicated in patients with allergies to soy products?

    A. Nimodipine (Nimotop)
    B. Clevidipine (Cleviprex)
    C. Nicardipine (Cardene)
    D. Sodium nitroprusside (Nipride)

33. In a hypertensive emergency, what is the recommended reduction in MAP during initial treatment in the first hour?

    A. 10%
    B. 15%
    C. 20%
    D. 25%

34. Which of the following is the best drug in managing a dissecting thoracic aortic aneurysm?

    A. Sodium nitroprusside (Nipride)
    B. Nicardipine (Cardene)
    C. Hydralazine
    D. Esmolol (Brevibloc)

35. Which class of antihypertensives is preferred in the perioperative period in high-risk cardiac patients?

    A. β-blockers
    B. α-antagonists
    C. Calcium channel blockers
    D. Dopaminergic-1 receptor agonist

36. A patient is admitted with a cocaine overdose. He is tachycardic and hypertensive. Which of the following drugs should be avoided when initially managing this patient?

    A. β-blockers
    B. α-antagonists
    C. Calcium channel blockers
    D. Dopaminergic-1 receptor agonist

37. Which drug therapy is recommended in patients with mitral stenosis to improve LV filling?

    A. α-antagonists
    B. Diuretics
    C. β-blockers
    D. Digitalis

38. A patient presents with a history of intermittent claudication. His femoral pulse is strong but his popliteal and dorsalis pedis are absent. At what level is the obstruction?

    A. Aortoiliac
    B. Femoropopliteal
    C. Distal veins
    D. Popliteal dorsalis

39. A patient is admitted for severe claudication in lower extremities. ABI was noted to be 0.38. The physician has discussed the possibility of a bypass procedure with the patient. What is a normal ABI?

    A. Greater than 1.40
    B. 1.00 to 1.40
    C. 0.80 to 1.00
    D. Less than 0.40

40. This question refers to the patient in Question 39. In the previous patient scenario, which of the following would you expect the physician to order at this time?

A. Cardiac catheterization
B. MRI
C. Doppler ultrasonography
D. Arteriogram

41. Which of the following strokes is more common in patients following CPB surgeries?

   A. Lacunar stroke
   B. Vasospasms
   C. Watershed stroke
   D. Subarachnoid hemorrhage

42. A patient in your unit is hypotensive following a cardiac procedure. He has a significant history of hypertrophied cardiomyopathy. Which of the following vasoconstrictors would be the most appropriate for this patient?

   A. Phenylephrine
   B. Norepinephrine
   C. Dopamine
   D. Epinephrine

43. Your patient has RV failure. Which of the following agents can be used to decrease pulmonary vascular resistance to improve RV function?

   A. Nitroglycerin
   B. Nipride
   C. Epoprostenol
   D. Nicardipine

44. Which of the following potential side effects is the biggest concern when administering recombinant factor VIIa (rVIIa) to a bleeding patient?

   A. A hypersensitivity reaction
   B. Thrombocytopenia
   C. Arterial thromboembolic events
   D. Hemolytic blood transfusion reaction

45. Which of the following statements best describes the clinical significance of a new right bundle branch block (RBBB) following cardiac surgery?

   A. It is usually temporary and of little clinical significance
   B. It requires an external pacemaker until it resolves
   C. Shifts of the axis are uncommon and should be reported immediately
   D. It indicates the need for a biventricular pacemaker

46. While monitoring a post-CABG patient, the ST-segment monitor alarms due to a change in the ST segment. What finding on a 12-lead ECG would indicate acute graft failure?

   A. ST elevation in all the leads
   B. ST elevation in two or more contiguous leads in the territory of the grafted artery
   C. ST elevation in all the anterior leads
   D. ST depression in the inferior leads

47. While turning your post-CABG patient, there is a sudden increase in dark bloody output from the mediastinal tubes. Which of the following would be the most appropriate response?

    A. Page the cardiovascular surgeon stat
    B. Continue watching the patient for any signs of hemodynamic compromise
    C. Prepare the patient immediately for return to the operating room
    D. Strip the mediastinal chest tubes

48. On admission to the ICU from open heart surgery, a patient's ACT level was 250 seconds. Protamine 25 mg IV was ordered. After administering the protamine, saturations decreased to 89% and the patient became hypotensive. What is the most likely cause for these sudden changes?

    A. Severe bleeding
    B. Pulmonary embolism
    C. Cardiac tamponade
    D. Protamine reaction

49. You have a patient with an implanted pacemaker. The patient does not know what type of pacemaker she has and is not carrying the pacemaker ID card with her. Which of the following is the best method of determining the type of pacemaker this patient has?

    A. Echocardiogram
    B. 12-lead ECG
    C. CXR
    D. Right-sided 12-lead ECG

50. Your patient has an AAI implanted pacemaker. The patient has developed a second-degree Mobitz Type II block. What would you expect the physician's actions to be at this time?

    A. Watch the patient for signs of development of third-degree heart block
    B. Place an external pacemaker and prepare to replace the current pacemaker
    C. Place a magnet over the pacemaker to assure pacing
    D. Nothing; the patient already has a pacemaker

51. An implantable pacemaker was placed due to a third-degree AV block. One week after placement, it was noted that the pacemaker was not consistently capturing the ventricles. What would be the most likely cause for the change in pacing threshold?

    A. Lead maturation
    B. Fracture of lead
    C. Loss of lead contact with the heart
    D. Kinked lead

52. Your patient has been diagnosed with a dissecting abdominal aortic aneurysm. He is awaiting surgery and during your assessment, you note that his BP is 190/98 and HR is 108. Which of the following medications is most likely to be ordered?

    A. Nitroprusside (Nipride)
    B. Esmolol (Brevibloc)

C. Norepinephrine (Levophed)
D. Dobutamine (Dobutrex)

53. Your patient has an SvO_2 PAC, and the physician has ordered for oxygen delivery (DO_2) and oxygen consumption (VO_2) to be calculated. You note an increase in VO_2 after the CO was improved with dobutamine (Dobutrex). What does this indicate?

A. Tissues are adequately perfused
B. The patient was supply independent
C. DO_2 was not sufficient for the tissue demands
D. VO_2 was not calculated correctly

54. When caring for a patient after abdominal surgery, you note that SvO_2 has decreased from 68% to 55%. On assessment, you find the following:

BP 124/64
HR 88
RR 20
S_vO_2 97%
Temperature 35.0°C
CO/CI 4.5 L/min/3.4 L/min/m²
Hgb/hct 9.5/28%

Which of the following would be the most likely cause of the decrease in SvO_2 reading?

A. Shivering
B. Agitation
C. Anemia
D. Hypoxia

55. A patient is admitted to the critical care unit (CCU) following an anterior wall MI. He is hypotensive (82/55) and tachycardic (102 bpm). The echocardiogram found severe LV dysfunction, high LV filling pressures, and aortic regurgitation. The patient was diagnosed with cardiogenic shock. Which of the following interventions would be indicated at this time?

A. Dopamine (Intropin)
B. Dobutamine (Dobutrex)
C. IABP counterpulsation
D. Norepinephrine (Levophed)

56. While caring for a patient with an IABP, you note that the urine output has significantly decreased in the past hour. What potential complication of IABP would be of concern at this time?

A. Balloon rupture and air embolus
B. Timing problems with balloon inflating during systole
C. Balloon migration
D. IABP is no longer effective, and the patient is hypoperfused

57. Passive leg raising may be used to determine which of the following:

    A. Presence of hypovolemia
    B. Fluid responsiveness
    C. Presence of jugular venous distention
    D. CVP

58. A patient is admitted for severe pneumonia. It is noted that she has a history of MI. The most current echocardiogram determined LV EF to be 55%. She is classified as a Stage B in HF, according to the ACCF/AHA staging system. Which of the following would be an appropriate drug therapy for this patient to have received?

    A. Ramipril (Altace)
    B. Digitalis (Digoxin)
    C. Isosorbide (Isordil)
    D. Furosemide (Lasix)

59. A patient is in the ICU for respiratory failure and is found to have a significantly elevated BNP level. An echocardiogram shows hypertrophied cardiomyopathy. The patient is diagnosed with CHF. Which of the following medications would you expect the physician to order at this time?

    A. Dobutamine (Dobutrex)
    B. Nifedipine (Procardia)
    C. Furosemide (Lasix)
    D. Digitalis (Digoxin)

60. Which of the following statements best describes the role of BNPs?

    A. BNPs initiate the rennin–angiotensin system and increase the release of aldosterone.
    B. A decrease in BNP levels indicates HF.
    C. BNPs block the release of renin and decrease reabsorption of sodium.
    D. Elevation of BNP works as a vicious cycle in worsening HF.

61. Which type of cardiomyopathy is associated with a normal to high EF?

    A. Restrictive
    B. Constrictive
    C. Dilated
    D. Hypertrophied

2

Pulmonary System Review

In this chapter, you will review:

- Acute respiratory failure
- Acute respiratory distress syndrome (ARDS)
- Pulmonary embolism (PE)
- Chronic obstructive pulmonary disease (COPD) exacerbations/severe asthma/status asthmaticus
- Acute respiratory infections
- Air leak syndromes
- Aspirations
- Pulmonary hypertension
- Thoracic trauma
- Mechanical ventilation
- Pulmonary therapeutic interventions

ACUTE RESPIRATORY FAILURE

■ *What are the two characteristics of respiratory failure found on an arterial blood gas (ABG)?*
■ **Hypercapnia and hypoxemia**

Respiratory insufficiency occurs when the patient is struggling to breathe but still able to maintain gas exchange. Respiratory failure is difficulty breathing and the inadequacy of the respiratory system to support gas exchange. Respiratory failure is characterized by hypercapnia ($PaCO_2 > 45$ mmHg) and hypoxemia ($PaO_2 < 55$ mmHg).

> ❯ HINT
> "Crossed blood gas" is an indicator of respiratory failure ($PaCO_2 > PaO_2$).

■ *In normal conditions, what does the $PaCO_2$ directly vary with?*
■ **Minute ventilation (MV)**

MV is respiratory rate (RR) multiplied by tidal volume (TV). The $PaCO_2$ measures ventilation. In normal conditions, there is a direct inverse relationship between MV and $PaCO_2$. As the MV increases (rate or volume), the $PaCO_2$ decreases. Elevated $PaCO_2$ is the hallmark of hypercapnic respiratory failure.

> ❯ HINT
> Increasing $PaCO_2$ in asthma patients is an ominous sign of impending respiratory failure.

PATHOPHYSIOLOGY

■ *What is a ventilation perfusion (VQ) mismatch in which there is perfusion without ventilation called?*

■ **VQ shunt**

A shunt is needed when the mixed venous blood from the right side of the heart enters the left side without being oxygenated. The primary problem is ventilation. The alveoli are not open and ventilating but are being perfused. A shunt is considered a low VQ state (Box 2.1).

> ❯ HINT
> Hypoxemia due to a shunt is not reversible with oxygen therapy.

Box 2.1 Common Causes of Shunts

Atelectasis	Central airway obstruction
Pneumothorax	Compressive atelectasis (pleural effusion)
ARDS	Chronic bronchitis
Pulmonary edema	Alveolar hemorrhage

■ *What is the compensatory mechanism in the lungs that occurs following onset of a VQ shunt?*

■ **Pulmonary vasoconstriction**

This hypoxic vasoconstriction reduces some of the blood flow to the areas of the lungs that are underventilated in an attempt to compensate.

> ❯ HINT
> This hypoxic response can result in pulmonary hypertension and right ventricular (RV) failure.

■ *What is alveolar dead space?*

■ **Ventilation without perfusion**

Dead space is the opposite end of the spectrum from a shunt. In dead space, the alveoli are open and being ventilated but without perfusion. The VQ mismatch is related to decreased blood flow through the pulmonary capillaries. This is most commonly caused by a PE. Dead space is a high VQ state (Box 2.2).

Box 2.2 Causes of Dead Space

Pulmonary embolism
Pulmonary hypertension (primary and secondary)
Emphysema/chronic obstructive pulmonary disease (COPD)

■ *What are two major conditions that lead to hypercapnic respiratory failure?*
■ **Hypoventilation and high dead space**

Hypoventilation, or decrease in MV, leads to accumulation of CO_2. Alveolar ventilation decreases as dead space increases, resulting in hypercapnia even with a high MV. Air trapping from obstructive lung disease can also result in high dead space and hypercapnic respiratory failure (Box 2.3).

Box 2.3 Causes of Hypercapnic Respiratory Failure

Hypoventilation	High Dead Space
Respiratory muscle fatigue	COPD
Obesity (i.e., obstructive sleep apnea, obesity hypoventilation syndrome)	Pulmonary embolism
Central nervous system (CNS) depressants (i.e., opioid, benzodiazepines, alcohol)	Pulmonary hypertension
Spinal cord injury	Pulmonary fibrosis
Neuromuscular disorders (i.e., myasthenia gravis, Guillain-Barré)	
CNS disorders (i.e., stroke, traumatic brain injuries)	
Chest wall disorders (i.e., kyphosis)	

The pattern of increasing dead space can cause a downward spiral into respiratory failure in obstructive airway disease such as COPD (Figure 2.1).

> **HINT**
> Any cause of increased RR in obstructive airway diseases can cause rapid decline into respiratory failure.

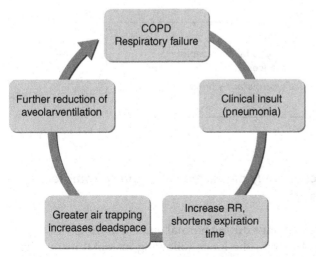

FIGURE 2.1 Respiratory failure due to dead space.

SYMPTOMS/ASSESSMENT

■ *On the ABG, which component should be used to determine whether hypercapnia is acute or chronic?*

■ pH

A patient with chronic respiratory failure with hypercapnia will have a high $PaCO_2$, but a normal pH due to metabolic compensation (elevated bicarbonate level). People with chronic respiratory failure appear to breathe comfortably, without dyspnea, with a low PaO_2.

> ❯ HINT
> A low pH in a COPD patient indicates "acute-on-chronic" respiratory failure.

■ *Which VQ mismatch results in uncoupling the relationship between MV and $PaCO_2$?*

■ Dead space

Dead space may be recognized on an ABG by the uncoupling of the relationship between the MV and $PaCO_2$. The relationship may actually move in the opposite direction. An increase in MV does not result in a significant decrease in $PaCO_2$ and may actually have a high $PaCO_2$ with the increase in MV.

> ❯ HINT
> An increase in end-tidal CO_2 (capnography) during normal ventilation may indicate the presence of dead space.

■ *What mental status change occurs with hypercapnic respiratory failure?*

■ Decreased level of consciousness

Hypercapnia results in a decreased level of consciousness. Hypoxia causes agitation, confusion, and delirium initially (Box 2.4).

Box 2.4 Other Signs of Respiratory Failure

Increased work of breathing (WOB)	Tachypnea
Use of accessory muscles	Inability to talk in complete
Flushed appearance (hypercapnia)	sentences
Central cyanosis	Tachycardia/arrhythmias
Abdominal breathing	

DIAGNOSIS

■ *Which lung volumes are most commonly measured using the spirometer?*

■ TV and forced vital capacity (FVC)

TV is the volume moved in and out of the lungs during normal quiet breathing. FVC is the maximal amount of air forcibly expelled from the lungs following maximal inspiration.

They are both measured by a spirometer. These tests are used to determine lung capacity during respiratory distress. A normal, spontaneous TV is 400 to 500 mL/breath and normal FVC is 3,700 to 4,800 mL (Box 2.5).

Box 2.5 Lung Volumes and Pulmonary Function Tests

Lung Volume Measurements	Description	Normal Findings
Vital capacity (VC)	Maximal breath in and maximal breath out (TLC – residual volume)	3,700–4,800 mL
Residual volume	Volume of air in lungs after maximal exhalation	1,200 mL
Functional residual capacity (FRC)	Volume of air in lungs after normal quiet exhalation	2,400 mL
Total lung capacity (TLC)	Volume of air in lungs at maximal inspiration (VC + residual volume)	4.7–6.0 L
Forced expiratory volume in 1 second (FEV1)	Amount of air exhaled at the end of 1 second of forced exhalation after maximal inspiration	>80% of the predicted FEV1 (based on age, gender, ethnicity of patient)
FEV1/FVC ratio	Ratio of FEV1 to the forced vital capacity (FVC)	75%–80%
Tidal volume (TV)	Amount of air moved in and out during normal quiet breathing	400–500 mL
FVC	Maximal amount of air forcibly exhaled from the lungs following maximal inspiration	3,700–4,800 mL
Peak expiratory flow rate (PEFR)	Highest forced expiratory flow (speed)	> 80% predicted value (predicted PEFR based on height and gender)

- **If FEV1 is decreased but the FVC is normal resulting in a decreased FEV1/FVC ratio, is this a restrictive or obstructive disease?**
- **Obstructive disease**

An obstructive disease (i.e., asthma, COPD) will result in a decrease in FEV1 with typically normal FVC resulting in a decrease in the FEV1/FVC ratio. In a restrictive disease (i.e., pulmonary fibrosis), both FEV1 and FVC are decreased resulting in a normal FEV1/FVC ratio (Box 2.6).

> **⟩ HINT**
> FEV1/FVC is used to differentiate an obstructive from a restrictive disease process.

Box 2.6 Severity of Obstruction Determined by FEV1

FEV1 > 80% predicted	Normal
FEV1 = 60%–79% predicted	Mild obstruction
FEV1 = 40%–59% predicted	Moderated obstruction
FEV1 < 40% predicted	Severe obstruction

MANAGEMENT

■ *What is the technique of applying positive pressure ventilation via a mask called?*

■ **Noninvasive ventilation (NIV)**

NIV is the technique of supplying positive pressure ventilatory support to the airways through a mask attached to a patient's nose or mouth. It is used in an attempt to avoid artificial airways and the complications associated with them. Continuous positive airway pressure (CPAP) and bilevel positive airway pressure (BiPAP) are forms of NIV.

■ *Which patients are most likely to be successfully treated with NIV?*

■ **Those with COPD**

Patients who present with exacerbation of COPD or hypercapnic respiratory failure are most likely to benefit from NIV. The ideal patient is one in whom impending respiratory failure is present but in whom cooperation with a mask system is still possible. Early application has shown to be more effective. Respiratory failure resulting in reduction in functional residual capacity (FRC) can cause an increase in work of breathing (WOB), leading to respiratory muscle fatigue. Increasing the FiO_2 alone without assisting the ventilation may not treat the respiratory problem.

> ❯ HINT
> NIV has been found to "buy time" for reversible pulmonary issues
> (Box 2.7).

Box 2.7 Indications for NIV

COPD	Immunocompromised patient
Status asthmaticus	Congestive heart failure (CHF) with pulmonary edema
Acute hypoxic respiratory failure	
End of life (refusing intubation)	Cystic fibrosis
Compromised lung function during conscious sedation	

■ *Would NIV be a potential option on an upper gastrointestinal bleeding (GIB) patient with a compromised airway?*

■ **No**

NIV with a mask does not protect the airway and can increase risk of aspiration with vomiting. A compromised airway in an upper GIB would be an indication for intubation and mechanical ventilation.

> ❯ HINT
> NIV is not recommended for patients with altered mental status,
> swallowing abnormalities, or an inability to control secretions due to risk
> of aspiration (Box 2.8). Do not use NIV in rapidly deteriorating patients
> at risk for respiratory arrest. These patients should be intubated and
> placed on mechanical ventilation (Box 2.9).

Box 2.8 Contraindications for NIV

Cardiopulmonary arrest	Pneumocephalus
Hemodynamic instability	Cardiogenic shock
Apnea	Extreme anxiety
Vomiting	Decreased level of
GIB	consciousness
Facial trauma or surgery	
Burns facial region or inhalation injuries	

Box 2.9 Advantages and Disadvantages of NIV

Advantage	Disadvantage
Avoid complications of endotracheal intubation (ventilator-acquired pneumonia, tracheal injury)	Does not provide airway protection or ready access for airway toiletry
Decreased length of stay	Increased risk of aspiration
Improved ability in communication	Facial skin abrasions
Decreased need for sedation or analgesia	Decreased ability to clear secretions
Less antibiotic use	Gastric distension
Reduced need for prolonged mechanical ventilation	Aspiration gastric contents

■ *Is CPAP or BiPAP a time-cycled, pressure-targeted mode of NIV?*
■ **BiPAP**

BiPAP applies pressure during inspiration and expiration. It is a time-cycled, pressure-targeted mode of ventilation. The pressure provided during inspiration can assist with the work overload of the respiratory muscles while the expiratory pressure can reduce the breath triggering resistance by the positive end-expiratory pressure (PEEP). CPAP raises the functional residual capacity, which may reduce the inspiratory work to breathe but does not provide ventilation.

> ❯ **HINT**
> BiPAP can further reduce the inspiratory workload over CPAP.

COMPLICATIONS

■ *In an awake patient with respiratory distress being placed on NIV, what should be restricted until the patient's tolerance increases and reverses acute ventilatory failure?*
■ **Oral intake**

Oral intake should be restricted during the initiation of NIV following acute ventilatory failure to prevent aspiration. Once the patient is tolerating NIV and the acute ventilatory failure is reversed, oral intake may be resumed unless there are other contraindications.

> ❯ **HINT**
> A nasal mask is better for oral intake because patients are able to take fluids without removing the mask and there is a lower incidence of aspiration (Box 2.10).

Box 2.10 Complications of NIV

Claustrophobia	Skin breakdown
Aspiration	Gastric distention
Air leaks	

ACUTE RESPIRATORY DISTRESS SYNDROME

■ *What type of pulmonary edema occurs with ARDS?*

■ **Noncardiogenic pulmonary edema**

ARDS is defined as a noncardiac pulmonary edema characterized by an increase in capillary permeability with interstitial and alveolar edema of the lungs.

> ❯ HINT
> A patient with congestive heart failure (CHF) can be diagnosed with ARDS if the clinical condition cannot be fully explained by cardiac failure or fluid overload.

■ *Is ARDS considered to be a primary or secondary lung disease?*

■ **Secondary**

ARDS is a secondary lung disease that develops as a result of a trauma or injury to the lung. The injury may be direct or indirect (through the bloodstream). ARDS is the pulmonary component of the generalized systemic inflammatory process affecting multiple organs and caused by circulating mediators in response to a major insult or injury.

> ❯ HINT
> ARDS is most commonly associated with sepsis/septic shock.

PATHOPHYSIOLOGY

■ *Is the excessive fluid in the lungs of an ARDS patient interstitial or intra-alveolar?*

■ **Both interstitial and intra-alveolar**

There is damage to the alveolar capillary endothelium resulting in an increase in capillary permeability leading to both interstitial and alveolar edema ("white out" of lung). The pathophysiology of ARDS centers on the processes of:

1. Increased microvascular permeability
2. Capillary endothelial damage
3. Neutrophil activation

■ *What lung cells make up the alveolar–capillary membrane and are responsible for gas exchange?*

■ **Type I pneumocytes**

The vascular endothelium and alveolar epithelium are made up of Type I pneumocytes and are responsible for integrity and gas exchange. Following injury, the Type I pneumocytes are damaged, which increases alveolar–capillary membrane permeability. The fluid in the lung is composed of sodium, water, and proteins that have crossed into the alveolar and interstitial compartments. Administration of albumin during a period of increased permeability may cause more protein extravasation in the lungs.

> ❯ HINT
> Damage to the capillary–alveolar membrane results in initial hypoxemia and chest x-ray (CXR) changes.

■ *What do Type II pneumocytes produce in the lungs?*
■ **Surfactant**

Damage to Type II pneumocytes results in a decrease and alteration in surfactant, leading to atelectasis, VQ mismatches, and further hypoxemia. Analysis of bronchial lavage after the development of ARDS found the surfactant to be low in phospholipids and proteins A and B, causing the surfactant to be ineffective.

> ❯ HINT
> Disruption in the production of surfactant results in further hypoxemia and increased WOB.

■ *What role does a surfactant have in the lungs?*
■ **Decreases alveolar surface tension**

A surfactant decreases surface tension in the alveoli, thus allowing the alveoli to inflate more readily and increase lung compliance. The surfactant "splints" alveoli open and allows for recruitment of alveoli, thus improving the FRC in the lungs. This correlates to WOB.

> ❯ HINT
> Balloon analogy: Take a balloon that is already filled with air, empty some of the air out, and then blow it back up. It is easy because of the FRC or "splinting" of the balloon walls open with the remaining air. That is alveoli with a normal surfactant. Now take a new balloon and blow it up. It is much harder to inflate because of the surface tension within the balloon without air. This is alveoli without a normal functioning surfactant.

■ *What does the release of pro-inflammatory cytokines and activation of neutrophils cause in the pulmonary vasculature?*
■ **Pulmonary hypertension**

Pro-inflammatory cytokines (i.e., tumor necrosis factor [TNF]) are released following a pulmonary injury. Pro-inflammatory cytokines recruit neutrophils into the lungs. Activation of the neutrophils in the lungs causes the release of toxic chemical mediators, further damaging the alveolar–capillary membrane, increasing capillary permeability and causing pulmonary vasoconstriction leading to pulmonary edema. The resulting pulmonary hypertension worsens hypoxemia and increases the workload of the right ventricle.

> ❯ HINT
> Pulmonary vasoconstriction creates a dead space, worsening the VQ mismatch.

■ *What is the chronic change that occurs in the lungs in ARDS patients?*
■ **Fibrosis**

Fibrosis of the lung occurs during the proliferative phase. The repair component involves proliferation and altered function of endothelial cells, Type II pneumocyte cells, and interstitial matrix cells. Type I cells are destroyed and are replaced with Type II cells, which leads to fibrosis.

> ❯ HINT
> The fibrosis contributes to a decrease in lung compliance of ARDS patients.

■ *Which two lung volumes significantly decrease in ARDS?*
■ **Vital capacity (VC) and FRC**

There is a decrease in lung capacity and FRC due to the collapsed airways. There is a nonuniform collapse of the functional lung units.

> ❯ HINT
> FRC correlates to WOB. As the FRC decreases, the WOB increases. PEEP applied to the ventilator will increase the FRC and lower the WOB and improve oxygenation (Box 2.11). The primary VQ mismatch is an alveolar shunt due to the decreased ability to ventilate.

Box 2.11 Physiological Effects of ARDS

Decreased FRC	Dead space with pulmonary vasoconstriction
Decreased total lung capacity	Abnormal gas exchange
Hypoxemia due to alveolar shunt	

SYMPTOMS/ASSESSMENT

■ *What are the initial symptoms in a patient during the early stages of ARDS?*
■ **Hypoxemia, tachypnea, and dyspnea**

The symptoms usually have a quick onset, within hours to days after the initial injury or insult to the lungs. The initial presentation is hypoxemia with tachypnea and dyspnea. CXR changes may also be an early sign of ARDS and can occur within 4 to 24 hours of the initial insult (Box 2.12).

> ❯ **HINT**
> A cardinal sign of ARDS is hypoxemia refractory to supplemental oxygen.

Box 2.12 Early Signs of ARDS

Use of accessory muscles	Course crackles
Shallow, rapid breathing	Restlessness
Respiratory alkalosis	Increased work of breathing

- ■ *What is the primary issue with ventilating a patient in the later stages of ARDS?*
- ■ **Decreased lung compliance**

The lung is considered a "baby lung" with only about one third of the lung being ventilated during the later stages of ARDS. The lung is filled with fluid, alveoli have collapsed, signaling the onset of pulmonary fibrosis. The characteristic problem associated with ventilating ARDS patients is decreased lung compliance (Box 2.13).

> ❯ **HINT**
> Peak inspiratory and plateau pressures increase on the ventilator due to decrease in lung compliance.

Box 2.13 Symptoms of ARDS at Later Stages

Increase peaked inspiratory pressures (PIP)	Tachycardia
Course crackles and rhonchi bilateral	Severe hypoxemia
Metabolic acidosis due to elevated lactate levels	Pallor and cyanosis
Respiratory acidosis due to hypercarbia	Bilateral pulmonary infiltrates
Use of accessory muscles and nasal flaring	Increased work of breathing

DIAGNOSIS

- ■ *What are the primary CXR criteria used to diagnose ARDS?*
- ■ **Bilateral fluffy infiltrates**

ARDS is a bilateral lung disease characterized by pulmonary infiltrates. It is commonly called "white out on CXR." A computed tomography (CT) scan may also be used to determine the presence of bilateral fluffy infiltrates (Box 2.14).

Box 2.14 Berlin Definition of ARDS

Acute onset	Within 7 days of a defined event
Impaired oxygenation	Abnormal PaO$_2$/FiO$_2$ ratio (PF ratio)
Bilateral fluffy infiltrates	CXR or CT scan

■ *Severe ARDS is defined by what PaO$_2$/FiO$_2$ ratio?*
■ **Less than 100**

The Berlin definition of ARDS includes categories of severity based on the PaO$_2$/FiO$_2$ ratio (also called the PF ratio).

> ❯ **HINT**
> Remember, when calculating the PaO$_2$/FiO$_2$ ratio, use the decimal point (40% is 0.40; Box 2.15).

Box 2.15 Severity of ARDS

Severity of ARDS	PaO$_2$/FiO$_2$ Ratio
Mild	200–300
Moderate	100–200
Severe	<100

For example:
If a patient's PaO$_2$ is 80 on 50% FiO$_2$,
80 ÷ 0.50 = 160

> ❯ **HINT**
> A normal PaO$_2$ is only normal on room air. If on a higher FiO$_2$, a normal PaO$_2$ (80–100 mmHg) may actually be abnormal. PF ratio calculation is used to determine severity of impaired oxygenation.

■ *What is the most common indirect injury to the lungs that can result in the development of ARDS?*
■ **Sepsis**

The development of respiratory failure following a clinical injury to the lungs, either directly or indirectly, leads to the diagnosis of ARDS. An indirect injury is usually the result of an inflammatory reaction to a certain disease or clinical state. Direct injury to the alveoli or lung parenchyma results in a loss of integrity of the alveolar–capillary membrane, leading to ARDS (Boxes 2.16 and 2.17).

Box 2.16 Indirect Lung Injury

Sepsis/septic shock	Diabetic ketoacidosis (DKA)
Pancreatitis	Drug overdose
Massive trauma	Cardiopulmonary bypass
Multiple blood transfusions	Amniotic fluid embolus
Prolonged severe shock	Tissue necrosis

Box 2.17 Direct Lung Injury

Excessive fluid resuscitation	Pneumonitis
Inhalation injuries (smoke or toxic gases)	Drug inhalation
Oxygen toxicity	Pulmonary contusions
Aspiration	Pneumococcal pneumonia
Near drowning	Pulmonary embolism

MANAGEMENT

- ▣ *Is the current management of ARDS aimed at reversing permeability abnormalities or maintaining ventilation and organ perfusion?*
- ▣ **Maintaining ventilation and organ perfusion**

The goal in managing an ARDS patient is to maintain acceptable gas exchange with minimal complications. Maintaining gas exchange and an aerobic metabolism will limit the hypoperfusion and organ dysfunction. When determining the appropriate ventilatory technique, the goal of oxygenation must be carefully weighed against the potential for further injury to the lungs.

- ▣ *What is trauma to the lungs caused by repeated cycles of recruitment and derecruitment called?*
- ▣ **Atelectrauma**

Atelectrauma is the injury caused by repeated cycles of recruitment and derecruitment of the alveoli. Damage to conducting airways may be secondary to the cyclical collapse and reopening of the terminal airways with shear stress.

> ❯ **HINT**
> Lung recruitment with PEEP can limit the injury of atelectrauma (Box 2.18). A high-pressure alarm sounding on the ventilator of an ARDS patient may indicate pneumothorax from barotrauma.

Box 2.18 Ventilatory Complications in ARDS Patients

Complication	Description	Prevention
Barotrauma	High ventilatory pressures cause air to mitigate out of alveoli into the extrapulmonary space	Maintain peak inspiratory pressure (PIP) < 40 cm H_2O and plateau pressures (PLP) < 30 cm H_2O
Atelectrauma	Hearing effect caused by repeated cyclic recruitment and derecruitment of alveoli	Utilize lung recruitment techniques to maintain alveoli open; PEEP
Volutrauma	Caused by overdistention and stretch-type injury with greater inflammatory response in lungs	Use small TVs for ventilating; recommended 6 mL/kg TV
Biotrauma	Release local mediators in lung and associated with large TV	Use small TVs, avoid overdistension on alveoli
Oxygen toxicity	Causes endothelial damage, decrease in surfactant, thickening of alveoli membrane, decreased macrophage activity	Maintain oxygenation on FiO_2 < 60%

■ *What is the recommended TV for a patient with ARDS?*
■ **6 mL/kg**

An ARDS net trial found that small TVs with lower plateau pressures (PLPs) improved outcomes. The recommendation from that trial was a TV of 6 mL/kg with PLP less than 30 to 35 cm H_2O. The high inspiratory pressure required to deliver traditional TVs (10 mL/kg) to the remaining normal lung tissue causes significant overdistension, barotrauma, and diffuse alveolar damage. Low TVs have also been associated with less intra-alveolar cytokines.

> **HINT**
> Use ideal body weight (in kg), not actual body weight, to calculate TV (Box 2.19).

Box 2.19 Goals of Ventilation

Oxygenation	Maintain > 88%–90%
FiO_2	< 60%–70%
Peak inspiratory pressure (PIP)	< 40–45 cm H_2O
PLP	< 30 cm H_2O
TV	6 mL/kg ideal body weight
RR	Up to 35 bpm (breaths per minute) (minute ventilation [MV] 7–9 L/min)

■ *Which lung volume does PEEP increase when ventilating a patient with ARDS?*
■ **FRC**

FRC is the volume in the lungs at the end of expiration. PEEP is used to increase FRC of acutely injured lungs, resulting in an increased alveolar size, holding the alveoli open, and recruitment of collapsed alveoli. This increases the surface area for gas exchange and decreases shunting.

> **HINT**
> Monitor hemodynamics closely because PEEP can have a paradoxical effect on oxygen delivery by reducing venous return and cardiac output.

■ *What is that point on a compliance curve below which the alveoli will collapse?*
■ **Lower inflection point**

A compliance curve in the lungs has two inflection points. The lower inflection point is the critical opening pressure of most alveoli that are available for recruitment. It is the minimal pressure required to begin to open the alveoli, below which the alveoli will collapse. The upper inflection point is the maximal pressure beyond which no more alveoli will be recruited and overdistension occurs. The pressure–volume curve is a method used to determine the amount of PEEP required to maximally recruit and maintain lung volumes without overdistension

■ *What is the ventilatory technique that is used to reduce a patent's ventilatory support to a minimally acceptable PaO$_2$ while allowing PaCO$_2$ to rise?*

■ **Permissive hypercapnia**

To achieve the low plateau and peak inspiratory pressures recommended, TVs may be very low with resulting elevations in the PaCO$_2$. Manipulation of the ventilator settings to lower the PaCO$_2$ may increase barotrauma, volutrauma, and/or atelectrauma. This strategy is a deliberate hypoventilation in an effort to reduce pulmonary overdistention and high pressures within the noncollapsed portion of the lung (Box 2.20).

> **❭ HINT**
> Ventilator changes usually made to correct hypercapnia include increasing the RR and/or TV.

Box 2.20 Permissive Hypercapnia Management

No upper limit of PaCO$_2$
Allow pH to decrease to at least 7.20 before treatment
If < 7.20, sodium bicarbonate or THAM may be administered

■ *What clinical condition would be contraindicated in performing permissive hypercapnia?*

■ **Increased intracranial pressure (ICP)**

Permissive hypercapnia is contraindicated in neurological patients with increased ICP. Hypercapnia causes cerebral vasodilation with an increase in cerebral blood volume, thus increasing ICP. Other conditions that may also be contraindicated are active coronary artery disease (hypercapnia causes a negative inotropic effect), arrhythmias, hypovolemia, and GIB.

■ *Which mode of ventilation is used to control peak inspiratory pressures?*

■ **Pressure-controlled ventilation (PCV)**

PCV sets an upper pressure limit on the ventilator (pressure control) that determines the end of the inspiratory cycle and inspiratory volume. The TV varies per breath, depending upon the compliance of the airway and lungs. This method of ventilation is used to limit excessive airway pressures and improve mean airway pressure. Inverse inspiratory to expiratory ration (I:E) ratios may be used in this mode of ventilation.

> **❭ HINT**
> The flow waveform used to deliver a breath in PCV is a decelerating waveform (volume control uses a square waveform).

■ *What change in the ventilator settings can be made to increase TV?*

■ **Increasing pressure limit**

The inspiratory volume stops being delivered at a preset inspiratory pressure. Within a static period of lung compliance and airway resistance, an increase in the set pressure limit will increase the TV delivered. It allows a greater airway pressure to be reached before the end of inspiration.

> ### ❯ HINT
> Remember, airway resistance and lung compliance affect the amount of inspiratory volume delivered per breath in pressure-controlled ventilation.

■ *Which mode of ventilation not only uses a pressure limit but also allows spontaneous breathing throughout the cycle?*

■ **Airway pressure release ventilation (APRV)**

APRV is a pressure-limited, time-cycled mode of ventilation used to manage ARDS patients. It allows for spontaneous breathing throughout the respiratory cycle. APRV is considered a lung-protective mode of ventilation that allows for the recruitment of alveoli and splints alveoli open to prevent injury from derecruitment. The proposed advantage is the ability to maintain a higher mean airway pressure while the peak alveolar pressure remains lower and allows for spontaneous breathing.

> ### ❯ HINT
> This mode of ventilation is also called bilevel, biphasic, and bi-vent.

■ *In the APRV mode of ventilation, is the majority of the time in the higher pressure (P high) or lower pressure (P low)?*

■ **Higher pressure (P high)**

A baseline high pressure (called P high) and a low pressure (called P low) are set. Mandatory breaths of the ventilator are delivered by releasing the high pressure briefly to the low pressure, which allows the lungs to partially deflate, then quickly return to the high pressure. The amount of time spent at the high pressure is about 80% to 95% of the cycle. Other parameters set in this mode are T high and T low. T high is the time spent in the high pressure, and T low is the amount of time in the low pressure.

> ### ❯ HINT
> Remember spontaneous breathing occurs throughout this cycle, increasing MV.

■ *What occurs when the expiratory time is limited in modes such as APRV or inverse I:E ratio with pressure control?*

■ **Auto-PEEP**

When using the inverse I:E ratio, the expiratory time is shorter than the inspiratory time, allowing a residual amount of air to remain in the lungs, called intentional auto-PEEP. In APRV, the release time from high P to low P is much shorter than the equilibrium time in high P, causing air trapping or intentional auto-PEEP. Auto-PEEP is used to prevent derecruitment of alveoli and is optimally above the level of the lower inflection point.

> ❯ **HINT**
>
> Auto-PEEP occurs by restricting expiratory flow time. Monitoring of the amount of auto-PEEP is necessary when using these modes of ventilation.

■ *What ventilator settings can be changed to improve oxygenation in the APRV mode besides FiO$_2$?*

■ **Prolong T high or increase P high**

Prolonging the time at the higher pressure (T high) or increasing the high pressure (P high) can improve oxygenation. These changes will increase the mean airway pressure and recruit more alveoli. Hypercapnia is an expected consequence of APRV ventilation and permissive hypercapnia is typically used in combination with the APRV. If severe, reduce the PaCO$_2$ by reducing the T high (this increases the frequency of releases).

> ❯ **HINT**
>
> Pressure support can be added to APRV to improve spontaneous breaths.

■ *What is the method of weaning the ventilator in APRV mode?*

■ **Decrease P high and prolong T high**

By decreasing the P high, there is less pressure splitting the alveoli, and lengthening the T high decreases the frequency of release allowing for more of the breaths to be spontaneous breaths over mechanical. The goal is for most or all of the MV to be from spontaneous breaths (Box 2.21).

> ❯ **HINT**
>
> APRV can be changed to CPAP once the spontaneous breaths are adequate to complete the weaning process.

Box 2.21 Advantages and Disadvantages of APRV

Advantage	Disadvantage
Spontaneous breaths, better ventilation for dependent regions of lungs	Potential overstretching of alveoli
Relatively comfortable form of ventilation and is well tolerated	Lack of ability to spontaneously breathe in this mode of ventilation
Less sedation	Increased ICP due to increase in mean airway pressures
Greater mean airway pressure	Increase in bronchopleural fistulas (worsening of air leaks)
Improved venous return and cardiac output	Patient maintains the work of breathing
Lower peak pressures	

■ *What is the method of delivering the MV in high-frequency oscillatory ventilation (HFOV)?*

■ **High frequencies and low TV**

High-frequency ventilation is the use of higher than normal frequencies of ventilation with very small TVs. An oscillator ventilator provides a continuous flow in the circuit and oscillates or moves the air back and forth with a piston. In theory, HFOV minimizes alveolar overdistension and recruitment–derecruitment injury. It has the unique benefit that both inspiration and expiration are active.

> **HINT**
> HFOV may be described as CPAP with a "wriggle."

■ *In HFOV, how is the frequency of ventilation measured?*

■ **Hertz (Hz)**

The frequency is measured in hertz on an oscillator ventilator. The piston-driven diaphragm delivers the small TVs at frequencies between 3 and 15 Hz. Lowering the frequency will increase TVs and CO_2 elimination. The power is also set, which means the piston pressure swings generating the TV. Increasing the power will increase CO_2 elimination by increasing the TV.

> **HINT**
> 15 Hz is equal to 15 breaths per second.

■ *In HFOV mode of ventilation, oxygenation is dependent on what settings?*

■ **Mean positive airway pressure (mPaw) and FiO$_2$**

The mPaw and FiO_2 can be titrated to improve oxygenation. Improvement in VQ matching and oxygenation is found to correlate well with high mPaw. The mPaw is set in this mode of ventilation. The initial setting is typically 5 cm H_2O pressure above the mPaw in a conventional ventilator.

> **HINT**
> Usually when the mPaw has been titrated down to less than 24 cm H_2O pressure and FiO_2 is 40% to 50%, the patient is ready to return to a conventional ventilator.

■ *A patient with ARDS demonstrating problems with maintaining saturations can be placed in what position?*

■ **Prone**

Lung infiltrates and damaged lung units in ARDS are not uniformly distributed. CT scans have found that dependent portions of the lungs are more affected and less dependent areas remain normal with normal compliance. The prone position can improve oxygenation by improving ventilation perfusion ratios in the dependent regions. The use of the intermittent prone position can improve oxygenation. It is recommended in refractory hypoxemic patients (Boxes 2.22 and 2.23).

Box 2.22 Risks of Prone Position

Inadvertent dislodgement of the endotracheal tube	Initial worsening in respiratory status
Inadvertent dislodgement of lines or tubes	Facial edema
Development of pressure ulcerations	Hemodynamic instability

Box 2.23 Other Experimental Therapies

Extracorporeal membrane oxygenation (ECMO)	Nitric oxide (NO) or prostacyclin
Surfactant	Perflourocarbons ("liquid ventilation")

COMPLICATIONS

■ *What is the first pharmacological intervention for ventilator dyssynchrony ("bucking the ventilator")?*

■ **Sedation**

Sedation is the first step to improve ventilator–patient synchrony. Neuromuscular blocking agents (NMBAs) can be used but are considered to be the last resort. If the patient continues to "fight" the ventilator, and ventilatory pressures remain elevated with sedation and analgesics alone, then adding an NMBA would be appropriate.

> ❯ **HINT**
> Assure adequate sedation and pain management before initiating NMBA.

■ *How are NMBAs monitored?*

■ **Peripheral nerve stimulation using the train-of-four (TOF)**

Patients receiving NMBAs should be monitored with both observation and TOF. The peripheral nerve stimulator is used to assess neuromuscular blockade, and the most common stimulation is called train-of-four. Frequently used sites for peripheral nerve stimulation include the ulnar and facial nerves. Count the number of twitches. If stimulating the ulnar nerve, observe the thumb and the facial nerve, watch the muscle above the eyebrow.

> ❯ **HINT**
> The goal for adjusting NMBA is typically to achieve one or two twitches (Box 2.24); 0/4 twitches indicate the need to lower the infusion rate to prevent prolonged paralysis.

Box 2.24 TOF Twitches

Number of Twitches	Amount of Blockade
4/4	0%–75% receptors blocked
3/4	At least 75% receptors blocked
2/4	80% receptors blocked
1/4	90% receptors blocked
0/4	100% receptors blocked

■ *What is the long-term complication of using neuromuscular blocking agents?*

■ **Critical illness polyneuropathy or myopathy**

Prolonged immobilization may contribute to the development of critical illness polyneuropathy and myopathy. The use of NMBA has been associated with long-term skeletal muscle weakness (Box 2.25). Long-term complications are more likely associated with neuromuscular, neurocognitive, and psychological rather than pulmonary dysfunction (Box 2.26).

> **HINT**
> A combination of NMBA and steroids may significantly increase the risk of skeletal muscle weaknesses.

Box 2.25 Acute Complications of ARDS

Cardiac dysrhythmias	Sepsis
Acute renal failure	Injury to lung with positive pressure ventilation
Thrombocytopenia	Chronic lung changes
Gastrointestinal bleed	

Box 2.26 Long-Term Complications of ARDS

Neuromuscular	Neurocognitive	Psychological
Critical illness polyneuropathy	Memory deficits	Depression
	Attention deficits	Anxiety
Myopathy	Decreased ability to concentrate	Posttraumatic stress disorder (PTSD)
	Alteration in higher cognitive functioning	

PULMONARY EMBOLISM

■ *What is the most common site of origin for thrombus in a PE?*

■ **Leg veins**

A PE is defined as a partial or complete obstruction of a branch in the pulmonary arterial system. The most common site of origin is the leg or pelvic thrombosis. Deep vein thrombosis (DVT) and PE are caused by the same underlying physiological event, and the combination is called venous thromboembolism (VTE). The actual frequencies of VTEs are underestimated and an unknown cause of death in the hospital may actually be a PE diagnosed on autopsy (Box 2.27).

Box 2.27 Origins of Thromboemboli

Leg veins (popliteal and calf)	Upper extremities
Pelvic	Right atrium (atrial fibrillation, tricuspid valve)
Inferior vena cava (iliac and femoral veins)	Right ventricle (myocardial contusion, right ventricular dysfunction)

> ❯ **HINT**
> Peripherally inserted central catheter (PICC) lines are a common cause of an upper extremity DVT. Assessing and monitoring for DVTs after placement of PICC lines is recommended.

■ *Which has a greater risk of embolization, DVT in the calf or popliteal veins?*
■ **Popliteal veins**

Calf DVTs involve the distal veins (i.e., peroneal, anterior tibial, posterior tibial), whereas the popliteal is a proximal vein. The proximal veins are more likely to extend or become an embolus. Distal DVTs may not require anticoagulation therapy.

■ *What is the highest risk for the development of a DVT?*
■ **Immobilization**

Critically ill patients are at high risk for the development of VTE. The majority of the patients are immobilized for long periods of time following their acute injury or disease process. Proactive nursing involves getting patients out of bed and ambulating as early as possible, based upon the stability of the patient (Box 2.28).

Box 2.28 Risk Factors for VTE

Immobilization	Trauma
Bed rest	Major trauma
Prolonged sitting position (traveling)	Orthopedic trauma
Casts	Spinal cord injury
Paralysis	Chronic venous insufficiency
Surgeries	Heart failure
Orthopedic	Central venous lines (PICC lines)
Vascular	Malignancy
Major general surgery	Pregnancy
Laparoscopic surgery	Oral contraceptives and estrogen replacement
Hypercoagulable predisposition	Obesity
Dehydration	Increasing age

PATHOPHYSIOLOGY

■ *What is the primary determinant of the severity of the PE?*
■ **Size of the embolus**

The hemodynamic consequence of a PE is determined by the size of the embolus and the amount of lung obstruction. Emboli range in severity from two to three pulmonary segments to 15 to 16 segments that are underperfused. Sudden death is caused by obstruction of the pulmonary trunk and/or both main pulmonary arteries. This is called a "saddle embolus."

> ❯ **HINT**
> Comorbidities and the degree of pulmonary vasoconstriction also affect the outcomes.

■ *With hemodynamically significant PE, what is the consequence of increased pulmonary resistance?*
■ **Right ventricular (RV) failure**

A sudden increase in pulmonary artery pressure due to a partial or complete obstruction and pulmonary vasoconstriction can cause RV dysfunction. RV failure causes the interventricular septal wall to deviate toward the left, resulting in a smaller left ventricular (LV) chamber. The pulmonary obstruction and RV failure cause less blood to flow to the LV, thus causing a decrease in cardiac output.

> ❯ **HINT**
> Symptoms of RV failure indicate a significant obstruction in the pulmonary vasculature and potential for hemodynamic instability.

SYMPTOMS/ASSESSMENT

■ *What is the most common initial presentation of a patient with a PE?*
■ **Sudden-onset dyspnea**

Sudden onset of dyspnea, tachypnea, and hypoxemia should raise the clinical suspicion of a PE. Symptoms of a PE are neither sensitive nor specific and require the clinician to consider the risk factors along with the presentation to recognize the PE (Boxes 2.29 and 2.30).

> ❯ **HINT**
> A PE can mimic other high-acuity disorders such as acute myocardial infarction.

Box 2.29 Symptoms of PE

Dyspnea	Hemoptysis
Tachypnea	Cough
Hypoxemia	Crackles
Chest pain	Feelings of "impending doom"

Box 2.30 Other Associated Signs of PE

Palpitations	Tachycardia
Low-grade fever	Systolic murmur
Development of S_3 or S_4	Crackles
Syncope	Wheezing
Diaphoresis	New-onset atrial fibrillation

DIAGNOSIS

■ *What 12-lead ECG finding is classic for PE with RV dysfunction?*

■ **$S_1Q_3T_3$**

The $S_1Q_3T_3$ is the ECG manifestation of acute pressure and volume overload of the RV. An S wave in lead I signifies a complete or more often incomplete right bundle branch block (RBBB). Lead III will have a Q wave, slight ST elevation, and an inverted T wave. These findings are due to the pressure and volume overload in the right ventricle, which causes repolarization abnormalities in leads correlating to the RV.

■ *What laboratory test may be used to assist with the diagnosis of PE?*

■ **D-dimer**

The fibrin fragment D-dimer is produced by the degradation of fibrin by plasmin (proteolytic enzyme that breaks down clots). If the D-dimer is negative, the possibility of a PE is very low. An elevated D-dimer though only determines the need for further diagnostic evaluation.

> ❯ **HINT**
> Immediate postoperative patients will have elevated D-dimer so a
> D-dimer test is not able to exclude PE in these patients.

■ *On a CXR, what is the presence of dilated pulmonary vessels with sharp cut-offs called?*

■ **Westermark sign**

A CXR is typically obtained to exclude other pulmonary and cardiac abnormalities. It is not used to diagnose a PE exclusively. A late sign that can sometimes be found on a CXR is a Westermark sign, which is the dilation of the pulmonary vessels with a sharp cut-off. Atelectasis, small pleural effusion, and elevated diaphragm may also be found, but are nonspecific for a PE.

■ *Which test can be performed to diagnose a DVT?*

■ **Ultrasound**

Compression ultrasound of the proximal leg veins or whole-leg ultrasonography may be performed to screen for a DVT in lower extremities. The presence of a known DVT in addition to clinical symptoms of a PE increases the likelihood of a positive PE diagnosis.

> ❯ **HINT**
>
> May have false negative findings in obese patients and require further testing (i.e., CT venography).

■ *Which diagnostic test is recommended in a suspected high-risk PE hemodynamically unstable patient?*

■ **CT arteriogram (CTA)**

A CTA is recommended to visualize the pulmonary arteries to confirm the diagnosis of PE in a high-risk patient suspected of PE. It is more accurate than a VQ scan and is replacing VQ scans and pulmonary angiograms as the gold standard for diagnosing PE.

> ❯ **HINT**
>
> If the patient is too unstable to transport for a CTA, then a bedside echocardiogram may be used (Box 2.31).

Box 2.31 Findings on Echocardiogram of PE

Abnormal right ventricular wall motion	Increased pulmonary artery pressure
Right ventricular dilation	Inferior vena cava congestion
Paradoxical septal motion	Dilated pulmonary artery
Tricuspid valve insufficiency	

MANAGEMENT

■ *What is the pharmacological therapy recommended for preventing VTE in a high-risk patient?*

■ **Heparin**

Heparin (unfractionated or low molecular), fondaparinux, or factor Xa inhibitors may be used to prevent a VTE in a high-risk patient as long as the patient is not at high risk for bleeding. Intermittent pneumatic compression devices (mechanical devices) may be used in patients with high bleeding risk instead of anticoagulation therapy.

> ❯ **HINT**
>
> All critically ill patients are considered a high risk for VTE and should have some type of prophylaxis.

■ *What is the pharmacological management recommended for a known DVT in the proximal leg veins or PE?*

■ **Heparin or fondaparinux and warfarin**

Heparin (unfractionated or low molecular) or fondaparinux is recommended as the initial treatment for a proximal DVT to prevent extension or a PE. Warfarin is recommended to be started on the same day as heparin or fondaparinux and both drugs are continued for 5 days or until the international normalized ratio (INR) is above 2.0 for longer than 24 hours. Then warfarin should be continued as the lone anticoagulation therapy, maintaining an INR between 2.0 and 3.0. If known PE, continue the heparin for the 5 days despite an INR of 2.0 or greater.

> **HINT**
> If the patient is at high risk for bleeding (i.e., postoperative patient), an inferior vena cava filter may be placed instead of anticoagulation therapy.

■ *Which of the anticoagulation therapies used in treating a PE is recommended if severe renal failure is present?*

■ **Unfractionated heparin**

Unfractionated heparin is recommended in renal-failure patients over low-molecular-weight heparin (LMWH) or Arixtra (fondaparinux). The therapeutic goal is 1.5 to 2.5 times the normal activated partial thromboplastin time (aPTT value). The recommended length of therapy with anticoagulants is a minimum of 5 days in combination with warfarin; then, warfarin is administered for 3 to 6 months.

> **HINT**
> Fondaparinux or argatroban (direct thrombin inhibitor) is the drug that may be used if the patient has developed heparin-induced thrombocytopenia (HIT) Type II.

■ *What would be the indication for administering a systemic thrombolytic to a patient diagnosed with a PE?*

■ **Hypotension**

A patient hemodynamically unstable (BP < 90 mmHg) may be treated with systemic thrombolytic therapy. It is not recommended in patients hemodynamically stable. The thrombolytic recommended is tissue plasminogen activator (tPA) due to its short infusion time. The infusion should be administered over 2 hours through a venous catheter. Heparin may be stopped during the infusion and restarted after the aPTT is less than 80 seconds. Thrombolytic therapy has shown improved pulmonary artery pressures, oxygenation, and RV performance but has a higher risk for bleeding. It is not recommended in stable patients with a PE.

> **HINT**
> In cardiac arrest caused by suspected PE, recommend administering thrombolytics even during resuscitation.

COMPLICATIONS

■ *Obstruction in the pulmonary artery can lead to what major complication of the lung tissue?*

■ **Pulmonary Infarction**

Obstruction of the pulmonary artery causes a loss of blood flow distal to the balloon and may result in a pulmonary infarction. This commonly presents with dyspnea and hemoptysis (Box 2.32).

Box 2.32 Symptoms of Pulmonary Infarction

Dyspnea	Pleural effusions
Hemoptysis	Decreased excursion of affected hemothorax
Pleuritic pain	Pleural friction rubs

■ *Sudden-onset dyspnea associated with hypotension and an S₃ gallop would indicate which complication of a PE?*

■ **RV failure**

RV failure caused by pulmonary hypertension can result in a decreased cardiac output (CO) and hypotension. The presence of RV involvement with a PE increases the risk of mortality. Elevated cardiac troponin and brain natriuretic peptides (BNP) are also predictors of risk of complications and mortality in a PE.

> **HINT**
> An S₃ gallop typically indicates the presence of heart failure and is the clue in this question (Box 2.33).

Box 2.33 Symptoms of Right Ventricular Failure

Sudden unexplained dyspnea	Cyanosis
Jugular distention	Systolic murmur (tricuspid regurgitation)
S₃ gallop	New or complete RBBB
Hypotension	

■ *What is the development of leg ulcer in the affected leg of a known DVT called?*

■ **Post-thrombotic syndrome (PTS)**

PTS develops in about 50% of the patients with a DVT in the lower extremity. The symptoms include chronic pain, redness, swelling, and ulcerations.

■ *What long-term complication can result in elevated pulmonary artery pressures?*

■ **Chronic thromboembolic pulmonary hypertension (CTPH)**

CTPH is defined as pulmonary artery (PA) pressures greater than 25 mmHg that persist for longer than 6 months after PE is diagnosed. Symptoms may not be present initially ("honeymoon period") even though pulmonary hypertension exists. It is usually recognized when the patient presents later with dyspnea, hypoxemia, and RV dysfunction. Surgical management of choice for symptomatic CTPH is vascular disobliteration with pulmonary endarterectomy. Medical management is similar to primary pulmonary hypertension (Box 2.34).

> ❭ **HINT**
> Fibrinolytic therapy has been found to reduce the risk of CTPH.

Box 2.34 Other Complications of PE

Sudden cardiac death	Atrial or ventricular arrhythmias
Shock	Pleural effusions
Pulseless electrical activity (PEA)	Severe hypoxemia

COPD EXACERBATIONS/SEVERE ASTHMA/STATUS ASTHMATICUS

■ *What is the most common cause of acute respiratory failure in a COPD patient?*

■ **Pulmonary infection**

COPD is defined as symptoms of airflow obstruction in the absence of an alternative explanation for symptoms. Airflow obstruction is defined as postbronchodilator FEV1 – FVC ratio less than 0.70. Frequently, pulmonary infections (i.e., pneumonia, infectious bronchitis) are the cause of acute exacerbation and admission into the intensive care unit (ICU) for ventilatory support. These can be bacterial or viral infections, bacterial being the most common. Other precipitating factors include CHF, PE, and worsening of chronic airflow.

■ *What is the most common factor that contributes to airway hyperresponsiveness in asthma patients?*

■ **Environmental allergens**

Exposure to environmental allergens is one of the most common factors contributing to bronchial hyperresponsiveness in asthma. Environmental allergens include cockroach allergens, dust mite allergens, pet allergens, mold spores, sulfur dioxide, ozone, and tobacco smoke (Box 2.35).

Box 2.35 Factors That Contribute to Airway Hyperreactivity

Environmental allergens	Examples: cockroaches, dust mites, pets, mold spores, fungi
Viral respiratory infections	Examples: history of viral pneumonia, rhinovirus
Environmental pollutants	Examples: smoke (tobacco or wood), dust, air pollution
Irritants	Examples: household sprays, paint fumes
Occupational exposure	Examples: coal mining, farmers, painters, plastic manufacture
Latex allergies	
Exercise induced	

(continued)

Box 2.35 Factors That Contribute to Airway Hyperreactivity *(continued)*

Gastroesophogeal reflux disease (GERD)
Chronic sinusitis
Stress or emotional induced
Aspirin or nonsteroidal anti-inflammatory
drug (NSAID) hypersensitivity
Obesity

PATHOPHYSIOLOGY

- **What is the underlying cause of the increased WOB that occurs in acute exacerbation of COPD?**
- **Greater limitations in airway flow**

COPD exacerbation is associated with increased limitations of airway flow, air trapping, and reduction of chest wall and lung compliance leading to an increased WOB. The increased pressure required for airflow may overload the respiratory muscles decreasing MV and worsening hypercapnia. Air trapping generates auto-PEEP, resulting in the patient requiring greater negative inspiratory pressures to initiate a breath and worsen the VQ mismatch and WOB. Acute asthma has the same physiological effects of limitations to airflow due to narrowing of the airways.

> **HINT**
> Use of accessory inspiratory muscles indicates an increasing severity of exacerbation (Figure 2.2).

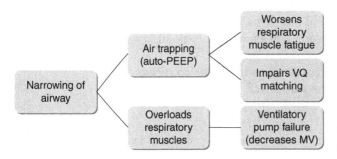

FIGURE 2.2 Airway obstruction in exacerbation of COPD and severe asthma.

- **What are three physiologic changes found in severe asthma that contribute to airway obstruction?**
- **Bronchoconstriction, airway inflammation, and mucus plugs**

Bronchoconstriction is a result of an immune-mediated response to an allergen. Airway edema is a response to the bronchoconstriction and may be present within 6 to 24 hours. Mucus plugs are exudate composed of cellular debris and eosinophils. Chronic asthmatics may also have some airway remodeling due to the effects of long-term inflammation.

> **HINT**
> The obstruction to airflow is both into the lung (during inspiration) as well as out of the lung (during expiration).

■ *Is the hypoxemia associated with asthma a shunt, a dead space, or both a shunt and a dead space?*

■ **Both**

Bronchospasm and inflammation are not uniform throughout. Some alveoli are under-ventilated in relation to perfusion (shunt), whereas others are overinflated in relation to perfusion (dead space). Hypoxic pulmonary vasoconstriction occurs due to VQ mismatch and will worsen the mismatch.

> **❯ HINT**
> This also increases the afterload (resistance) of the right ventricle, which interferes with the filling of the left ventricle.

SYMPTOMS/ASSESSMENT

■ *What is a clinical sign of diaphragmatic fatigue that may indicate imminent ventilatory failure?*

■ **Paradoxical breathing**

Paradoxical breathing occurs when the diaphragm becomes fatigued and is no longer the primary muscle of the inspiratory effort. Normally, the diaphragm drops during inspiration pushing the abdominal wall outward. In paradoxical breathing, the fatigued diaphragm rises and the abdominal wall sinks inward. Another sign of impending respiratory failure is respiratory alternans (cyclic alternation between abdominal and thoracic breathing).

■ *What typically brings a patient to the hospital in an exacerbation of COPD?*

■ **Increased dyspnea**

The presentation of exacerbated COPD involves a worsening or a change in the person's typical symptoms. The decrease in airflow experienced with the exacerbation results in increased dyspnea and typically results in the person seeking medical attention (Box 2.36).

Box 2.36 Other Signs of an Acute Exacerbation of COPD

Coughing is more severe	Increased wheezing and rhonchi
Increase in sputum production	More predominant use of accessory muscles
Sputum color changes form whitish to yellow-green	Orthopnea
Purulent sputum with streaks of blood	Paroxysmal nocturnal dyspnea

■ *What clinical sign indicates a life-threatening presentation of an acute asthma attack?*

■ **Speaking in incomplete sentences**

The current classification of severity of asthma describes a subset of severe acute asthmatic patients who present with a life-threatening attack. These patients are more likely to be admitted to the ICU for management. The clinical sign used to differentiate severity is the degree of dyspnea. Assessing a patient's ability to talk is an objective assessment of dyspnea. An inability to talk accompanied by diaphoresis indicates a more severe episode of asthma, which may be life threatening. Other signs include a decreased level of consciousness or apnea (Box 2.37).

> ❯ HINT
> Dyspnea that interferes with conversation may also indicate a more severe asthma.

Box 2.37 Signs of Exacerbation of Asthma

Wheezing (expiratory and inspiratory)	Anxiety
Cough	Tachypnea
Chest tightness or pain	Tachycardia
Dyspnea	Supraclavical and intercostal retractions
Diaphoresis	Nasal flaring and abdominal breathing
Hypoxemia	

■ *In the early presentation of acute severe asthma, is the patient hypercarbic or hypocarbic?*

■ **Hypocarbic**

In the early stages of an acute asthmatic crisis, the patient will hyperventilate. This increase in MV lowers the CO_2 levels. The patient may have hypoxemia with hypocarbia due to the greater diffusion of CO_2 than O_2 across the pulmonary bed. Respiratory alkalosis will be present initially. As the airway obstruction increases and the patient's ventilatory effort fatigues, the patient will start to retain CO_2 and develop hypercarbia and respiratory acidosis.

> ❯ HINT
> Normalization of the CO_2 (called pseudonormalization) and the development of hypercapnia may be ominous signs indicating respiratory failure.

■ *What is it called when the systolic BP decreases during inspiration due to large changes in intrapleural pressures?*

■ **Pulsus paradoxus**

Pulsus paradoxus is defined as a systolic decrease of more than 10 mmHg during inspiration. It can indicate the presence of an obstructed airway disease. During periods of limited airflow and air trapping with asthmatic patients, there is an increase in negative pressure in the intrapleural space during inspiration. This increase in negative pressure increases venous return and filling of the RV. The septal wall displaces toward the LV, limiting the filling of the LV and decreases the stroke volume during inspiration. Arterial waveforms will demonstrate a decrease in waveform amplitude during inspiration.

> **HINT**
> Pulsus paradoxus is not a good indicator of the severity of acute asthma.

■ *Can hypercapnia be detected by monitoring oxygen saturations with a pulse oximetry?*

■ **No**

Pulse oximetry is recommended while managing acute exacerbation of asthma but it does not monitor changes in CO_2 levels. Hypercapnia is a sign of worsening of asthma with a potential need for intubation. Saturations of less than 92% (regardless of the FiO_2) are associated with an increased chance of hypercarbia and indicate the need to obtain an ABG.

> **HINT**
> May use end-tidal CO_2 (capnography) monitoring while managing acute exacerbation of asthma to monitor trends of CO_2.

DIAGNOSIS

■ *What finding on the ABG is used to determine whether there is an acute worsening of COPD?*

■ **Respiratory acidosis**

Patients who present with chronic respiratory acidosis will have a fully compensated blood gas with a normal pH. $PaCO_2$ and bicarbonate levels will be high. If the patient has an "acute on chronic" respiratory acidosis, the pH will be below the normal range. $PaCO_2$ and bicarbonate levels will also be high but now they are only partially compensated due to an acute increase in CO_2.

■ *What test is needed to establish the diagnosis of asthma?*

■ **Spirometry**

A pulmonary function test (spirometry) is used before and after the patient inhales a short-acting bronchodilator. This determines the presence of airflow obstruction, its severity, and whether it is reversible with short-term management (Box 2.38).

Box 2.38 Pulmonary Function Tests (PFTs) With Spirometry

FEV1	FVC
FEV6 (forced expiratory volume in 6 seconds)	FEV1/FVC (FEV1 to FVC ratio)

MANAGEMENT

■ *What would be the priority of care in a COPD patient with a saturation of 87% on room air?*

■ **Administer oxygen**

Oxygen should be administered to maintain the oxygen saturation of more than 90% to 92% and PaO_2 of 60 to 65 mmHg. Withholding oxygen during severe hypoxemia can increase complications and mortality.

> ❯ HINT
> Higher levels of oxygen will increase dead space and $PaCO_2$ levels, so use the lowest FiO_2 to accomplish goals. The use of nonselective β-adrenergic agonists (i.e., theophylline) is not recommended due to frequently associated cardiac comorbidities of COPD patients (Box 2.39).

Box 2.39 Other Medications Used to Manage Acute Exacerbation COPD

Corticosteroids	Bronchodilators (i.e., Albuterol)
Antibiotics	Anticholinergics (i.e., Ipratropium)

■ *Between acute exacerbation of COPD and severe asthma, which would more likely require antibiotics?*

■ **COPD**

Antibiotics may be useful in COPD patients presenting with pulmonary infections or who show changes in sputum production, color, or amount, even in the absence of pneumonia.

> ❯ HINT
> Antibiotics are not usually recommended in acute asthma.

■ *What can be used as a first-line intervention for patients with acute exacerbation of COPD to provide short-term rest of their respiratory muscles?*

■ **NIV**

NIV through a nasal or face mask might provide time to manage the acute pulmonary infection and prevent the need for intubation. This allows the respiratory muscles a "rest period" while the underlying pathology that caused the exacerbation is being treated. It decreases WOB and increases alveolar ventilation (Box 2.40).

> ❯ HINT
> The decision to discontinue NIV and intubate is clinical. It involves monitoring hypercapnia/respiratory acidosis and assessing for fatigue or discomfort during NIV. The clinical benefit of NIV in COPD patients will typically be seen within the first few hours. Absence of improvement may be an indication for intubation.

Box 2.40 Potential Physiological Benefit of NIV in COPD

Increased TV	Improved oxygenation
Decreased RR	Better ventilation and gas exchange (lowering $PaCO_2$)
Decreased HR	Lower air trapping (decrease auto-PEEP)

■ *A patient with COPD is intubated and mechanically ventilated. His initial PaCO₂ is 58 mmHg. Should the PaCO₂ be normalized while the patient is being mechanically ventilated?*

■ **No**

Normalization of $PaCO_2$ while on mechanical ventilation will cause difficulties with weaning from the ventilator in the future. Correcting the respiratory acidosis causes metabolic alkalosis (due to high compensatory bicarbonate levels) and the kidneys will "dump" the bicarbonate in the urine. During weaning, the patient will begin to retain CO_2 and develop uncorrected respiratory acidosis.

■ *What is the most common PFT used to determine airway responsiveness to interventions during asthma treatment?*

■ **FEV1/FVC ratio**

FEV1 is the forced expiratory volume in 1 second and is expressed as a percentage of predicted value or the proportion of FVC.

> ❯ **HINT**
> The initial assessment goal is to determine the severity of the attack and follow-up assessments are to determine control of the asthma or responsiveness of the patient to interventions.

■ *What is the first-line pharmacological agent used to manage acute exacerbation of asthma?*

■ **Short-acting β-agonists**

Inhaled β-agonists are used to relieve bronchoconstriction. The use of short-acting, β_2-selective agonists is preferred due to fewer cardiovascular side effects. Repeat doses of the β-agonist can be administered at 15- to 30-minute intervals until an adequate response is obtained. Steroids should also be administered to all acute asthma patients to manage the airway inflammation. Oxygen should be administered to maintain saturations more than 94% to 98%.

> ❯ **HINT**
> The earlier the steroids are given in an acute attack, the better the outcome.

■ *What is the electrolyte abnormality commonly associated with the administration of a β-agonist?*

■ **Hypokalemia**

B-agonist drugs cause a shift of potassium from the intravascular to the intracellular space. This lowers the plasma potassium levels. Patients being treated with frequent intervals of β-agonists need to have K^+ levels drawn and closely monitored for complications of hypokalemia.

> **〉 HINT**
> A treatment for hyperkalemia is nebulized β-agonist agents to drive the
> K⁺ back into the cells.

■ *What nebulized drug can be added to β-agonist while managing severe or life-threatening asthma?*

■ **Ipratropium bromide**

Ipratropium bromide, an anticholinergic drug, can produce greater bronchodilation in a shorter time than a β-agonist alone. It may not be needed in mild to moderate asthma but it has been found to improve outcomes in severe and life-threatening attacks. Intravenous (IV) magnesium may also be considered as adjunctive therapy with a β-agonist.

> **〉 HINT**
> Mg⁺ levels need to be monitored if a magnesium infusion is
> administered to manage the asthma. Symptoms of hypermagnesemia
> can be muscle weakness and respiratory failure.

COMPLICATIONS

■ *A patient remains unresponsive to short-acting bronchodilator therapy. A CXR is ordered. What is the potential complication?*

■ **Pneumothorax**

A routine CXR is not recommended in the treatment of exacerbation of asthma. If the patient is unresponsive to interventions with short-acting bronchodilators, a CXR may be used to diagnose the presence of a pneumothorax. The increase in negative pressure for inspiration may cause barotrauma and the development of pneumothorax.

ACUTE RESPIRATORY INFECTIONS

■ *How long after intubation in which pneumonia develops would the infection be called a ventilator-acquired pneumonia (VAP)?*

■ **More than 48 to 72 hours**

VAP is defined as a pneumonia that develops more than 48 hours after endotracheal intubation that was not already present or incubating prior to intubation. VAP is considered a subset of hospital-acquired pneumonia (HAP) or nosocomial pneumonia. Community-acquired pneumonia (CAP) is defined as pneumonia that develops in a nonhospitalized patient or within 48 hours of hospitalization.

> **〉 HINT**
> If the patient's clinical symptoms of pneumonia occur before 48 hours,
> it is not considered to be associated with intubation and mechanical
> ventilation.

PATHOPHYSIOLOGY

■ *What is the greatest risk of HAP?*
■ **Endotracheal intubation**

Endotracheal intubation and mechanical ventilation significantly increase the risk of pneumonia. The endotracheal tube (ETT) provides a direct access of oral secretions colonized by bacteria into the lungs. The ETT cuff is not completely occlusive and secretions can pool above the cuff and leak into the lower airways.

> ❯ **HINT**
> Bacteria lining the ETT (biofilm) can become dislodged and embolized distal into the lungs from instillation of saline into the tube, suctioning, or repositioning the tube (Box 2.41).

Box 2.41 Risks of an ETT for VAP

Secretions pool in the subglottic region	Stimulates increase in sputum production
Compromises cough	Injuries to tracheal epithelium
Prevents mucociliary clearance	Bacteria aggregates on the tubing (biofilm)

■ *Which patient position can lower the risk of aspiration and VAP?*
■ **Head of bed (HOB) elevated 30 to 45 degrees**

Supine position with the HOB flat can increase the risk of aspiration. A recommendation is to keep the patient's HOB elevated at 30° to 45° to prevent VAP, especially during enteral feeding (Box 2.42).

Box 2.42 Risk of VAP

Unintentional extubations/reintubations	Oropharyngeal bacterial colonization
Enteral feeding	Contaminated ventilator circuit
Elevated gastric pH (i.e., H_2 receptor blockers)	Naso-orogastric tubes
Bronchoscopy	Cross-contamination by health care providers

SYMPTOMS/ASSESSMENT

■ *A patient has been on the ventilator for 72 hours. What CXR change would increase the suspicion of a VAP?*
■ **New or progressive infiltrates**

The occurrence of new or progressive infiltrates on CXR should increase suspicion of a HAP/VAP. A complete blood count (CBC) should be performed and the patient assessed for other signs of pneumonia. The diagnosis of VAP is determined by the CXR changes and one or more of the clinical findings of VAP/HAP, indicating that the infiltrate is infectious (Box 2.43).

> **HINT**
Infiltrates may be caused by other pathologies in the lung (i.e., atelectasis).

Box 2.43 Clinical Findings of HAP/VAP

Fever > 100.4°F (38°C)	Decrease oxygenation
Purulent secretions	Unexplained hemodynamic instability
Leukocytosis or leukopenia	

DIAGNOSIS

- *Which route of obtaining sputum for a culture is the best to diagnose pneumonia and determine the causative agent?*
- **Bronchoalveolar lavage (BAL)**

A BAL or protected specimen brush (PSB) can be obtained either by bronchoscopy or blindly without a bronchoscopy (distal airway sample). It is considered a quantitative culture that isolates fewer microorganisms growing above the threshold and allows more specific determination of the causative micro-organism. A qualitative culture can be obtained by suctioning the ETT but this sample grows a greater number of bacteria with a high false positive. Suctioning the artificial airway remains the most commonly used route for obtaining sputum cultures.

> **HINT**
Diagnosis is based on clinical criteria, including the CXR findings and clinical findings.

- *What other pulmonary infection may present with clinical findings but without the new or progressive infiltrate on CXR?*
- **Ventilator-associated tracheobronchitis (VAT)**

VAT is characterized by clinical findings of pulmonary infections (i.e., purulent secretions, fever, leukocytosis) without evidence of pneumonia on CXR (pulmonary infiltrates). VAT is a bacterial infection of the tracheobronchial tree following intubation. Diagnosis and treatment are similar to VAP.

MANAGEMENT

- *What is a nursing intervention that has been found to lower the incidence of VAP?*
- **Oral care**

Oral decontamination with tooth brushing (includes gums, teeth, and tongue) and rinsing of the oral cavity to remove plaque and bacteria lowers the incidence of VAP. The use of oral antimicrobials, such as chlorhexidine, has been found to lower bacterial colonization in the oral cavity. Meticulous hand washing, routine turning of patients, and aspiration prevention are also correct for nursing interventions in the prevention of VAP (Box 2.44).

> ### ❯ HINT
> Avoid the use of saline lavage when suctioning the ETT. It increases the risk of VAP and has not been found effective in preventing mucus plugs.

Box 2.44 Prevention of HAP/VAP

Proper hand washing	Subglottic suctioning
Oral decontamination	Selective decontamination of digestive tract
Frequent turning of patient	Daily interruption from sedation
Keep HOB elevated 30° to 45°	Avoid unintentional extubations and reintubations
Prevention of aspiration	Silver-coated ETT
Maintain adequate cuff pressures	Prevention of stress-related mucosal disease
Wean and extubate as soon as possible	Prevention of VTE
Avoid saline lavages	

■ *VAP caused by a multidrug-resistant (MDR) pathogen would most likely occur as an early or late infection?*
■ **Late infection**

Typically, MDR pathogens are found to cause infections, including VAP, in patients with longer than 5 days hospitalization. An early presentation of VAP is most commonly caused by pathogens more susceptible to antibiotics. Late presentation is commonly associated with MDR and is more difficult to manage. Antibiotics are the treatment of VAP and may be administered aerosolized in combination with IV.

> ### ❯ HINT
> Initiation of appropriate antibiotics prior to culture results depend on the length of hospitalization and other risk factors for MDR pathogens.

COMPLICATIONS

See Box 2.45.

Box 2.45 Complications

Longer ICU and hospitalized days
Greater mortality
Greater costs

AIR-LEAK SYNDROMES

■ *Which of the air-leak syndromes is considered the most life threatening?*
■ **Tension pneumothorax**

An air leak is defined as any extrusion of air from normal gas-filled cavities, including lungs, tracheobronchial tree, sinuses, and GI tract. Of all the air-leak syndromes, a pneumothorax is considered to be the most serious complication and a tension pneumothorax is the most life threatening. If a patient presents with or develops subcutaneous emphysema and/or pneumomediastinum, a pneumothorax should be ruled out.

> ❯ **HINT**
> Pneumopericardium can also be life threatening but is less common than a pneumothorax (Box 2.46). Subcutaneous emphysema and pneumomediastinum are not life threatening except in rare cases and must be observed.

Box 2.46 Air-Leak Syndromes

Pneumothorax	Pneumopericardium
Pneumomediastinum	Subcutaneous emphysema
Pneumoperitoneum	

■ *A pneumothorax can develop due to which ventilatory complication?*
■ **Barotrauma**

Positive pressure ventilation can result in barotrauma and air-leak syndromes. The patient can develop a pneumothorax, pneumomediastinum, or pneumoperitoneum following institution of positive pressure ventilation with high pressures. A pneumothorax is caused by the pressure gradient between the interstitium and the alveoli reaching a critical point followed by rupture of alveoli. Air then enters the interstitial space and pleural space (Box 2.47).

Box 2.47 Other Causes of Pneumothorax

Iatrogenic	Traumatic	Spontaneous	Underlying Lung Pathology
Subclavian central-line placement	Barotrauma	Subpleural blebs	Asthma
Transthoracic needle biopsy	Penetrating chest trauma	Smokers	COPD
Lung resection	Blunt chest trauma	Valsalva maneuver	ARDS
Cardiopulmonary resuscitation	Tracheo-bronchial rupture	Coughing	Lung cancer
Misplaced tracheostomy tube			Sarcoidosis
			Cystic fibrosis
			Pulmonary infections

PATHOPHYSIOLOGY

■ *What may keep the lung from collapsing in a patient with chronic lung disease following pneumothorax?*
■ **Adhesions**

Adhesions can develop between the parietal and visceral layers of the pleural space in chronic lung disease patients. When a pneumothorax occurs, it may be a very localized, loculated area of the pleural space. Typically, pneumothoraces are widespread throughout the pleural space and result in the collapse of the lung.

> **HINT**
> A patient may require more than one chest tube to drain the different locations of loculated air.

SYMPTOMS/ASSESSMENT

- *What are the two most common initial symptoms of a pneumothorax in an awake patient?*
- **Chest pain and dyspnea**

A sudden-onset pleuritic chest pain and severe dyspnea are most commonly the initial symptoms of a patient who is awake and is developing pneumothorax. The patient will typically also experience significant hypoxemia with a respiratory alkalosis (Box 2.48).

Box 2.48 Symptoms of Pneumothorax

Dyspnea	Absent or diminished breath sounds and affected lung
Pleuritic chest pain	Asymmetrical chest wall movement
Hypoxemia	Subcutaneous emphysema
Respiratory alkalosis	Tracheal deviation (away from affected side)
Tachypnea	Hypotension
Tachycardia	

- *What change on the ventilator could be a sign of a new pneumothorax on a ventilated patient?*
- **Acute increase in PIP**

A sudden increase in the PIP on a ventilated patient can be an indication of a new pneumothorax. It is commonly associated with a sudden decrease in oxygen saturation and tachycardia. A CXR should be obtained and further assessment performed.

> **HINT**
> The increase in PIP may be the initial symptom of a pneumothorax in ventilated patients not awake or unable to communicate.

DIAGNOSIS

- *Which diagnostic radiographic procedure is best to determine the size of the pneumothorax?*
- **CT and ultrasonography**

An anterior-posterior (AP) or posterior-anterior (PA) CXR generally underestimates the size of the pneumothorax. The PA view of a pneumothorax measuring 2 cm may actually be almost half of the hemithorax. Ultrasonography is more accurate for determining the size of the pneumothorax and is able to identify small collections of air. A CT scan is considered the gold standard to verify a pneumothorax if the diagnosis is doubted.

> ❯ HINT
>
> CXR remains the first diagnostic test of choice to be obtained with a suspicion of a pneumothorax.

MANAGEMENT

■ *If the pneumothorax is smaller than 2 cm and the patient is asymptomatic, what is the primary treatment?*

■ **Administer 100% FiO_2**

A small pneumothorax (< 2 cm on a chest radiograph) on an asymptomatic patient is usually observed closely for signs of hypoxemia or respiratory distress. Administering oxygen at 100% FiO_2 will assist with increasing the absorption of air more rapidly. Serial CXRs will be required to monitor the resolution of the pneumothorax.

> ❯ HINT
>
> If the patient is on positive pressure ventilation (a CPAP or mechanical ventilator), then chest tube placement would be required. Positive pressure ventilation can increase the size of the pneumothorax.

■ *Your patient has a chest tube for a pneumothorax that was inserted 24 hours ago. Upon earlier assessment, you noted intermittent bubbling. While the radiology technician was obtaining a CXR, the chest drainage system was broken. What would be the best nursing action to manage the chest tube system?*

■ **Place chest tube in water**

Because the chest tube was recently placed and had intermittent bubbling, this is an indication that the pneumothorax has not been resolved yet. Clamping this tube is not a good option since a tension pneumothorax can occur, which is life threatening. The patient is in the unit so a sterile cup of saline is readily available to put into the tube to make a water seal. Leaving the tube open until a new drainage system is prepared and then placing it back to suction would also be an option in this situation.

> ❯ HINT
>
> If a chest tube is clamped, the patient needs to remain under close observation. On any sign of hemodynamic instability, the tube should be quickly unclamped.

■ *A patient inadvertently dislodged his chest tube when turning in the bed. The last CXR showed complete resolution of the pneumothorax. What would be the best nursing intervention at this time?*

■ **Cover with Vaseline gauze and an occlusive dressing**

The pneumothorax has resolved based on the most recent CXR. Covering the incision with Vaseline gauze and an occlusive dressing will prevent air from re-entering the pleural space. If the pneumothorax was unresolved based on CXR and clinical assessment, a three-sided dressing would be indicated to prevent a tension pneumothorax. The taping of the dressing on three sides only allows the air to exit but it cannot re-enter into the pleural space (one-way valve).

> **❯ HINT**
> Continue to monitor the patient closely for deterioration, indicating a pneumothorax or tension pneumothorax.

COMPLICATIONS

■ *What can be injected into the pleural space to treat a recurring pneumothorax?*

■ **Talc**

The instillation of talc or bleomycin through the chest drainage tube can be used to treat recurring pneumothoraces or a continuous air leak. This is called medical pleurodesis. There is also a surgical pleurodesis in which the parietal pleura is abraded. These techniques produce fibrosis and scarring to allow the visceral layer to adhere to the chest wall, preventing further pneumothoraces.

■ *What could be the cause of a significant air leak and loss of delivered TV on a ventilated patient after chest tube insertion?*

■ **Bronchopleural fistula**

A bronchopleural fistula is a communication between the pleural space and the bronchial tree. It presents as a persistent air leak or failure to reinflate the lung after chest tube placement. Management requires a lower TV, RR, PEEP level, and lower pressures to allow the fistula to heal. This may require accepting a lower oxygenation and permissive hypercapnia. Refractory cases may require surgical repair (Box 2.49).

> **❯ HINT**
> Assess exhaled TV on the ventilator. It should be within 100 mL of the preset TV. More than 100 mL indicates a loss of delivered TV.

Box 2.49 Causes of Bronchopleural Fistula

Chest trauma	Complications with mechanical ventilation
Chest tube inadvertently placed into lung parenchyma	Complication with diagnostic or therapeutic thoracic interventions

ASPIRATIONS

■ *What type of aspiration is the most common in a critically ill patient?*
■ **Microaspirations**

Small volume (microaspirations) is the most common form of aspiration in critically ill patients. Small aspirations of contaminated oropharyngeal secretions and gastric contents frequently occur in intubated critically ill patients and play a major role in VAP.

PATHOPHYSIOLOGY

■ *What is the intervention most likely to contribute to aspirations in a critically ill patient?*
■ **Tube-feeding infusion**

Tube feeding has been found to increase the risk of both large-volume aspirations and small-volume microaspirations in more than 50% of the patients receiving tube feeds (Box 2.50).

Box 2.50 Risk Factors for Aspiration

Mechanically ventilated	Sedation
Decreased level of consciousness	Tube feeding
Presence of a feeding tube	No PEEP with mechanical ventilation
Abnormal gag or swallow reflex	

SYMPTOMS/ASSESSMENT

■ *What should be assessed after extubation following a prolonged intubation prior to feeding the patient?*
■ **Swallow evaluation**

Intubation, especially prolonged, may affect the ability of the patient to swallow after extubation. Performing a swallow evaluation prior to feeding the patient is recommended. If the patient is found to have a swallowing abnormality, then obtaining a consultation with a speech therapist for a complete dysphagia evaluation is recommended to lower the risk of aspiration.

> ❯ HINT
> High-risk patients for dysphagia may have silent aspirations and should still have a speech consultation for swallow evaluation.

■ *How often should assessment of gastric residuals be performed during tube feeding through a nasogastric tube?*
■ **Every 4 hours**

In critically ill patients, it is recommended that gastric residuals be assessed every 4 hours to assess for gastric distention and increased risk of regurgitation. Small-bore feeding tubes are more likely to collapse during aspiration and are not as reliable for checking residuals. Clinical assessment of tolerance to tube feeding should be used in conjunction with the volume to determine proper response to large residuals (Box 2.51).

> ❯ **HINT**
>
> Injection of air into the small-bore tube prior to aspiration may prevent some of the collapsing to improve accuracy.

Box 2.51 Signs of Intolerance With Tube Feeds

Large gastric residuals	Vomiting or regurgitation
Abdominal pain	No abnormal bowel sounds
Distended abdomen	Nausea
No flatus or stool passage	

DIAGNOSIS

■ *What measurement may be used to diagnose microaspiration of gastric contents?*

■ **Pepsin**

Quantitative pepsin in tracheal secretions is accurate in diagnosing microaspirations of gastric contents. Methylene blue has been used but requires a bronchoscopy to diagnose aspiration of blue dye, which is not always visible with suctioning. Dye in the enteral feed has been found to have side effects of diarrhea, gastric bacterial colonization, and systemic absorption with death. Glucose testing is not recommended as a method for testing for tube-feed aspirates.

MANAGEMENT

■ *What degree of the HOB elevation is recommended to prevent aspiration?*

■ **30° to 45°**

A sustained supine position (0°) has been shown to increase gastroesophageal reflux and increased risk of aspiration. To prevent aspiration elevating the HOB to a semirecumbent position of 30° to 45° is recommended in high-risk patients. If unable to elevate the backrest, one may use the reverse Trendelenburg position to elevate the head unless contraindicated (Box 2.52).

> ❯ **HINT**
>
> High-risk patients include those mechanically ventilated and/or with a feeding tube in place.

Box 2.52 Prevention of Aspiration

Maintain HOB elevated to 30° to 45°	Assess swallowing ability
Avoid oversedation	Maintain endotracheal cuff at the appropriate level
Assure correct placement of feeding tube	Subglottic suctioning
Avoid bolus feeding	Postpyloric feeding

■ *Between bolus and continuous tube feeding, which has been found to have a higher risk of reflux and aspiration?*

■ **Bolus tube feeding**

Bolus tube feeding typically administers a 4-hour volume over a short time period causing greater gastric distention and increased risk of regurgitation. It is also proposed that bolus feeding may lower esophageal pressure and predispose the patient for reflux.

■ *What is the recommendation for minimal ETT cuff pressure?*

■ **20 cm H$_2$O**

The ETT cuff pressure needs to be within a particular range to maintain preset TVs and reduce the risk for aspiration secretions that accumulate above the cuff. A range of 20 to 30 cm H$_2$O is recommended. Less than 20 cm H$_2$O is inadequate to protect from aspiration. Hypopharyngeal suctioning prior to deflating the cuff is used to minimize aspiration of secretions.

> ❯ HINT
> The addition of supraglottic suctioning can assist in the prevention of aspiration of pooled secretions.

COMPLICATIONS

■ *What complication is of the highest risk following aspirations?*

■ **Pneumonia**

Microaspirations and large-volume aspirations are associated with VAP and HAP.

PULMONARY HYPERTENSION

■ *Which ventricle is involved with pulmonary arterial hypertension (PAH)?*

■ **Right ventricle**

PAH is a syndrome that results from restricted blood flow through the pulmonary arterial bed, increasing pulmonary vascular resistance (PVR) and resulting in RV failure (Box 2.53).

Box 2.53 Causes of PAH

Idiopathic PAH	Connective tissue disease
Familial PAH	Drugs and toxins
HIV	Portal hypertension

- *Is elevated PVR caused by left ventricular failure called PAH or pulmonary hypertension (PH)?*
- **Pulmonary hypertension**

PAH is a subcategory of PH. PH is defined as abnormally high pulmonary vascular pressure. It affects both precapillary and postcapillary pressures (arterial and venous side pulmonary circulation), whereas PAH affects precapillary (arterial) pressures only (Box 2.54).

Box 2.54 Causes of PH

Left ventricular failure	Chronic obstructive pulmonary disease
Left-sided valvular heart disease	Pulmonary fibrosis
Pulmonary embolism	Sarcoidosis

> **HINT**
>
> PAH (primary pulmonary hypertension) primarily involves the pulmonary arteries, whereas PH (secondary pulmonary hypertension) can be caused by left-sided failure or lung abnormalities.

- *What hemodynamic findings define PAH?*
- **mPAP more than 25 mmHg and PAOP less than 15 mmHg**

Mean pulmonary artery pressure (mPAP) is elevated but the left atrial or left ventricular end diastolic pressure (LVEDP) remains relatively normal. PH caused by left-sided failure or pulmonary diseases would elevate the pulmonary artery occlusive pressure (PAOP) in addition to the mPAP.

PATHOPHYSIOLOGY

- *What are the pathological changes that occur within the pulmonary artery resulting in increase in resistance?*
- **Vascular remodeling**

Vascular remodeling produced by excessive cell proliferation affects the small pulmonary arteries. The vascular changes can include intimal hyperplasia, medial hypertrophy, and adventitial proliferation. Pulmonary artery vasoconstriction can contribute to the pulmonary hypertension.

SYMPTOMS/ASSESSMENT

- *What are common symptoms of patients presenting with PH?*
- **Dyspnea, chest pain, and syncope**

Primary symptoms of PH include dyspnea, chest pain, and syncope. Symptoms may also include history of fatigue and peripheral edema. Assessment for signs of RV failure should be performed to determine the degree of RV involvement (Box 2.55).

Box 2.55 Symptoms of PH

Dyspnea	Murmurs/extra heart sounds
Fatigue	Increased jugular distention
Chest pain	Hepatomegaly/splenomegaly
Syncope	Ascites
Cyanosis	Crackles
Clubbing of fingers	

■ *What type of murmur is most likely to develop with severe PH?*

■ **Systolic murmur**

Development of a new-onset tricuspid regurgitation can occur following the onset of PH. The murmur is heard during systole because of the valve's incompetency to maintain intactness. Pulmonary regurgitation can also occur and presents with a diastolic murmur.

> **❯ HINT**
> The presence of right ventricle S_4 can also indicate RV heart failure (HF) (Box 2.56).

Box 2.56 Heart Sounds With PH

Early systolic click	Sudden interruption in the opening of the pulmonic valve due to high arterial pressure
Midsystolic ejection murmur	Turbulent flow through the pulmonic valve
Right ventricular S_3 and S_4	Volume overload in the right ventricle due to heart failure or noncompliance of the ventricle
Holosystolic murmur	Tricuspid regurgitation
Accentuated pulmonary component S_2	High arterial pressure closed the pulmonic valve with greater force
Diastolic murmur	Pulmonic regurgitation

DIAGNOSIS

■ *What diagnostic test is frequently used to identify pulmonary hypertension with RV involvement?*

■ **Echocardiogram**

An echocardiogram is used to screen for pulmonary hypertension and right-sided involvement (right ventricle and atrium). Suspicion of pulmonary hypertension is based on presenting symptoms and history. In order to treat effectively, the underlying associated disease or cause should be identified.

> **HINT**
Etiology dictates treatment of the PH. For example, etiology of CHF causing PH, requires treatment aimed at improving HF.

■ *What is considered the confirmative diagnosis for PAH?*
■ **Right heart catheterization (RHC)**

Right heart catheterization can confirm the hemodynamic measurements that verify the diagnosis of PAH. Other diagnostics include history and physical, CXR, and echocardiogram.

> **HINT**
Echocardiogram can assist with identifying right atrial and ventricular enlargement and tricuspid regurgitation (Box 2.57).

Box 2.57 Findings of RHC Indicative of PAH

Transpulmonary gradient (PA mean – PAOP) is high	Normal to low PAOP
Elevated pulmonary vascular resistance (PVR)	Increased "A" and "V" waves

■ *Which of the hemodynamic parameters is the best diagnostic reading to differentiate between primary PAH and secondary PH?*
■ **Pulmonary vascular resistance (PVR)**

PVR may be more important than the mean PAP because it reflects influence of the transpulmonary gradient and is only elevated if vascular obstruction occurs on the precapillary side. It is useful to obtain whether the mean PAP is elevated.

> **HINT**
PAH caused by pulmonary vascular pathology will elevate both PVR and mPAP, whereas PH caused by other disorders, including left-sided failure, will elevate the mPAP but not the PVR.

MEDICAL MANAGEMENT

■ *What is the primary contraindication for testing vasoreactivity in patients with PAH?*
■ **Hemodynamic instability**

Administration of a vasodilator is used to test vasoreactivity to consider potential patients for long-term calcium channel blocker therapy. Patients with hemodynamic instability and overt right ventricular failure should not be tested with a vasodilator. A positive responder to the administration of a vasodilator includes a decrease in mPAP by at least 10 mmHg or absolute reduction less than 40 mmHg without a decrease in cardiac output. The vasodilators frequently used to test vasoreactivity include inhaled nitric oxide, epoprostenol, or adenosine.

> **HINT**
Close hemodynamic monitoring should be performed during testing
with a vasodilator to determine reactivity in PAH.

■ **Which of the calcium channel blockers is not indicated in managing PAH even
with good reactivity testing?**

■ **Verapamil**

Calcium channel blockers are frequently used to vasodilate the pulmonary arteries and
lower the pulmonary artery vascular resistance. Verapamil causes a decrease in myocardial contractility and can worsen RV failure in PAH patients.

■ **What medical management is recommended for all patients
with idiopathic PAH?**

■ **Warfarin**

Anticoagulation therapy with warfarin is recommended for all patients with idiopathic
PAH. Calcium channel blockers are indicated in those patients found to be responsive
to vasodilator therapy. Diuretics may be used if there are signs of acute right-side HF.
Calcium channel blockers are used only in PAH patients shown to have positive reactiveness to vasodilator therapy. Phosphodiesterase (PDE)-5 inhibitors have improved exercise
tolerance and hemodynamics.

> **HINT**
INR goal for patients on warfarin for PAH is 1.5 to 2.5.

■ **Which drug has been found to increase survival in PAH?**

■ **Epoprostenol**

Epoprostenol, a prostanoid, is the preferred treatment for critically ill patients and has
been found to improve survival. Prostanoids are vasodilators with antiproliferative
effects. PAH causes a reduction in prostacyclin synthase, thus resulting in lower levels
of prostacyclin.

> **HINT**
Eposprostenol may be administered as a continuous infusion through a
long-term catheter (Box 2.58). Treprostinil administered SC may cause
pain and erythema at the sites of injection. IV route has possibly been
associated with a higher risk of catheter sepsis (Box 2.59).

Box 2.58 Routes of Prostanoids

Prostanoid	Route of Administration
Epoprostenol	Continuous IV
Treprostinil	SC or continuous IV
Iloprost	Aerosolized devices

Box 2.59 Common Side Effects of Epoprostenol

Headache	Diarrhea
Jaw pain	Nausea
Flushing	Musculoskeletal pain

■ *What laboratory value needs to be monitored monthly and indefinitely when on endothelin receptor antagonists?*

■ **Liver function tests (LFTs) and hemoglobin and hematocrit (H&H)**

Endothelin receptor antagonist (Bosentan, Sitaxsentan) is administered orally. The significant side effect is elevated liver enzymes. It also requires close monitoring of liver enzymes monthly and hematocrit every 3 months. Endothelin-1 is a vasoconstrictor that contributes to PAH. This class is used to inhibit or block endothelin-1 resulting in vasodilation. Other drugs that may be used to treat PAH include PDE-5 inhibitors (Sildenafil).

> ❯ **HINT**
> Due to the different mechanism of action, a combination of drugs is usually used to medically manage PAH.

SURGICAL MANAGEMENT

■ *What surgical procedure can be performed in patients experiencing worsening of symptoms on multiple medications for PH?*

■ **Atrial septostomy**

Atrial septostomy creates a right-to-left shunt that decreases right heart filling pressures and improves right heart function. This procedure increases LV filling and improves cardiac output. It will cause a greater systemic hypoxia but the goal is for the increase in CO to improve systemic oxygen delivery.

■ *What is the potential surgical option for end-stage pulmonary disease?*

■ **Lung transplant**

Lung transplant is an option in select patients with worsening of symptoms despite maximal pharmacological treatments. The transplant may include single lung, double lung, or heart/lung transplant. The decision is made on the severity of the decompensated heart failure. Extracorporeal membrane oxygenation (ECMO) is also gaining popularity with unstable patients with end-stage pulmonary disease refractory to adequate oxygenation while on mechanical ventilation.

> ❯ **HINT**
> RV assist device may be used as a "bridge" for transplantation.

■ *Following a large PE, a patient can develop chronic PH. What surgical intervention can be used to lower the PVR in such a patient?*

■ Pulmonary thromboendarterectomy

The diagnosis of chronic PH following a PE is perfusion scanning and, potentially, pulmonary angiogram. If PH develops and the patient is an acceptable surgical risk, removal of the fiber strands and material from the pulmonary artery with pulmonary thromboendarterectomy can lower the PVR.

COMPLICATIONS

■ *What is the most common cause of death in a patient with PAH?*

■ RV failure

RV failure is a common complication of PAH. The initial response of the RV when pumping against the high resistance is to develop hypertrophy. This compensatory mechanism can reduce wall stress and improve cardiac output. Second, the RV begins to dilate and less blood flows to the LV. Prolongation of RV contraction encroaches on the LV filling. The effect is a decrease in LV filling and cardiac output causing cardiovascular collapse. Atrial arrhythmias are caused by RV failure and include paroxysmal atrial tachycardia, atrial flutter, and atrial fibrillation.

> ❯ HINT
> Increased RV tension may lead to RV ischemia and acute myocardial infarction.

THORACIC TRAUMA

■ *What is the most common mechanism of injury for a pulmonary contusion (PC)?*

■ Blunt trauma

The most common mechanism of injury for pulmonary contusion is a blunt, high-impact trauma to the chest producing a compression–decompression effect. The most common cause is a motor vehicle collision. PC can also be caused by penetrating trauma with high-velocity missiles to the chest.

PATHOPHYSIOLOGY

■ *What is the physiological change in the lungs following a high-impact blunt trauma to the chest?*

■ Disruption of alveolar–capillary integrity

The disruption of the alveolar–capillary integrity results in hemorrhage and edema in both the interstitial and intra-alveolar spaces in the lungs. Reflexive increase in bronchial mucus secretions result in early development of atelectasis and ventilation/perfusion defects. The combination of atelectasis, blood and fluid, and interstitial edema produces a decrease in pulmonary compliance and an increase in airway pressures.

- ■ *What is the most common site of injury for tracheobronchial tear following blunt trauma?*
- ■ **Bifurcation mainstem bronchus**

The most common site of injury is at the bifurcation of the mainstem bronchus, approximately 1 inch from the carina. The injury may not be evident for up to 5 days after the injury.

SYMPTOMS/ASSESSMENT

- ■ *Following blunt trauma to the chest, a patient develops productive cough. What would you expect the sputum to look like?*
- ■ **Blood streaked (hemoptysis)**

Hemoptysis may occur after a blunt injury to the chest wall due to the rupture of the alveolar–capillary membranes. The blunt force causes damage to the pulmonary vasculature, allowing blood to enter the alveoli and interstitium. This causes a "bruise" in the lung tissue and manifests as blood-tinged or -streaked sputum (Box 2.60).

Box 2.60 Symptoms of PC

Dyspnea	Wheezing over affective area
Tachypnea	Labored respirations
Chest pain	Tachycardia
Hemoptysis	Pallor or cyanosis
Crackles or rhonchi	Hypoxemia

> **❯ HINT**
> The onset of symptoms with PC occurs within 6 to 48 hours following the injury.

- ■ *A nurse finds subcutaneous air when assessing a patient 24 hours after a blunt trauma to the chest. The patient also demonstrates noisy breathing. What is the most likely cause of these findings?*
- ■ **Tracheobronchial tear**

Tracheobronchial tears may not be recognized immediately following the trauma but can present 24 to 48 hours later. The typical presentation is pneumothorax or unresolved pneumothorax and subcutaneous air (Box 2.61).

Box 2.61 Symptoms of Tracheobronchial Tear

Noisy breathing	Progressive mediastinal emphysema
Hemoptysis	Pneumothorax
Cough	Air leak in chest
Subcutaneous air	

DIAGNOSIS

■ *What CXR changes occur with a PC?*
■ **Diffuse infiltrates**

The infiltrates are diffuse and do not conform to segments or lobes of the lung. Findings on CXR may not appear until 4 to 6 hours after injury and up to 48 hours later.

> **❭ HINT**
> CXR findings are similar to those found in ARDS.

■ *Which radiograph is the most sensitive in determining the extent of the pulmonary contusion?*
■ **Computed tomography (CT)**

A CT scan is highly sensitive to findings of pulmonary contusion and the volume of lung involvement. CT scanning may be used to determine the clinical outcomes. PC involving more than 18% of the lung is considered a significant injury, associated with poorer outcomes.

> **❭ HINT**
> Occult PC is defined as changes seen on initial CT but not visible on CXR. This has a good prognosis.

■ *What is a finding on CXR that may indicate tracheobronchial injury?*
■ **Pneumomediastinum**

A tracheobronchial tear results in air introduced into the mediastinum. The air can be recognized on CXR if the tear is below the level of the carina.

■ *What test is considered to be the definitive diagnosis for a tracheobronchial tear?*
■ **Bronchoscopy**

Bronchoscopy can be used to visualize the actual tear, whereas CXR only identifies mediastinal air.

MANAGEMENT

■ *What emergency management of a hemodynamically unstable trauma patient may affect PC outcomes?*
■ **Volume overload**

Too much volume used in resuscitation can worsen the PC, increasing lung fluid, and worsening hypoxia. Adequate resuscitation to improve blood flow to the organs is important but over-resuscitation can cause pulmonary complications (Box 2.62).

Box 2.62 Overall Management of PC

Good pulmonary toiletry
Avoid volume overload
Adequate ventilation

> **HINT**
Current research does not support the use of corticosteroids or antibiotics when treating PC.

■ *What mode of ventilation may benefit a patient with severe unilateral lung injury following a blunt chest trauma?*
■ **Independent lung ventilation (ILV)**

If the PC involves a single lung, the lung compliance becomes unequal. This results in asymmetrical ventilation. Airflow will take the path of least resistance, causing an overinflation of the noninjured lung and underinflation of the injured lung. ILV uses a double-lumen ETT allowing for separate ventilation of each lung (Box 2.63).

Box 2.63 Ventilator Modes for PC

PEEP	Pressure release ventilation
Pressure controlled ventilation	Independent lung ventilation
High-frequency oscillator/jet ventilation	

> **HINT**
Ventilator management is similar to that used for patients with ARDS.

COMPLICATIONS

■ *What is a major complication of a severe PC?*
■ **Adult respiratory distress syndrome (ARDS)**

ARDS is a complication of a severe PC. An injury to the alveolar capillary membrane causes noncardiogenic pulmonary edema, which is one criterion for the diagnosis of ARDS. VAP can also be a complication of PC.

■ *What is a life-threatening complication of tracheobronchial injury?*
■ **Tension pneumothorax**

Air can be introduced into the mediastinum and pleural space. A tension pneumothorax can occur due to air being forced into the pleural space and unable to leave, developing tension.

> **HINT**
Assess for tension pneumothorax by palpating trachea to determine if midline. A deviate trachea indicates a tension pneumothorax.

MECHANICAL VENTILATION

▪ *Which measured pressure is considered to be equal to the alveolar pressure?*
▪ **Plateau pressure (P$_{plat}$)**

Plateau pressure is obtained after inspiration and before exhalation by delaying the expiration on the ventilator. This equalizes the pressures in the alveoli to the mouth and correlates to the pressure within the alveoli.

> ❯ **HINT**
> Plateau pressures are measured by holding inspiratory time.

▪ *Which measured pressure, when elevated, causes barotrauma to the lungs?*
▪ **PIP**

PIP is the amount of pressure required by the ventilator to deliver the set TV. This is the highest pressure recorded at the end of inspiration. Pressures that are too high may cause barotraumas. Pressures greater than 35 to 40 may be damaging to the lungs (Box 2.64).

Box 2.64 Measurement Compliances in Lungs

Calculated Compliance	Measures	Causes of Decreased Compliance	Calculation

Dynamic compliance	Measurement of the total compliance (lung and chest wall)	▪ Bronchoconstriction
		▪ Increase in airway resistance
		  – Secretions
		  – Mucus plug
		▪ Flail chest
		▪ Muscle tension
			TV ÷ PIP – PEEP
			Normal 100 mL/cm H$_2$O

Static compliance	Measurement of the lung compliance reflects changes within the alveoli	▪ Air trapping ▪ Pulmonary edema ▪ Atelectasis ▪ Pneumonia ▪ Pneumothorax/hemothorax ▪ Loss of surfactant ▪ Abdominal distension	TV + P$_{plat}$ – PEEP Normal 70–100 mL/cm H$_2$O Goal > 50 mL/cm H$_2$O

> ❯ **HINT**
> Static compliance takes resistance airway and compliance of the chest wall out of the equation and looks only at the alveoli.

▪ *Which measured pressure may improve oxygenation when increased?*
▪ **mPaw**

Paw is the sum of the amount and duration of pressure applied to the chest on the intrathoracic structures. A lower mean pressure will have less negative cardiovascular effects. But an increase in Paw may increase oxygenation.

■ *Auto-PEEP occurs when the I:E ratio does not allow what to occur?*
■ **Adequate expiratory time**

After a breath is delivered, if the next breath is delivered before all the air leaves the lungs, it causes "stacking of breaths" or auto-PEEP. If breaths continue to be delivered without adequately allowing the complete exhalation of air, the end-expiratory pressure and volumes increase and can result in a lung injury called barotrauma. Auto-PEEP is not set on the ventilator but it has an additive effect in increasing end-expiratory pressure with the actual set PEEP.

> ❯ HINT
> Total PEEP = set PEEP + auto-PEEP.

■ *How is auto-PEEP typically measured on the ventilator?*
■ **Occlusion of expiratory time**

It is measured by temporarily occluding the expiratory circuit in the ventilator, which equalizes pressures in the lungs and ventilator circuit.

> ❯ HINT
> This measurement is most accurate if the patient is sedated or paralyzed.

■ *What is the best method to manage auto-PEEP?*
■ **Decrease breaths per minute**

The best method to decrease the inspiratory time is to decrease the total breaths per minute. This allows for greater exhalation times. A lowering of the TV may also be used but is not as efficient as changing the ventilatory rate. Increasing the inspiratory flow rate is not effective at lowering total inspiratory time unless inappropriately set in the beginning.

> ❯ HINT
> Many patients are breathing over the set RR and may require sedation or neuromuscular blocking agents to lower the total ventilatory rate.

■ *What is the adverse effect of auto-PEEP on ventilation?*
■ **Increases WOB**

The inspiratory effort of the patient must not just equal the sensitivity setting on a demand ventilator but must now overcome the level of auto-PEEP to initiate the airflow into the lungs. This increases WOB.

> ❯ **HINT**
> Decrease WOB by setting the PEEP level slightly below the total PEEP level to decrease the amount of inspiratory effort needed to trigger the ventilator breath.

PULMONARY THERAPEUTIC INTERVENTIONS

WEANING FROM THE VENTILATOR

- ■ *What is the primary point when clinicians suspect that a patient may be ready to wean?*
- ■ **Disease process improved**

One of the clinical changes that indicate the timing to begin weaning is the adequate treatment of the disease process that caused the respiratory failure. The decision to attempt weaning and discontinue the ventilator is also based on the patient being hemodynamically stable, awake, and meeting the minimal ventilator dependency criterion (Box 2.65).

> ❯ **HINT**
> Shortening the weaning process is an important goal to prevent VAP and other ventilation complications.

Box 2.65 Minimal Ventilator Dependency

$FiO_2 < 40\%$	$PaO_2 > 60$
PEEP < 8 cm H_2O	No vasopressors
PF ratio > 200 mmHg	No continuous sedation
Arterial saturation > 90%	

- ■ *What are the most common techniques used to perform a spontaneous breathing test (SBT)?*
- ■ **T-Bar (or flow-by), CPAP, and pressure support ventilation (PSV)**

A T-bar spontaneous breathing test involves taking the patient off the ventilator, whereas CPAP and PSV modes can be performed while the patient remains on the ventilator. A CPAP of 5 cm H_2O is frequently used for weaning. Higher CPAP levels defeat the purpose of spontaneous breathing.

> ❯ **HINT**
> Close observation of the patient during SBT is needed to recognize respiratory fatigue or failure.

- ■ *What is the rapid shallow breathing index (RSBI) used to determine readiness for extubation?*
- ■ **RR/TV**

The RSBI is used to predict successful weaning from a ventilator. RSBI can be calculated after 5 to 10 minutes of initiation of a weaning trial (Box 2.66).

Box 2.66 RSBI Scores

≤ 80 predicts successful weaning
80–100 predicts weaning may or may not be successful
≥ 100 predicts weaning unsuccessful

- *During an SBT, which is used to wean patients, what is the primary cause for an increase in airway resistance?*
- **ETT**

The ETT has a smaller diameter than the patient's own airway. This narrowing of the upper airway increases the airway resistance and WOB.

> **HINT**
> CPAP and/or PSV can be used during spontaneous breathing trials to overcome the resistance of the ETT.

- *Which of the weaning parameters most closely correlates with inspiratory muscle strength?*
- **Negative inspiratory pressure (NIP)**

NIP is also known as negative inspiratory force (NIF). The NIP is the maximal inspiratory pressure and is used to assess muscle strength. An NIP value of less than –20 to –25 cm H_2O is predictive for successful weaning.

> **HINT**
> Remember, spontaneous inspiration is a negative pressure. A greater negativity of the NIP correlates to a stronger inspiratory effort (Box 2.67).

Box 2.67 Weaning Parameters

RR < 35 bpm	VC > 10 mL/kg
NIP < –20 to –25 cm H_2O	RR/VT < 105 bpm/L
TV > 5 mL/kg	

- *What is the most common arrhythmia associated with failure of weaning from the ventilator?*
- **Sinus tachycardia**

Sinus tachycardia is the most common arrhythmia caused by a failure to wean from the ventilator. Failure of weaning includes the failure of spontaneous breathing test or reintubation within 48 hours after extubation (Box 2.68).

Box 2.68 Signs of Failed Weaning

Objective Signs	Subjective Signs
Tachypnea (> 35 bpm)	Anxiety
Tachycardia (increase > 20)	Dyspnea
Hypertension (increase > 20)	Increased WOB
Hypotension	
Hypoxemia	
▪ PaO$_2$ < 50 mmHg	
▪ SaO$_2$ < 90%	
Acidosis	
New arrhythmias	
Agitation	
Diaphoresis	
RSBI > 100	
Depressed mental status	
Increased use of accessory muscles	

▪ *Immediately following extubation, a patient develops audible wheezing and increased difficulty in breathing. What would be the most likely cause?*

▪ **Laryngospasm**

Laryngospasm is a prolonged protective reflex of the vocal cords. It is seen immediately post extubation and is due to airway irritation, presence of a foreign body, or secretions (saliva, blood, vomitus). It may also be associated with emergence anesthesia, airway trauma, or a difficult intubation. There are certain factors that increase the risk of laryngospasm and include the history of smoking, COPD, airway irritability, and asthma.

> **HINT**
> Inability to speak indicates a complete airway obstruction (Box 2.69).

Box 2.69 Symptoms of Laryngospasm

High-pitched inspiratory stridor	Wheezing
Anxiety	Chest and abdominal paradoxical movement
Tracheal tug	Tachypnea

▪ *What is the initial management of laryngospasm?*

▪ **Apply oxygen 100% FiO$_2$**

If stridor develops or if the patient begins to exhibit other signs of laryngospasm, place the patient in a lateral position unless contraindicated to promote drainage of secretions. Apply supplemental oxygen using 100% FiO$_2$ and humidification. Administer racemic epinephrine to decrease the edema and consider the administration of succinylcholine at a low dose in an attempt to relax the laryngeal muscles. Severe cases may require intubation and positive ventilation.

■ *Prior to extubation, what intervention can be performed to assess for airway edema?*

■ **Deflate the cuff to assess for an air leak**

Prior to extubation, assess for the presence of airway edema by deflating the cuff and ensuring an audible air leak is heard around the deflated cuff. If no audible air leak is present, this indicates airway swelling, and extubation should be delayed. Management of airway edema following extubation is similar to laryngospasm with the addition of steroid treatments.

> **❯ HINT**
> Prevention of airway swelling includes limiting the amount of trauma to the airway such as limiting ETT movement and prevention of coughing or "bucking" of the ventilator.

RESPIRATORY MONITORING DEVICES

■ *What is the technique used to continuously measure exhaled CO_2?*

■ **Capnography**

Capnography is the continuous measurement of end-tidal CO_2 ($ETCO_2$). Capnography is used to verify ETT placement, confirming that the tube is in the trachea. $ETCO_2$ can determine changes in pulmonary circulation and respiratory status before pulse oximetry. Substantial hypercarbia must occur before the patient demonstrates hypoxemia.

■ *Which VQ mismatch demonstrates a greater discrepancy between $PaCO_2$ and $ETCO_2$?*

■ **Dead space**

The difference between $PaCO_2$ and $ETCO_2$ increases as dead space volume increases.

> **❯ HINT**
> An acute discrepancy in arterial and end-tidal CO_2 with sudden-onset dyspnea increases the suspicion of a PE.

■ *What affects the accuracy of the capnography?*

■ **High breathing rates**

High breathing rates can exceed capnography capabilities and may decrease the accuracy of the readings. Increased airway resistance may also affect the accuracy of the reading.

■ *A patient is admitted with carbon monoxide poisoning. The pulse oximetry reading is 99% to 100% saturation, but the ABG sent to the lab revealed an 86% saturation. Which of the two is more accurate in this situation?*

■ **ABG saturation**

Carbon monoxide diffuses faster and binds to hemoglobin and forms carboxyhemoglobin in the blood. This reduces the oxygen-carrying capacity of the hemoglobin, resulting in hypoxia. The pulse oximetry measures bound hemoglobin, whether bound with oxygen or any other substance, whereas an ABG analyzed in the laboratory can differentiate between oxygen and carbon monoxide.

> ❯ **HINT**
> This discrepancy also occurs with Nipride (nitroprusside) toxicity of cyanide poisoning.

BIBLIOGRAPHY

ACCP's guidelines for diagnosis and management DVT/PE/VTE (9th ed.). (2012). *Chest*, 141(Suppl 2), 1S. doi:10.1378/chest.1412S1

American College of Cardiology Foundation/American Heart Association (ACCF/AHA). (2009). Expert consensus document on pulmonary hypertension. *Circulation, 119*, 2250–2294.

Modrykamien, A., Chat-Burn, R. L., & Ashton, R. W. (2011). Airway pressure release ventilation: An alternative mode of mechanical ventilation in acute respiratory distress syndrome. *Cleveland Clinical Journal of Medicine, 78*(2), 101–110.

Questions

1. A patient presents with labored breathing and an RR of 40 beats per minute (bpm). The following ABG is obtained:

   PaO_2 68 mmHg
   $PaCO_2$ 50 mmHg
   pH 7.34
   SaO_2 91%
   HCO_3 22

   Which of the following is the most accurate interpretation of the above situation?

   A. Normal ABG for COPD patient
   B. Respiratory failure due to metabolic acidosis
   C. Obstructive upper airway most likely causing respiratory failure
   D. Respiratory failure due to dead space

2. What is the compensatory mechanism for VQ shunting?

   A. Decrease MV
   B. Bronchoconstriction
   C. Pulmonary vasoconstriction
   D. Increase cardiac output

3. Which of the following findings would indicate the presence of obstructive airway disease?

   A. FEV1/FVC ratio of < 60%
   B. FEV1/FVC ratio 75% to 80%
   C. FEV1/FVC ratio > 80%
   D. Normal FEV1/FVC ratio

4. A patient in the ICU is diagnosed with ARDS. The following are the ventilator settings and ABG results:

   SIMV
   550 mL TV
   Rate 16
   FiO_2 40%
   PEEP 5
   7.46 pH
   48 $PaCO_2$
   82 PaO_2
   94% SaO_2

   What is the calculated PaO_2/FiO_2 ratio?

   A. 120
   B. 20
   C. 235
   D. 205

5. A patient on a ventilator diagnosed with ARDS experiences a worsening hypoxia. On obtaining an ABG, it is noted that the patient has a PaO_2/FiO_2 ratio of 84. What does this ratio indicate regarding the severity of the patient's impaired oxygenation?

A. Normal oxygenation
B. Mild impairment
C. Moderate impairment
D. Severe impairment

6. Shearing injury to the lung during mechanical ventilation of an ARDS patient, which is a result of repeated cycles of recruitment and derecruitment, is called

A. Barotrauma
B. Volutrauma
C. Atelectrauma
D. Biotrauma

7. A patient is on pressure-controlled ventilation for ARDS. The physician has stated that he wants the patient's TVs to be more than 250 mL/breath. On assessment, it is noted that the average TV is 200 mL/breath. Which of the following ventilator settings can be changed to increase the TV?

A. Increase pressure limit
B. Decrease RR
C. Decrease the flow rate
D. Increase PEEP levels

8. A patient with ARDS is being ventilated in APRV mode. His oxygen saturation has decreased to 87%. The following are the ventilator settings:

P high 26 cm H_2O
P low 0 cm H_2O
T high 4 seconds
T low 0.6 seconds
FiO_2 100%

What ventilator change can be made to improve the oxygen saturation of this patient?

A. Increase P high
B. Shorten T high
C. Increase P low
D. Prolong T low

9. An ARDS patient is changed from a conventional ventilator to a HFOV. After 6 hours, the $PaCO_2$ on the ABG was 54. Which of the following ventilator changes can be made to increase elimination of CO_2?

A. Decreasing the power
B. Increasing FiO_2
C. Increasing mean airway pressure (mPaw)
D. Lowering the frequency (Hz)

10. Mr. M is on a pressure-control mode of ventilation. He is currently on versed and morphine infusion. He continued to "buck the ventilator" and vecuronium (Norcuron) was ordered with a goal of TOF of 2/4 twitches. Which of the following percentages of neuromuscular blockade would you expect with a 2/4 twitch?

    A. 0% to 75%
    B. 80%
    C. 90%
    D. 100%

11. Which of the following signs would be the most significant finding in a COPD patient indicating the need for ventilatory support?

    A. $PaCO_2$ > 55 mmHg
    B. Production of purulent sputum
    C. Inspiratory wheezing
    D. Paradoxical breathing

12. High levels of FiO_2 administered to a COPD patient can cause ventilatory abnormalities. Which of the following best describes these abnormalities?

    A. Results in bronchoconstriction and wheezing
    B. Increases WOB
    C. Increases dead space and $PaCO_2$ levels
    D. Increases production of sputum

13. A patient presents with respiratory insufficiency and is admitted to the ICU. He has a significant history of cigarette smoking and COPD. An ABG is obtained. Which of the following would indicate an acute on chronic respiratory failure requiring intubation?

    A. $PaCO_2$ of 64 mmHg
    B. PaO_2 of 60 mmHg
    C. SaO_2 of 90%
    D. pH 7.28

14. Your mechanically ventilated patient is on the following ventilator settings: assist control (AC) rate of 10, TV of 350, FiO_2 of 40%, and PEEP 5. The patient has been agitated and breathing 18 to 20 bpm. He is now hypotensive and is noted to have excessive auto-PEEP. Which of the following would be the best method to treat the auto-PEEP?

    A. Decrease TV
    B. Sedate the patient with propofol
    C. Increase flow rate
    D. Administer bronchodilators

15. Which of the following presentations of acute asthma would most likely be admitted to the ICU for close monitoring and treatment?

    A. Dyspnea that interferes with daily activities
    B. Presence of inspiratory wheezes
    C. Inability to communicate in full sentences
    D. Requiring corticosteroid treatment

16. What is the first-line pharmacological treatment recommended for severe or life-threatening asthma?

A. Anticholinergic
B. Heliox
C. Leukotriene receptor antagonist
D. β_2-selective agonist

17. A patient develops a pneumothorax from a central line. The patient is asymptomatic. Which of the following patients would be best to observe and place on 100% FiO_2 without placing a chest tube?

A. Spontaneously breathing and pneumothorax > 2 cm
B. Mechanically ventilated and pneumothorax < 1 cm
C. CPAP patient and pneumothorax < 2 cm
D. Spontaneous breathing and pneumothorax < 2 cm

18. Which of the following would be an indication for the removal of the chest drainage tube that was placed for a pneumothorax?

A. No subcutaneous emphysema present
B. < 50 mL of chest drainage in 12 hours
C. Intermittent bubbling only present in the chest drainage system
D. Bubbling has ceased in the chest drainage system

19. What is the minimal endotracheal tube cuff pressure required to prevent aspiration of secretions?

A. 10 cm H_2O
B. 20 cm H_2O
C. 30 cm H_2O
D. 40 cm H_2O

20. Which of the following causes of elevated pulmonary vascular resistance is classified as PAH?

A. Idiopathic
B. Left ventricular failure
C. COPD
D. PE

21. Which of the following procedures is used to determine potential effectiveness of long-term calcium channel blockers in managing PAH?

A. Fluid challenge
B. Vasodilator reactivity test
C. Stress test
D. Dobutamine stress test

22. While performing a spontaneous breathing test on a patient being assessed for potential extubation, an RSBI is calculated. Which of the following correlates best to prediction of successful weaning?

    A. < 80 breaths per minute (bpm)
    B. Between 80 and 100 breaths-min-L
    C. Between 100 and 150 breaths-min-L
    D. > 150 breaths-min-L

23. Following extubation, a patient immediately developed audible stridor and wheezing. Which of the following interventions would be the priority care?

    A. Reintubate the patient immediately
    B. Administer 100% FiO_2 oxygen and racemic epinephrine
    C. Administer small dose succinylcholine
    D. Provide heliox treatments

24. Following a large PE, which of the following statements is most correct regarding the effect on the LV?

    A. Obstruction increases the pressure load of the LV
    B. Decreases LV preload
    C. Increases LV distensibility
    D. Lowers the coronary perfusion gradient of the LV

25. Which of the following pulmonary disorders results in an elevated central venous pressure and a normal to decrease in PAOP?

    A. Pulmonary edema
    B. Pneumonia
    C. Atelectasis
    D. PE

26. Which of the following 12-lead ECG changes is considered to be a classic finding of a PE?

    A. $S1Q_3T_3$ pattern
    B. ST segment depression inferior leads
    C. Peaked T waves
    D. New onset RBBB

27. Which of the following is considered to be an absolute contraindication for anticoagulation therapy in managing a VTE?

    A. Hypertensive patient
    B. Intracranial hemorrhage
    C. Postoperative patient
    D. Presence of epidural catheter

28. Which of the following weaning parameters most closely correlates to respiratory muscle strength?

A. NIP
B. VC
C. MV
D. Spontaneous TV

29. After 10 minutes of a weaning trial of pressure support, the patient is noted to have an RSBI of 110. Which of the following statements is most accurate?

A. Predicts a successful weaning
B. Indicates the need for immediate extubation
C. Predicts unsuccessful weaning
D. Indicates the patient requires sedation and paralysis

30. A patient is admitted following a blunt chest trauma. Within 24 hours of admission, the CXR demonstrates bilateral fluffy infiltrates and the patient's saturations are decreasing. Which of the following statements is most accurate regarding this patient's current presentation?

A. This patient is developing early-onset ARDS due to sepsis.
B. This patient is volume overloaded from resuscitation that is too aggressive.
C. This patient has a pulmonary contusion.
D. This patient is developing a HAP.

Endocrine System Review

In this chapter, you will review:

■ Diabetic ketoacidosis (DKA)/hyperglycemic hyperosmolar nonketotic syndrome (HHNS)
■ Diabetes insipidus (DI)/syndrome of inappropriate antidiuretic hormone (SIADH)/cerebral salt wasting syndrome (CSWS)

DIABETIC KETOACIDOSIS/HYPERGLYCEMIC HYPEROSMOLAR NONKETOTIC SYNDROME

■ *An insulin-dependent patient is more likely to have which of these diabetic complications: diabetic ketoacidosis (DKA) or hyperglycemic hyperosmolar nonketotic syndrome (HHNS)?*

■ **DKA**

Clinically, we do not refer to diabetes as type 1 or 2 anymore. In the past, the thought was that type 1 diabetics required insulin and type 2 diabetics did not; this has changed because as we have seen clinically, many type 2 diabetics require insulin. We now refer to patients as insulin-dependent diabetic mellitus (IDDM) or noninsulin-dependent diabetic mellitus (NIDDM). (Note: Some references still use type 1 and 2.) Insulin-dependent diabetics are more likely to develop DKA whereas noninsulin-dependent diabetics will develop HHNS. HHNS is hyperglycemia with hyperosmolar states but without ketonemia and ketoacidosis. HHNS may occur over days to weeks, whereas DKA tends to have a shorter time to symptoms.

> ❯ **HINT**
> Noninsulin-dependent diabetics still produce some insulin (although inadequate for glucose control) allowing for control of the ketone bodies.

■ *Between DKA and HHNS, which has a higher mortality?*
■ **HHNS**

DKA and HHNS are both life-threatening complications of diabetes mellitus, but HHNS has greater mortality. Symptoms of HHNS may persist for several days resulting in higher glucose and osmolality levels. HHNS causes hyperglycemia and hyperosmolar states similar to DKA but without the increase in ketones, which are responsible for inducing nausea and vomiting in DKA patients and requires seeking medical assistance. Symptoms of HHNS are less severe, which can result in the delay of treatment.

> ❯ HINT
> The serum osmolality correlates to mortality. Other predictors include the extremes of age, coma, and hypotension.

■ *What is the most common precipitating factor for the development of DKA or HHNS?*

■ **Infection**

The most common cause for the development of life-threatening complications of diabetes is infection. Another common cause of DKA is new-onset type 1 diabetes or noncompliance with use of insulin (Box 3.1).

Box 3.1 Precipitating Factors

Infection	Treatment errors (inadequate insulin or noncompliance)
New-onset diabetes	Abdominal disorders
Alcohol abuse	Acute myocardial infarction
Pancreatitis	Hyperthyroidism
Stroke	Stress induced
Trauma	Emotional factors
Drug induced	

PATHOPHYSIOLOGY

■ *The basic underlying physiology of DKA is a decrease in insulin and an increase in which hormones?*

■ **Counterregulatory hormones**

The combination of a decrease in insulin and an increase in counterregulatory hormones causes an increase in glucose production and impaired utilization in the peripheral tissue cells.

> ❯ HINT
> The role of counterregulatory hormones is opposite that of insulin (Box 3.2).

Box 3.2 Counterregulatory Hormones

Glucagon	Growth hormone
Catecholamines	Cortisol

■ *Is insulin an anabolic hormone or a catabolic hormone?*

■ **Anabolic hormone**

Insulin, being an anabolic hormone, synthesizes or builds proteins from amino acids and triglycerides from free fatty acids. It allows for the use of glucose in the peripheral tissues and controls glucose levels in the serum. Without the suppressive effects of insulin and the catabolic effects of the counterregulatory hormones, a patient will develop proteolysis and lipolysis. As muscles break down, they release amino acids and the adipose tissues release fatty acids.

> ❯ HINT
>
> Anabolic hormones build, whereas catabolic hormones break things down (Box 3.3). A decrease in insulin allows K^+ to leave the cells and enter the serum, resulting in an initial increase in K^+ levels.

Box 3.3 Actions of Insulin

Promotes	Inhibits
Glycogen synthesis in muscle and liver	Glucagon
Peripheral use of glucose by muscle	Lipolysis of triglycerides in adipose tissue
Uptake of amino acids by muscle and liver	Mobilization of stored fatty acids
Protein synthesis (builds amino acids to proteins)	Proteolysis
Synthesis of free fatty acids from glucose	Hepatic glucose production
Conversion of free fatty acids to triglycerides	Fatty acid oxidation
Movement of extracellular K^+, PO_4^+, Mg^+ into cells	

■ *As the glucose levels increase in both DKA and HHNS, what happens to the serum osmolality levels?*

■ **Elevate**

Glucose is a component of serum osmolality. Hyperglycemia increases osmolality in a progressive manner. Every 100 mg/dL increase in glucose will increase serum osmolality by 5.5 mOsm/kg. The increases in osmolality causes fluid shifts from the intracellular to extracellular spaces, resulting in cellular dehydration.

> ❯ HINT
>
> Fluid resuscitation includes administering "free water" after vascular resuscitation to replace the cellular losses. Free water losses are typically about 6 L.

■ *What is the primary cause of hypovolemia in DKA and HHNS patients?*

■ **Hyperglycemic osmotic diuresis**

Hyperglycemia stimulates the renal excretion of glucose when it exceeds the resorptive capacity of the proximal tubules. Glycosuria occurs with serum glucose levels of 170 to 200 mg/dL. Osmotic diuresis causes hypovolemia and primary losses of Na^+, Cl^-, K^+, Ca^{++}, PO_4^+, and Mg^+.

> ❯ HINT
>
> Even though the initial K^+ values do not reflect the extent of potassium deficit, there is an overall depletion of K^+. Potassium losses average 400 to 600 mEq/L, which is a combined loss of intracellular and extracellular K^+ (Figure 3.1).

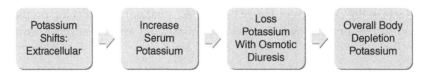

FIGURE 3.1 Effects of potassium on DKA and HHNS.

> ❯ HINT
> Patients with initial hypokalemia have a severe depletion and require cardiac monitoring for arrhythmias.

■ *What causes the increase in ketones in patients with DKA?*

■ **Lipolysis**

The breakdown of adipose tissue (lipolysis) to free fatty acids results in oxidation by the ketogenic pathway to ketone bodies (β-hydroxybutyrate and acetoacetate). Ketones uncontrolled by the insulin feedback loop will result in ketonemia and ketoacidosis. Ketones are excreted by kidneys (ketonuria) and neutralized by bicarbonate, causing a greater metabolic acidosis. HHNS results in a decrease in insulin, causing inadequate utilization of glucose but patients with this syndrome may make enough insulin to prevent lipolysis and control the production of ketone bodies.

> ❯ HINT
> Remember, both DKA and HHNS have hyperglycemia and hyperosmolality, but only DKA develops elevated ketones with the development of ketoacidosis.

■ *What is the primary compensatory mechanism for ketoacidosis?*

■ **Kussmaul's respiration**

The primary compensatory mechanism for ketoacidosis is Kussmaul's respiration. Increased minute ventilation (respiratory rate and depth of ventilation) will "blow off" carbon dioxide, which decreases ketones through the respiratory tract. A DKA patient's breath develops a fruity or musty odor because of the ketones (acetone breath).

SYMPTOMS/ASSESSMENT

■ *What are the classical "Ps" that patients with both DKA and HHNS may present with in their recent history?*

■ **Polyuria and polydipsia**

Both DKA and HHNS develop a hyperosmolar state and osmotic diuresis resulting in increased urine output (polyuria) and dehydration.

■ *What is the triad of symptoms of DKA?*

■ **Hyperglycemia, acidosis, and ketonemia**

Both DKA and HHNS result in hyperglycemia and hyperosmolar states, but only DKA presents with elevated ketones and metabolic acidosis caused by the ketones.

■ *Which is more likely to present in a coma: DKA or HHNS?*
■ **HHNS**

The level of consciousness (LOC) can range from being alert to a decrease in LOC or coma. HHNS patients are more likely to develop a decrease in LOC or progress to a coma (Box 3.4).

Box 3.4 Symptoms of DKA Compared to HHNS

DKA	HHNS
Polyuria, polydipsia	Polyuria, polydipsia
Abdominal pain	Dehydration
Nausea and vomiting	Decreased level of consciousness or coma
Anorexia	Normal ventilation
Hypotension (vasodilation)	
Tachycardia	
Dehydration	
Hypothermia	
Decreased level of consciousness	
Kussmaul's respiration	
Acetone breath	
Ketonemia, ketonuria	

DIAGNOSIS

■ *What level of serum bicarbonate meets the criteria for DKA?*
■ **Less than 18 mEq/L**

The American Diabetes Association (ADA) has set criteria to define DKA. These include acidosis with a serum bicarbonate level of less than 18 mEq/L (Box 3.5).

Box 3.5 ADA Criteria for DKA

Blood glucose > 250 mg/dL	Anion gap > 10
pH < 7.30	Ketone presence in serum
Bicarbonate < 18 mEq/L	

■ *Which patient is more likely to have a higher glucose level: one with DKA or HHNS?*
■ **HHNS**

The higher serum glucose concentration is due to underrecognition of the hyperglycemia because of lack of ketones. Serum glucose can get extremely high before the person becomes symptomatic, which usually presents as a decrease in LOC. HHNS can be diagnosed with a blood glucose level greater than 600 mg/dL.

> ### ❯ HINT
> Remember that ketones are what causes the patient to feel "bad."

■ *What is a normal anion gap?*

■ **Less than 10 mEq/L**

DKA develops a high-anion gap metabolic acidosis (> 10 mEq/L). To calculate, subtract major anions from the cations. Omission of K^+ in the daily calculation is acceptable clinically because the number is so low that it has little effect on clinical decisions (Box 3.6).

> ### ❯ HINT
> Ketoacids are unmeasured anions and therefore will elevate the anion gap.

Box 3.6 Calculation of Normal Anion Gap

$$(Na^+) - (Cl + CO_2)$$

■ *Why is the initial serum potassium normal to high when the overall body potassium is depleted?*

■ **Potassium shifts**

Despite the initial potassium level being normal to elevated, the overall body potassium is depleted. Potassium continually shifts from the intracellular to the extracellular space due to lack of insulin, acidosis, and hyperosmolality. When fluids and insulin are initiated, potassium concentrations may fall quickly because of shifts back into the cells resulting in hypokalemia and arrhythmias. During fluid resuscitation, serum potassium should be measured frequently (minimum of every 4 hours).

> ### ❯ HINT
> Presence of hypokalemia initially is a significant finding and requires potassium replacement prior to insulin replacement.

■ *In hyperglycemic emergencies (DKA and HHNS), is the patient hypernatremic or hyponatremic?*

■ **Hyponatremic**

Hyponatremia is usually associated with hypo-osmolality. Severe hyperglycemia causes hyperosmolality with concurrent hyponatremia (called translocational hyponatremia). The altered Na^+ level does not reflect the change in total body water (TBW). The hyperosmolar state (due to the added glucose) causes fluid shift from the intracellular space to the extracellular space. Sodium and chloride are severely lost during osmotic diuresis in an attempt to maintain normal osmolality.

> **HINT**
The hint in the question will be hyponatremia in the presence of hemoconcentration.

Correcting the sodium level is recommended when replacing fluid and sodium during the management of hyperglycemia (Box 3.7).

Box 3.7 Corrected Serum Sodium Calculation

For each 100 mg/dL of glucose over 100 mg/dL, add 1.6 mEq to Na^+ value

■ ***The depletion of which three electrolytes is usually masked by initial hemoconcentration?***

■ **Phosphorous, calcium, and magnesium**

The hemoconcentration that occurs with hyperglycemic, hyperosmolar serum of diabetic emergencies masks the depletion of electrolytes. Once hypovolemia is corrected, the depletion becomes apparent (Boxes 3.8 and 3.9).

> **HINT**
Initial lab results may appear to have normal electrolytes. Frequent metabolic profiles are required during fluid and insulin replacement.

Box 3.8 Laboratory Values for DKA

Leukocytosis (hemoconcentration)	Urine ketones positive
Plasma glucose > 250 mg/dL (typically between 250 and 800 mg/dL)	Increased hematocrit (hemoconcentrated)
Serum osmolality elevated but usually < 320	Hyponatremia
Glycosuria	Elevated amylase and lipase
Metabolic acidosis pH < 7.30	Hypophosphatemia
Low bicarbonate < 18 mEq/L	Hypocalcemia
Anion gap elevated > 10 mEq/L	Hypomagnesemia
Positive serum ketones > 5 mEq/L	

Box 3.9 Laboratory Values for HHNS

Leukocytosis (hemoconcentration)	Slight elevation in urine ketones
Anion gap normal to variable (due to lactic acidosis)	Increased hematocrit (hemoconcentrated)
Plasma glucose > 600 mg/dL (typically between 900 and 1100)	Hyponatremia
	Hypophosphatemia
Serum osmolality ≥ 320	Hypocalcemia
Glycosuria	Hypomagnesemia
Normal pH (unless lactic acidosis)	
Normal anion gap	

■ ***What laboratory test can be used to determine whether the DKA is a result of an acute process or progressive, undiagnosed diabetes?***

■ **Hemoglobin $A1_c$ test**

The hemoglobin $A1_C$ test measures the percentage of hemoglobin to which glucose molecules have become attached (glycosylated). As plasma glucose levels rise, more hemoglobin molecules become glycosylated. Red blood cells (RBCs) are replaced after about 4 months so the amount of glycosylated hemoglobin at any one time reflects the average plasma glucose level over the last 2 to 3 months. Normal levels of plasma glucose produce an $A1_C$ value of about 5% or less.

> **HINT**
> A 1% change in an $A1_C$ value reflects a change of about 30 mg/dL in average plasma glucose.

MANAGEMENT

■ *Which intravenous (IV) fluid is recommended initially to resuscitate patients with DKA and HHNS?*

■ **Normal saline (0.9% NaCl)**

The initial resuscitation of fluid is aimed at replacing the intravascular losses and restoring renal perfusion. Normal saline may be infused at a rate of 1 L/hr in the first 1 to 2 hours and adjusted to 15 to 20 mL/kg over the first several hours. About 50% of the fluid deficit should be replaced within the first 8 to 12 hours and the remaining fluid within the following 12 to 16 hours, as tolerated (Box 3.10).

> **HINT**
> Fluid replacement must be done with caution in patients with renal or cardiac impairment and requires close monitoring. Serum glucose levels will begin to decrease with volume replacement alone.

Box 3.10 Average Fluid Deficit

DKA	HHNS
5–9 L	9–12 L

■ *What value should be used to determine when to administer 0.45% sodium chloride (NaCl) versus 0.9% NaCl after the initial fluid replacement?*

■ **Corrected serum sodium**

After initial fluid replacement with 0.9% sodium chloride, corrected sodium is used to guide the type of fluid in the remaining resuscitation. If the corrected sodium is normal or elevated, 0.45% NaCl is recommended. If it is low, then 0.9% NaCl is continued.

> **HINT**
> Note 0.45% NaCl is "free water," which is used to replace extravascular fluid losses (Figure 3.2).

■ *At what rate should glucose be lowered per hour?*

■ **Between 50 and 75 mg/dL**

A low-dose continuous infusion of regular insulin is administered with the goal of decreasing blood glucose levels by 50 to 75 mg/dL/hr. The rate of insulin infusion can be started at a dose of 0.1 U/kg/hr and is adjusted to maintain this steady rate of decline in glucose levels. An initial bolus of insulin may be administered prior to the initiation of the infusion.

> **HINT**
> Do not bring the blood glucose levels down too rapidly. A blood glucose level of 600 mg/dL may require 8 hours to lower.

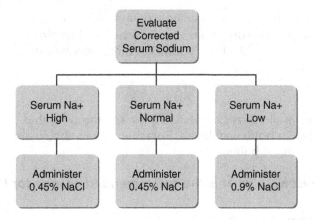

FIGURE 3.2 Guide for determining type of intravenous fluids.

■ ***What level of blood glucose would indicate the need to add glucose into the infusion?***
■ **250 to 300 mg/dL**

When the serum glucose reaches 250 mg/dL in DKA and 250 to 300 mg/dL in HHNS, the insulin infusion may be decreased and glucose may be added to the IV fluids to prevent hypoglycemia until acidosis in DKA is resolved. This is done to avoid severe hypoglycemia as a result of fluid resuscitation and insulin administration. Intravenous administration of serum glucose is recommended unless the DKA is considered to be mild, in which case it may be administered subcutaneously.

> **HINT**
> Insulin and glucose infusion may be continued in HHNS until an increase in mental awareness is achieved.

■ ***What is the primary treatment of ketoacidosis in DKA?***
■ **Insulin therapy**

Insulin is the primary treatment of ketoacidosis. Sodium bicarbonate is not recommended unless the pH remains less than 7.0 after initial fluid replacement. The correction of ketones usually takes longer than glucose so the insulin infusion will continue until the metabolic acidosis and anion gap are normalized. Venous pH may also be monitored frequently to evaluate for continued or improving acidosis.

> ❯ HINT
> Adding glucose to the IV fluids will prevent hypoglycemia during correction of ketones.

- **What potassium levels must be established before insulin may be administered?**
- **Greater than 3.3 mEq/L**

Insulin administration should be delayed until potassium levels are greater than 3.3 mEq/L to prevent complications of arrhythmias, cardiac arrest, and respiratory weakness. Adding 20 to 30 mEq of potassium to the liter IV infusion fluids may be sufficient to maintain normal potassium levels.

> ❯ HINT
> Remember, insulin drives potassium back into the cells, thus causing a drop in serum potassium levels. Potassium levels should also be monitored every 4 hours.

- **Once DKA is resolved, what is the recommended change for the insulin routine?**
- **Initiate subcutaneous route**

Once DKA has resolved, continue IV infusion of insulin and supplement with subcutaneous regular insulin as needed every 4 hours. Once the patient starts taking food by mouth, changing the insulin regimen to intermediate or long-acting insulin in addition to short-acting insulin may be indicated. Continuing the IV infusion for several hours after subcutaneous injections have been initiated is important to continue to maintain adequate plasma insulin levels (Box 3.11).

> ❯ HINT
> Abrupt discontinuation of intravenous insulin may result in rebound hyperglycemia because of erratic absorption through the subcutaneous route.

Box 3.11 Criteria for Resolution of DKA

Glucose < 200 mg/dL
Bicarbonate > 18 mEq/L
Venous pH > 7.3

COMPLICATIONS

- **If the osmolality decreases too rapidly, what life-threatening complication can occur?**
- **Cerebral edema**

Correction of osmolality by reducing blood glucose and sodium that is too rapid quickly results in interstitial fluid shifts. Cerebral edema is a rare complication but is usually fatal. Neurological deterioration may be rapid, with a decrease in LOC, pupillary changes, and seizures.

> **HINT**
> Frequent glucose monitoring is needed to prevent rapid reduction of blood glucose and potentially fatal complications.

■ *What is the most common complication of DKA and HHNS?*
■ **Hypoglycemia**

The most common complication of DKA and HHNS is hypoglycemia from overzealous treatment with insulin and not adding glucose into the fluids during resuscitation.

> **HINT**
> Remember, glucose needs to be added to the fluids when the blood glucose reaches 250 to 300 mg/dL to avoid hypoglycemia.

■ *Use of 0.9% NaCl in fluid resuscitation of patients with DKA/HHNS may cause what complication?*
■ **Hyperchloremic acidosis**

Use of large amounts of 0.9% NaCl and electrolyte replacements can result in hyperchloremic acidosis. Chloride replaces ketoanions lost as sodium and potassium salts during osmotic diuresis, resulting in transient hyperchloremic acidosis (Box 3.12).

> **HINT**
> Hyperchloremic acidosis is a nonanion gap metabolic acidosis compared to ketoacidosis, which produces an anion gap.

Box 3.12 Complications of DKA/HHNS

Hypoglycemia	Refractory shock
Rebound hyperglycemia	Acute respiratory distress syndrome (ARDS)
Cerebral edema	Electrolyte abnormalities
Hypokalemia	Seizures
Arrhythmias	Mucormyosis
Acute kidney injury	Hyperchloremic acidosis

DIABETES INSIPIDUS/SYNDROME OF INAPPROPRIATE ANTIDIURETIC HORMONE/CEREBRAL SALT WASTING SYNDROME

■ *Do patients with SIADH have an increase or a decrease in the antidiuretic hormone (ADH)?*

■ **Increase**

Patients with SIADH have too much ADH and will conserve water. DI patients do not have enough ADH and will lose water. The negative feedback that normally controls the ADH release does not function, and water imbalances occur (Box 3.13).

Box 3.13 Water Imbalances

DI	Syndrome of Inappropriate ADH	CSWS
Not enough ADH	Too much ADH	No effect on ADH

■ *Overall, what type of patient is most likely to develop water abnormalities such as DI, SIADH, or CSWS?*

■ **A patient with a neurological disorder**

Neurological disorders are most likely to involve water abnormalities because of abnormal levels of ADH. This disorder is a neuroendocrine abnormality that involves the hypothalamic–pituitary axis. DI can be neurogenic or nephrogenic. In nephrogenic DI, ADH is produced and released into the circulation normally, but the kidneys do not respond appropriately to the ADH by conserving water (Boxes 3.14 and 3.15).

> ❯ **HINT**
>
> DI occurring in neurological patients is commonly called central neurogenic DI. In oat cell carcinoma, there is an ectopic production of ADH from the malignant tissue.

Box 3.14 Common Causes of DI/SIADH/CSWS

Traumatic brain injury	Intracranial hypertension
Postcraniotomy	Subarachnoid hemorrhage
Primary brain tumors	Ischemic strokes
Meningitis	Hemorrhagic strokes

Box 3.15 Nonneurological Causes of SIADH

Bronchogenic carcinoma	Lung abscess
Oat cell carcinoma of lungs	Positive pressure ventilation
Pneumonia	Certain medications

■ *Which of the ADH abnormalities occurs following brain death?*

■ **DI**

ADH is synthesized, stored, and released from the brain. Following brain death, the brain does not produce or release ADH and will develop DI.

PATHOPHYSIOLOGY

■ *What area of the brain is responsible for the production of ADH?*

■ **Hypothalamus**

The hypothalamus synthesizes ADH, which is then stored in the posterior pituitary in the brain and is responsible for water balance. ADH works on the distal convoluted tubules and collecting ducts in the kidneys. ADH is also called vasopressin and increases the reabsorption of water.

> ❯ HINT
>
> Thinking of "anti" can get confusing when taking the test so when you read ADH, think "water-saving hormone" (Figure 3.3).

■ *What is the primary role of ADH in the body?*

■ **Maintain osmolality and blood volume**

ADH is controlled by osmoreceptors and baroreceptors. Osmoreceptors are sensitive to changes in serum osmolality, and baroreceptors are affected by changes in pressure or blood volume. For example, as the osmolality increases, ADH is released to conserve water and lower the osmolality (Box 3.16).

Box 3.16 ADH Regulation

Increases ADH Release	Decreases ADH Release
Increases serum osmolality	Decreases serum osmolality
Decreases circulating blood volume	Increases circulating blood volume
Hypotension	Hypertension

> ❯ HINT
>
> Positive pressure ventilation can also stimulate the release of ADH and increase water reabsorption in ventilated patients.

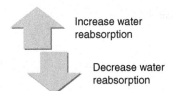

Increase water reabsorption

Decrease water reabsorption

FIGURE 3.3 Effects of the ADH.

■ *What is the cause of hyponatremia in CSWS?*

■ **Renal loss of Na⁺**

The hyponatremia of CSWS is a true loss of sodium through the renal system. There is a loss of sodium and fluid, resulting in hypovolemia (volume-contracted) and hyponatremia. It is not associated with an abnormal ADH level as are SIADH or DI.

> ❯ HINT
>
> SIADH is dilutional hyponatremia whereas CSWS constitutes a true loss of Na⁺.

SYMPTOMS/ASSESSMENT

■ *What is the initial clinical sign of DI?*

■ **Diuresis**

DI is associated with an abnormally large urine output, typically more than 250 mL/hr. If the patient is awake and able to take oral fluids, he will have an increase in thirst and fluid intake (polydipsia). This large diuresis will lead to hypovolemia and hemoconcentration.

> ❯ HINT
>
> Both DI and diuresis begin with a "D." So, remember DI causes diuresis.

■ *Which of the three water abnormality disorders (DI, SIADH, or CSWS) produces hypernatremia?*

■ **DI**

In DI, there is a loss of fluid that results in total body depletion of water, causing hemoconcentration. The total body sodium is normal but the serum sodium will be increased due to the hemoconcentration. The other two water abnormalities, SIADH and CSWS, result in hyponatremia.

■ *In DI, is the urine diluted or concentrated?*

■ **Diluted**

Because of high urine output and the kidneys' inability to conserve water, the urine is diluted. This is measured by urine osmolality and urine specific gravity.

> ❯ HINT
>
> Remember the 3Ds: DI, diuresis, and diluted urine (Box 3.17).

Box 3.17 Symptoms of DI

Polyuria	Decreased urine osmolality
Polydipsia	Decreased urine specific gravity
Thirst	Low urine sodium
Hypernatremia	Weight loss (prolonged or chronic)
Hypokalemia	Signs of dehydration
Hypomagnesium	Hypotension
Increased serum osmolality	Tachycardia

■ *What is typically the first sign of SIADH?*

■ **Hyponatremia**

In SIADH, the abnormally high levels of ADH cause renal reabsorption and retention of water. This water retention results in hemodilution and lowers the serum sodium levels. TBW increases but total body sodium is normal. This results in a dilution of hyponatremia. A decrease in urine output occurs but may not be initially recognized as SIADH.

> ❯ HINT
>
> The 24-hour intake/output records will show a positive fluid balance (Box 3.18).

Box 3.18 SIADH Symptoms

Decreased urine output (400–500 mL/ 24 hours)	Increased urine specific gravity
	Increased urine sodium
Hyponatremia	Generalized weight gain
Decreased serum osmolality	
Increased urine osmolality	

■ *SIADH patients are at risk for neurological complications, including altered mentation and seizures. Which electrolyte abnormality causes this complication?*

■ **Hyponatremia**

Hyponatremia and fluid overload (water intoxication) can cause neurological complications (Box 3.19).

Box 3.19 Symptoms of Hyponatremia and Water Intoxication

Headache	Confusion
Nausea and vomiting	Lethargy progresses to coma
Muscle twitching	Seizures
Fatigue	

■ *Does volume overload or volume depletion cause the clinical signs of CSWS?*
■ **Volume depletion**

In CSWS, there is a loss of sodium and water by the kidneys. This leads to a hypovolemic state as well as hyponatremia. The symptoms of CSWS are due to this combination (Box 3.20).

Box 3.20 Symptoms of CSWS

Orthostatic hypotension	Dry mucus membranes
Tachycardia	Lethargy
Dehydration	Decreased level of consciousness
Weight loss	Seizures

> **〉 HINT**
> The primary difference between SIADH and CSWS is fluid status.

DIAGNOSIS

See Boxes 3.21 and 3.22.

Box 3.21 Diagnosis of DI

Urine output > 250 mL/hr	Serum Na$^+$ > 145 mEq/L
Urine specific gravity < 1.005	Urine Na$^+$ normal to low (< 20 mEq/L)
Urine osmolality < 300 mOsm/kg	Blood urea nitrogen (BUN) is elevated
Serum osmolality > 295 mOsm/L	

Box 3.22 Diagnosis of SIADH

Urine output < 20–30 mL/hr	Serum osmolality < 275 mOsm/L
Urine sodium > 25 mEq/L	Serum Na$^+$ < 135 mEq/L
Urine osmolality > the serum osmolality	Urine Na$^+$ high (> 25 mEq/L)

> **〉 HINT**
> Urine osmolality is greater than serum osmolality (Box 3.23).

Box 3.23 Diagnosis of CSWS

Hyponatremia	Increased blood urea nitrogen (BUN)
Serum osmolality < 275 mOsm/L	Increased hematocrit
Elevated urine osmolality	Increased urine specific gravity
Urine sodium > 25 mEq/L	

MANAGEMENT

■ *What is the primary fluid management issue when treating a patient with DI?*
■ **Fluid replacement**

An awake and alert patient taking oral fluids may increase intake to replace the losses. Patients with impaired mental status or those unable to receive oral fluids will need IV fluids to replace these losses. The volume and rate of IV fluid replacement can be calculated using the milliliter per milliliter replacement rule or by calculating the free water deficit. The mL/mL replacement rule uses the previous hour's urine output to determine the next hour's rate of infusion. Replace IV fluid mL/mL of urine loss plus maintenance fluid. For example, if maintenance fluid was at 60 mL/hr and at 10:00, the urine output was 300 mL; at 11:00 IV fluid rate should be 300 mL plus 60 for a total of 360 mL/hr. If water loss occurs over a greater time period, then replacement may need to be corrected at a slower rate. The calculation of the free water deficit determines the total amount to be replaced. The first half of the calculated deficit is replaced within the first 12 hours and the second half is replaced over the next 24 to 48 hours (Box 3.24).

Box 3.24 Free Water Deficit Calculation

$[0.6 \times \text{Total body weight}] \times [(\text{Measured } [Na^+]/140) - 1]$

■ *What is the medical management of DI?*
■ **Replace ADH**

In DI, the patient does not have enough of ADH, so replacement is the primary medical management. Exogenous replacement of ADH can be with either desmopressin (DDAVP) or vasopressin (aqueous Pitressin).

■ *What is the fluid management recommended for SIADH?*
■ **Fluid restrictions**

The treatment of SIADH is to restrict fluids because the underlying cause of the hyponatremia is volume overload (dilutional). Diuretics may also be used in combination with the fluid restrictions. In the case of symptomatic hyponatremia, therapy may include replacing the sodium carefully with a hypertonic 3% NaCl. Chronic management of SIADH includes medications to either suppress ADH activity (demeclocycline hydrochloride) or to inhibit renal response to ADH (lithium carbonate).

> ❯ **HINT**
> Fluid restrictions and diuresis are usually enough when managing SIADH acutely.

■ *What is the fluid recommendation to manage CSWS?*
■ **Administer fluids**

Management of CSWS requires fluid replacement because of renal losses of fluid. Replacement fluid is 0.9% NaCl with the addition of hypertonic 3% NaCl to correct the hyponatremia. Treatment may also include fludrocortisone acetate to increase absorption of sodium from the renal tubules.

> **HINT**
> Fluid management of CSWS is opposite to that of SIADH.

■ *What is a complication of administering hypertonic 3% NaCl too rapidly?*
■ **Central pontine myelinolysis (CPM)**

The administration of a hypertonic solution too fast can cause a rapid shift in serum osmolality to a hyperosmolar state. This results in irreversible demyelination of the neurons in the brain, particularly in the pons (Box 3.25).

Box 3.25 Symptoms of CPM

Confusion	Quadriplegia
Dysarthria	Pseudobulbar palsy
Gaze disturbances	

■ *What is the recommended correction of sodium in a 24-hour period?*
■ **10 mEq/L in 24 hours**

To prevent this complication, Na^+ should not be corrected at a rate exceeding 1.3 mEq/L/hour with a total correction of no more than 10 mEq/L in 24 hours. Assure serum sodium levels are obtained every 4 to 6 hours depending on whether the patient is symptomatic or not.

> **HINT**
> Remember, give 3% NaCl in small amounts very slowly to correct
> sodium over a longer time (Box 3.26).

Box 3.26 Differentiating SIADH from CSWS

CSWS	SIADH
Serum sodium < 135 mEq/L	Serum sodium < 135 mEq/L
Decreased extracellular fluid volume	Increased extracellular fluid volume
Increased hematocrit (hct)	Normal hct
Increased albumin levels	Normal albumin levels
Normal or Increased K^+	Normal K^+
Normal or decreased plasma uric acid	Decreased plasma uric acid
Increased BUN/creatinine	Decreased BUN
Signs of dehydration	Urine Na^+ > 25 mEq/L
	Serum osmolality < 280 mOsm/kg
	Urine osmolality > serum osmolality
	Concentrated urine
	Signs of hypervolemia

COMPLICATIONS

See Box 3.27.

Box 3.27 Complications of DI/SIADH/CSWS

Hypo- or hypernatremia	Central pontine myelinolysis
Volume overload or dehydration	Acute renal failure

BIBLIOGRAPHY

John, C., & Day, M. (2012). Central neurogenic diabetes insipidus, syndrome of inappropriate secretion of antidiuretic hormone and cerebral salt wasting syndrome in traumatic brain injured patients. *Critical Care Nurse, 32,* e1–e7.

Kitabchi, A. E., Umpierrez, G. E., Murphy, M. B., Barrett, E. J., Kreisberg, R. A., Malone, J. I., Wall, B. M., & American Diabetes Association. (2004). Hyperglycemic crises in diabetes. *Diabetes Care, 27*(Suppl. 1), S94–S102.

Questions

1. Which of the following interventions is considered to be the first-line treatment in a patient with a hyperglycemic emergency?

   A. Insulin replacement
   B. Fluid administration
   C. Administer sodium bicarbonate
   D. Replace magnesium losses

2. A patient presents with an altered LOC and blood glucose level of 650 mg/dL. The following lab values were obtained on admission:

   K^+ 3.1
   Na^+ 126
   Mg^+ 3.0
   PO_4^+ 4.0

   Based on the above findings, which of the following interventions should be the initial treatment?

   A. Administer bolus dose of insulin
   B. Initiate continuous low-dose infusion of insulin
   C. Bolus 1/L IV fluids over 30 minutes
   D. Administer potassium IV

3. Which of the following disorders can cause hypernatremia?

   A. DI
   B. SIADH
   C. CSWS
   D. Diabetes mellitus (DM)

4. During treatment of stress-induced hyperglycemia, what is the most significant complication of strict glycemic control of 80 to 110 mg/dL?

   A. Cerebral edema
   B. Hypoglycemia
   C. Hyponatremia
   D. Hyperkalemia

5. What is the clinical finding most commonly associated with hypoglycemia in critically ill patients?

   A. Paroxysmal supraventricular tachycardia (SVT)
   B. Muscle twitching
   C. Fatigue
   D. Cognitive impairment

6. Which of the following statements best explains the lack of ketoacidosis in HHNS?

A. Become sicker faster than DKA patients and will seek medical assistance before ketones are produced

B. Higher osmolality of HHNS blocks fatty acid oxidation preventing ketone production

C. HHNS patients have the presence of small amounts of insulin, which prevents ketone production

D. The kidneys retain a greater amount of bicarbonate in HHNS patients to correct the metabolic acidosis

7. A 46-year-old male is admitted for a subarachnoid hemorrhage and aneurysm clipping. Three days after admission, the following labs and vital signs are obtained:

Blood pressure (BP) 124/64
Heart rate (HR) 72
Respiratory rate (RR) 16
Urine output (UO) 75 to 100 cc/hr
Na^+ 124 mEq/L
K^+ 3.6
Glucose 145 mg/dL
Serum osmolality 280 mEq/L
Urine Na^+ 35 mmol/L

Which of the following is the most likely cause for the hyponatremia?

A. DI
B. SIADH
C. CSWS
D. DM

8. A patient is diagnosed with CSWS following a traumatic brain injury. His current sodium level is 120 mEq/L. The physician has ordered 3% NaCl to be administered at a rate of 30 mL/hr and sodium levels checked every 4 hours. Which of the following is a complication of administering hypertonic normal saline?

A. Cerebral edema
B. Central pontine myelinolysis (CPM)
C. Abdominal compartment syndrome (ACS)
D. Acute respiratory distress syndrome (ARDS)

9. A patient with traumatic brain injury voided 350 mL/hr in the previous hour. Which of the following would be the most likely result of the sudden diuresis?

A. Over-use of Lasix
B. Volume overload
C. DM
D. DI

10. Which of the following laboratory findings would indicate a diuresis following a brain tumor resection as a result of DI?

    A. Low serum osmolality

    B. Low urine osmolality

    C. Hyponatremia

    D. High urine specific gravity

Hematology/Immunology System Review

In this chapter, you will review:

- Coagulopathies
- Heparin-induced thrombocytopenia (HIT)
- Idiopathic thrombocytopenia purpura (ITP)
- Blood transfusion monitoring

COAGULOPATHIES

DISSEMINATED INTRAVASCULAR COAGULATION

- *What type of coagulopathy is disseminated intravascular coagulation (DIC)?*
- **Consumptive**

DIC is an acquired syndrome characterized by intravascular activation of coagulation factors. It can originate from and cause damage to microvasculature, which, if sufficiently severe, can cause organ dysfunction and bleeding. The bleeding is caused by the consumption of the clotting factors as well as the activation of the fibrinolytic system. DIC is called a consumptive coagulopathy.

> **HINT**
> DIC begins as a clotting problem but manifests itself as a bleeding disorder.

- *What is the most common cause of death in DIC patients?*
- **Multisystem organ failure**

Occlusion in the microcirculation by the clots may manifest as multisystem organ failure. The deposits of fibrin and clots in the microcirculation result in ischemia to organs, skin, and limbs.

Pathophysiology

■ *What is the material that increases clotting in microcirculation and activates the coagulation system?*

■ **Procoagulants**

Procoagulants are factors that can increase clotting in microcirculation and initiate the release of tissue factor. Procoagulants include bacterial toxins, free hemoglobin, fragments of cancer or placental tissue, acidosis, and the release of tissue factor into the blood. Tissue factor is found on the surface of endothelial cells, macrophages, and monocytes and are not usually in contact with general circulation but can be exposed after vascular damage. Once activated, it binds to coagulation factors, which then trigger the extrinsic pathway (via factor VII) and then the intrinsic pathway (initially via XII).

> ❯ **HINT**
> The most common cause of DIC is bacteremia, either gram negative or gram positive (Box 4.1).

Box 4.1 Clinical Conditions Associated With DIC

Sepsis and septic shock	Snake bites
Traumatic injuries/crush injuries	Abruptio placentae
Hypoxia	Amniotic fluid embolism
Acidosis	Intrauterine fetal demise
Burns	Eclampsia
Transplant rejections	Recreational drugs
Transfusion reactions	Cancerous tumors
Hemorrhagic pancreatitis	Rocky Mountain spotted fever

■ *What is the normal process for fibrinolysis following clot formation?*

■ **Plasminogen converts to plasmin**

Plasminogen circulates in an inactive form in the blood. Following fibrin clot formation, plasminogen is activated and converts to plasmin, a proteolytic enzyme. Plasmin lysis or dissolves the fibrin to restore blood flow through the vessel. In DIC, the process of clot formation and degradation is accelerated, and the complete process leads to consumption of circulating clotting factors. In DIC, there is suppression of the fibrinolysis system due to elevated plasminogen activator inhibitor-1.

■ *What is the byproduct of a fibrin clot?*

■ **Fibrin degradation products (FDPs)**

Following fibrinolysis, the byproducts of fibrin breakdown are FDPs. As the body forms clots and breaks the clots down, it releases more FDPs, which work as an anticoagulant to prevent further clot formation. Other causes of anticoagulation effects in DIC include a reduction in antithrombin III and protein C.

> **HINT**
D-dimer test is used to measure FDPs.

Symptoms/Assessment

■ *What is the most obvious sign of DIC?*

■ **Bleeding**

Overt bleeding may occur from old intravenous (IV) puncture sites or present as bruising, purpura, ecchymosis, and expanding hematoma. Bleeding can occur from mucous membranes, hemoptysis, hematuria, or the intracranial and gastrointestinal tracts.

■ *What is the systemic finding of microvascular occlusion and organ dysfunction in DIC?*

■ **Elevated serum lactate levels**

The microvascular occlusion that occurs in DIC results in the conversion of aerobic to anaerobic metabolism with the elevation of lactate levels and metabolic acidosis. Respiratory rates may increase to buffer the increase in H^+ ions by lowering the $PaCO_2$ levels.

Diagnosis

■ *Which laboratory finding distinguishes a diagnosis of DIC?*

■ **Elevated D-dimer**

The D-dimer measures FDPs. The FDPs are byproducts of fibrin and will elevate when fibrin clots are formed and then lysed. A coagulopathy that does not clot first will not elevate FDPs. Multiple coagulopathies will produce elevated clotting times and thrombocytopenia, but DIC is the primary coagulopathy that forms clots and then consumes the clotting factors thereby in turn leading to bleeding complications.

> **HINT**
Elevated D-dimer is not specific to DIC. There are many causes of elevated FDPs but D-dimer assists with the differential diagnosis in DIC (Box 4.2). The decreasing platelet count is due to consumption of the platelets in an attempt to form clots.

Box 4.2 Laboratory Findings of DIC

Prolonged prothrombin time (PT) and partial thromboplastin time (PTT)	Thrombocytopenia
Decreased fibrinogen levels	Decreased antithrombin III
Increased D-dimer	

Management

■ *What is the most accepted intervention in managing patients with DIC?*
■ **Treat the underlying cause**

The most accepted treatment of DIC is to identify the underlying cause and to treat or remove it. DIC is an acquired syndrome caused by another underlying disease process that works as a procoagulant. The best method of treating DIC is to remove the procoagulant material.

■ *When would transfusion of red blood cells (RBCs) and components be indicated in a DIC patient?*
■ **Active hemorrhage**

Administration of blood and blood components in DIC patients has been controversial; however, during periods of active bleeding, acute decline in clotting factors, or a deterioration in the clinical status, transfusion therapy is recommended.

> ❯ HINT
> Administering clotting factors while the procoagulant is still active may "fuel the fire" and produce more clots (worsen ischemia) and FDPs (work as anticoagulants).

■ *What blood component may be indicated if fibrinogen levels are below 100 mg/dL and the patient is not responding to fresh frozen plasma (FFP)?*
■ **Cryoprecipitate**

Cryoprecipitation is recommended for symptomatic bleeding patients with fibrinogen levels less than 100 mg/dL. It may be used when the patient does not respond to FFP in elevating fibrinogen levels. The disadvantage is that cryoprecipitate is rich in fibrinogen and can increase FDPs and coagulopathy if the patient is still clotting in the microcirculation.

> ❯ HINT
> FFP is used in bleeding patients with prolonged bleeding times to replace clotting factors and fibrinogen.

■ *When would platelets most likely be transfused?*
■ **Active bleeding patient with platelets less than 50,000**

Platelets may be transfused for symptomatic bleeding patients with platelet count less than 50,000 or less than 10,000 to 20,000 without signs of bleeding.

> ❯ HINT
> Replacement therapy is only recommended if the patient is symptomatic; it is not used to treat laboratory abnormalities only.

- *What is the physiological effect of heparin that in theory may benefit the patient in DIC?*
- Indirect thrombin inhibitor

The administration of heparin or low-molecular-weight heparin (LMWH) in treating DIC remains controversial. In theory, heparin interacts with antithrombin to inactivate factor X, thus preventing conversion of prothrombin to thrombin. This will alter the ability of the clot to become stable.

Complications

- *What are the two primary complications of DIC patients?*
- Bleeding and multisystem organ failure

The consumption of the platelets and clotting factors lead to abnormal bleeding. Clots forming in the microcirculation, due to the release of a procoagulant, cause obstruction and hypoperfusion of organs (Box 4.3).

Box 4.3 Symptoms of Multisystem Organ Failure

Organ Involved	Symptoms
Lungs	PaO_2/FiO_2 ratio < 150, ARDS (acute respiratory distress syndrome)
Kidneys	Elevated creatinine, blood urea nitrogen (BUN), decreased urine output
Liver	Elevated liver enzymes
Brain	Altered level of consciousness
Gastrointestinal tract	Stress-related ulcerations

HEPARIN-INDUCED THROMBOCYTOPENIA (HIT)

- *What is the most common drug-related immune thrombocytopenia?*
- HIT

HIT is a drug-related immune thrombocytopenia. There are two classifications of HIT. HIT type I is a nonimmune reaction to heparin that decreases the platelet count. It is a reversible form of HIT. Type II is a more serious, immune-related form of HIT. HIT with thromboembolic syndrome (HITTS) includes patients who develop thromboembolic complications.

> ❯ HINT
> More patients develop thrombocytopenia alone than thrombocytopenia with thromboembolic complications.

- *Which anticoagulation therapy, unfractionated heparin (UFH) or low molecular weight heparin, has a greater risk of developing HIT?*
- Unfractionated heparin

UFH has a greater incidence of HIT than LMWH. UFH has approximately 2% to 3% risk, whereas LMWH is less than 1%. There is a lower frequency if heparin is used primarily as a flush. HIT occurs more frequently in patients receiving higher doses of heparin than standard prophylaxis doses.

> ❯ HINT
> Once HIT occurs, the patient should not receive either UFH or LMWH.

PATHOPHYSIOLOGY

- ■ *What antigen complex do the antibodies react with to cause platelet aggregation?*
- ■ **Heparin-platelet factor 4 complex**

Antibodies recognize complexes between heparin and platelet factor 4 (PF4). Heparin elicits a platelet-active antibody that specifically interacts with the GP IIb/IIIa receptors on the platelets. Following administration of heparin (antigen), heparin-platelet factor 4 stimulates the platelets and causes them to aggregate.

> ❯ HINT
> Platelet aggregation leads to thrombotic events and thrombocytopenia.

SYMPTOMS/ASSESSMENT

- ■ *What is the most common timing for the presentation of HIT after heparin exposure?*
- ■ **5 to 10 days**

This syndrome usually occurs within 5 to 10 days of heparin therapy. It may be present as early as 24 to 48 hours in patients with previous exposure to heparin within the past 100 days. The first day of immunizing heparin exposure is equal to day 0. Exposure to heparin within the previous 100 days indicates that antibodies may still be circulating and can cause abrupt thrombocytopenia after starting heparin.

- ■ *Which type of onset is the least common for the presentation of HIT?*
- ■ **Delayed onset**

Delayed-onset HIT is uncommon. Symptoms occur 2 weeks after being exposed to heparin. It is typically associated with very high-titer anti-PF4/heparin antibodies and requires a high dose and prolonged alternative anticoagulation to control massive thrombin generation.

DIAGNOSIS

- ■ *What finding is the most common reason for suspicion of HIT?*
- ■ **Decrease in platelet count greater than 50%**

The hallmark sign is a significant decrease in platelet count (> 50%) over a 24-hour period without any other known cause of thrombocytopenia within 5 to 10 days after starting heparin.

> ❯ **HINT**
> Another sign is a thromboembolic event within 5 to 10 days after starting heparin.

■ *Which laboratory test has a high negative predictive value but may be positive in patients without HIT?*

■ **Anti-PF4/heparin antibody**

The anti-PF4/heparin antibody test has a high negative predictive value; if it is negative, the patient has a very low possibility of having HIT. Not all positive anti-PF4/heparin antibodies are pathogenic and elevate due to exposure to heparin. The test is unable to clearly distinguish between pathogenic and nonpathogenic antibodies. Antigen assay (ELISA) is a quantitative test that increases in specificity relative to the magnitude of a positive test.

> ❯ **HINT**
> It is not recommended to routinely screen for the antibodies unless the patient exhibits clinical symptoms (Box 4.4).

Box 4.4 Four Ts Probability Scores

Four Ts	2 Points	1 Point	0 Point
Thrombocytopenia	Platelet count decrease > 50% and platelet nadir ≥ 20,000	Platelet count decrease 30%–50% (>50% decrease resulting from surgery) or platelet nadir 10,000–19,000	Platelet count decrease <30% or platelet nadir <10,000
Timing of platelet count decrease	Clear onset between days 5 and 10 or platelet decrease within 1 day (heparin exposure within 30 days)	Consistent with immunization but unclear history; onset after day 10; < 1 day (heparin exposure 1–3 months ago)	Platelet count decrease < 4 days of recent exposure
Thrombosis or other sequelae	New thrombosis (confirmed); skin necrosis; acute systemic reaction post-IV UFH bolus	Progressive or recurrent thrombosis; non-necrotizing (erythematous) skin lesions; suspected thrombosis not yet proven	None
Other causes of thrombocytopenia	None apparent	Possible	Definite

High probability: 6–8 points (HIT is likely); intermediate probability: 4–5 points (HIT is possible); and low probability: ≤ 3 points (HIT is unlikely)

MANAGEMENT

■ *Once the diagnosis of HIT is established, what is the priority of care?*
■ **Stop heparin administration**

Once this syndrome is suspected or diagnosed, heparin must not be given to the patient because of the potential life-threatening effects. All heparins need to be stopped, including LMWH, heparin catheter flushes, IV, or SC routes of heparin. High cross-reactivity occurs with LMWH once the patient develops the pathogenic antibody to heparin.

> **❯ HINT**
> Recommend placing a heparin allergy in the chart and post a sign at the bedside.

■ *After stopping heparin, what intervention is recommended to prevent thromboembolism complications?*
■ **Administer nonheparin anticoagulation therapy**

Nonheparin anticoagulation should be initiated promptly to limit thrombosis complications. Upon discontinuation of heparin, platelet counts start to recover within 4 days but may take longer than 2 weeks in patients with high-titer HIT antibodies. Heparin is replaced with either a direct thrombin inhibitor (DTI) or fondaparinux (Box 4.5).

> **❯ HINT**
> Remember, there are no antidotes for DTIs.

Box 4.5 Anticoagulants

Drug	Classification	Half-Life	Elimination
Arganova (Argatroban)	Synthetic direct thrombin inhibitor (DTI)	45 min	Liver
Lepirudin (Refludan)	Recombinant bivalent DTI	1.5 hr	Renal
Angiomax (Bivalirudin)	Bivalent DTI	30 min	Renal
Fondaparinux (Arixtra)	Pentasaccharide	17 hr	Renal

■ *What is the laboratory test recommended to monitor a DTI?*
■ **Activated partial thromboplastin time (aPTT)**

Frequent aPTT monitoring is recommended when starting these patients on DTIs. aPTT may underestimate the bleeding time and an ecarin clotting time may be required.

> **❯ HINT**
> Arganova (Argatroban) can erroneously elevate the PT/INR (prothrombin time/international normalized ratio), but it is not accurate for determining bleeding times.

■ *Which anticoagulant is recommended for more long-term management of HIT after alternative anticoagulant is started?*
■ **Warfarin (Coumadin)**

American College of Chest Physician's guidelines recommend warfarin therapy in patients requiring more long-term management to prevent thrombosis. The initial effect of warfarin, however, is a transient procoagulation. It is not recommended to start warfarin therapy in acute HIT as long as thrombocytopenia persists due to the risk of warfarin-induced microthrombosis. Initiate warfarin after the alternative anticoagulation therapy and overlap with the DTIs. Discontinue DTI only after a 5-day overlap and when the platelet count is stable.

> ❯ **HINT**
> Obtain an initial PT/INR as baseline before warfarin is started. After the desired overlap days and the goal INR is reached, withhold DTI for 48 hours and recheck PT/INR.

COMPLICATIONS

■ *What is the most common thromboembolic complication of HIT?*
■ **Venous thromboembolisms (VTEs)**

Approximately 50% to 75% of patients with HIT develop symptomatic thrombosis, which can occur even if platelet count remains greater than 150,000, but usually, the risk of thrombosis correlates with the magnitude of decrease in platelets. The thrombosis may occur 1 to 3 days before thrombocytopenia is recognized. Thromboembolic events are defined as thrombosis during therapy or worsening of thrombosis as confirmed by invasive or noninvasive diagnostic techniques.

> ❯ **HINT**
> Thrombotic events can be venous and/or arterial. This may occur as a single event or multiple thromboses (Boxes 4.6 and 4.7).

Box 4.6 Venous Thrombotic Complications

Venous thromboembolism (VTE)
Axillary vein thrombosis
Renal vein thrombosis
Adrenal vein thrombosis

Box 4.7 Arterial Thrombotic Complications

Limb ischemia/infarction
Mesenteric artery thrombosis
Stroke
Acute coronary syndrome (ACS)

IDIOPATHIC THROMBOCYTOPENIA PURPURA (ITP)

■ *What is the other name for ITP?*
■ **Immune thrombocytopenia**

ITP is an autoimmune disorder characterized by a decrease in platelet count and an increased risk of bleeding. The new term is recommended to emphasize the underlying immune pathophysiology. Primary ITP refers to occurence without the underlying disease process, and secondary ITP refers to ITP associated with other disease processes (Box 4.8).

Box 4.8 Secondary ITP-Associated Disease Processes

Human immunodeficiency virus (HIV)
Hepatitis C virus (HCV)
Lymphoproliferative disorder
Systemic lupus erythematosus

> HINT
ITP is commonly chronic in adult patients (Box 4.9).

Box 4.9 Classification of ITP

Classification	Duration of Findings
Newly diagnosed	< 3 months
Persistent	3–12 months
Chronic	> 12 months

PATHOPHYSIOLOGY

■ *Does ITP involve humoral or cellular immunity?*
■ **Both**

ITP is a complex syndrome that involves both humoral and cellular immunity causing the destruction of the platelets and also a decrease in production. Autoantibodies are developed against the platelet membrane glycoprotein IIb/IIIa (humoral immunity). Patients with ITP also have CD4+ T cells that react to GP IIb/IIIa and produce antiplatelet antibodies (cellular immunity).

> HINT
Antibody-coated platelets are rapidly cleared by the spleen and liver, resulting in a decrease in platelets.

SYMPTOMS/ASSESSMENT

■ *What underlying physiological change causes the clinical findings of ITP?*
■ **Thrombocytopenia**

The clinical features of ITP are due to thrombocytopenia and microvascular bleeding. These signs include petechiae (microvascular hemorrhage) and purpura (bruising). ITP may just present with a low platelet count and no other features of thrombocytopenia (Box 4.10).

Box 4.10 Symptoms of Thrombocytopenia

Petechiae	Gum bleeding
Purpura	Fatigue
Epistaxis	

DIAGNOSIS

■ *What is the primary finding used in the diagnosis of ITP?*
■ **Low platelet count**

ITP is primarily a diagnosis of exclusion. It may or may not be associated with clinical findings of bleeding. Other causes of thrombocytopenia are ruled out before the diagnosis of ITP is made. A peripheral blood smear may be used to assist with the differential diagnosis. In some patients, a bone marrow aspirate may be used if there are abnormalities on blood smear.

■ *What is the most common drug associated with drug-induced thrombocytopenia?*
■ **Heparin**

Other drugs that can cause an acute drop in platelets include antiepileptic agents, sulfonamides, interferon, and quinine. The decrease in platelet count within 5 to 10 days of initiating drug therapy should alert the practitioner of a potential, secondary, drug-induced thrombocytopenia.

■ *What is another cause of thrombocytopenia that causes acute anemia and fever?*
■ **Thrombotic thrombocytopenia purpura (TTP)**

The presence of fragmented RBCs on a peripheral blood smear helps make the differential diagnosis of ITP and TTP. TTP complications include renal failure and neurological involvement.

> **HINT**
Plasmaphoresis is the treatment of choice for TTP.

MEDICAL MANAGEMENT

■ *What platelet level would platelets most likely be administered to prevent bleeding complications of thrombocytopenia?*
■ **30,000**

If the platelets are low, but the patient is asymptomatic, then the patient may not necessarily require platelet transfusion. If the count is less than 30,000, platelets may be administered to prevent spontaneous hemorrhage, which can occur with platelet counts less than 20,000.

■ *What drug therapy is considered the primary treatment for ITP?*

■ **Steroids**

Oral corticosteroids are considered the initial treatment for ITP. This includes oral prednisone or high-dose dexamethasone (Decadron). IV administration of immunoglobulin is recommended in patients who do not respond to steroids or who demonstrate active bleeding. This therapy is typically successful at increasing the platelet count but it may have a transient effect and require multiple infusions. IV immunoglobulins are usually well tolerated but may have significant side effects and the rare complication of anaphylaxis.

> ❯ HINT
>
> Remember ITP is considered to be an autoimmune disorder. Steroids and immunosuppressants are typically first-line treatments for autoimmune disorders (Box 4.11). Secondary ITP is treated by managing the underlying infection or disease process.

Box 4.11 Side Effects of IV Immunoglobulin

Fever	Headache
Chills	Mylagias
Back pain	Arthralgesias (joint pain)

■ *A second-line drug may be given if steroids are ineffective in managing ITP. What is this drug?*

■ **Rituximab (Rituxan)**

Rituximab is a monoclonal antibody that targets B cells responsible for the production of antiplatelet antibodies. Side effects include infusion reactions and a rare complication of progressive multifocal leukoencephalopathy. Other drugs that have been used include thrombopoietin receptor agonists and immunosuppressants such as azathioprine (Imuran).

SURGICAL MANAGEMENT

■ *If patients do not respond to medical management, what surgical procedure may be performed to manage ITP?*

■ **Splenectomy**

A splenectomy may be performed if the patient is not responsive to medical management of ITP with primary and secondary pharmacological management. It still maintains the most durable, best response of the platelets in the long term.

> ❭ HINT
> The spleen is responsible for removing the platelets from circulation. Following a splenectomy, the platelets will remain in circulation longer and increase the platelet count.

■ *What vaccinations are recommended in a patient with splenectomy?*

■ **Pneumococcal, *Hemophilus influenzae*, and meningococcal**

Vaccinations may be administered 2 weeks prior to a planned splenectomy. Following the removal of the spleen, the patient is at a higher risk for certain systemic illnesses, including pneumococcal and meningococcal infections.

> ❭ HINT
> Early antibiotic therapy is recommended in post-splenectomy patients, with fever and signs of systemic infections.

COMPLICATIONS

■ *What is the biggest risk associated with ITP?*

■ **Intracerebral hemorrhage**

Bleeding is the biggest complication of ITP, especially intracerebral bleeding. However, major bleeding is uncommon with ITP and most complications are due to the pharmacological and surgical management of ITP.

TESTABLE NURSING ACTIONS

MONITORING BLOOD TRANSFUSIONS

■ *One unit of blood transfused should be expected to increase the hematocrit by how much?*

■ **3% increase**

One unit of blood should increase the patient's hemoglobin by 1.0 g/dL or hematocrit by 3%.

■ *What is the most common reason for an acute hemolytic transfusion reaction (AHTR)?*

■ **Administering incompatible blood**

AHTRs are almost always due to an error with administering incompatible blood. The reaction is caused by the activation of a complement system by inherited immunoglabulin M (IgM) anti-A, or anti-B antibodies. The result is a massive intravascular hemolysis. The complications and cause of death include DIC and acute kidney injury (AKI).

> HINT

The first intervention is to stop the transfusion immediately (Box 4.12).

Box 4.12 Symptoms of AHTR

Fever	Hypotension
Chills	Hemoglobinemia
Pain at infusion site	Hemoglobinuria
Back/flank pain	

■ *Following an AHTR, what laboratory test would one expect to send?*

■ **Direct antiglobulin**

Direct antiglobulin (Coomb's test) is used to detect antibodies or proteins that are bound to the transfused RBCs causing agglutination and hemolysis. Other laboratory tests include sending a new hemoglobin, type and crossmatch (T&C), and urine to assess hemoglobinuria.

> HINT

Do not throw away the blood bag; send it back to the blood lab to retype.

■ *What blood transfusion reaction can occur after the patient receives multiple units of antigen-specific uncross-matched blood?*

■ **Delayed hemolytic transfusion reactions (DHTRs)**

This delayed hemolytic reaction occurs due to the production of antibodies (usually of IgG class) to RBC antigens to which they have been previously exposed (such as pregnancy, previous transfusions, etc.). The antigens may not have been recognized in the first type and crossmatch due to the low titers. The result is a decrease in hemoglobin over the following 5 to 10 days due to hemolysis.

> HINT

Any time large amounts of uncross-matched blood are administered, a new T&C is recommended to prevent DHTR.

■ *What is the most common type of reaction a patient will have to blood transfusions?*

■ **Febrile nonhemolytic transfusion reaction (FNHTR)**

Fever is the most common type of reaction a patient will have to the administration of blood. Always respond and treat fever as the "worst case scenario" and test for AHTR. Once ruled out, continue with the transfusion. FNHTR is a febrile reaction caused by the effects of cytokine interleukin (IL)-6, IL-8, and tumor necrosis factor (TNF), which are produced by the donor leukocyte store within the blood product.

> HINT
Treat with antipyretics.

■ *During the administration of packed red blood cells (PRBCs), the patient develops dyspnea, hypoxia, angioedema, and hypotension. What is the most likely cause?*
■ **Anaphylactic reaction**

Anaphylactic transfusion reactions (ATRs) are due to the development of anti-IgA antibodies after a blood or blood product transfusion (PRBC, FFP, platelets, IV immunoglobulin). This occurs in patients who are IgA-deficient and is a rare reaction. The symptoms occur within minutes of initiating the transfusion.

> HINT

Stop the transfusion, administer epinephrine, antihistamine, and IV fluids.

■ *What is the transfusion reaction that can result in pulmonary failure and the development of acute respiratory distress syndrome (ARDS)?*
■ **Transfusion-related acute lung injury (TRALI)**

TRALI is the most commonly reported cause of transfusion-related deaths. The theory behind TRALI is that it is a "two hit" insult. The first hit is a stressful situation (such as trauma, sepsis, massive transfusion, cardiopulmonary bypass surgery), which causes the neutrophils to be "primed" and adhere to the pulmonary endothelial bed. The second hit is the actual transfusion of the blood. The transfused blood contains donor antibodies against neutrophil antigens and these antibodies activate the "primed" neutrophils and monocytes, resulting in increased capillary permeability and noncardiogenic pulmonary edema.

> HINT

Manifestations of TRALI may occur within hours of the transfusion.

■ *An acute decrease in blood pressure after the initiation of a blood transfusion can be due to the patient being on which medication?*
■ **Angiotensin-converting enzyme (ACE) inhibitor**

Acute hypotensive transfusion reactions present as a rapid and sudden decrease in blood pressure (BP) soon after the initiation of the transfusion. It is often a severe hypotension of systolic BP less than 70. Bradykinin is metabolized by ACE. Inhibiting ACE elevates bradykinin, causing the hypotension.

> HINT

Immediately stop the transfusion. Do not administer that unit of blood and hold the ACE inhibitor.

Questions

1. A patient admitted post–abdominal surgery develops acute renal failure. He is currently on low-molecular-weight heparin (LMWH) for VTE prevention, and the physician wants to monitor the effectiveness of the LMWH. Which of the following lab tests would be the best for monitoring LMWH?

   A. Platelet aggregometry
   B. Activated partial thromboplastin time (aPTT)
   C. PT with INR
   D. Anti-Xa assay

2. A patient on Coumadin presents with an intracranial hemorrhage and INR of 3.5. Which of the following interventions would be most appropriate at this time?

   A. Oral vitamin K and FFP
   B. Protamine sulfate and platelets
   C. IV vitamin K and FFP
   D. IV vitamin K and cryoprecipitate

3. Which of the following laboratory tests is considered to be the most specific to DIC?

   A. aPTT
   B. PT with INR
   C. Fibrinogen levels
   D. D-dimer

4. A patient has been in the intensive care unit (ICU) for 7 days after intubation for severe pneumonia. She has been receiving VTE prophylaxis with subcutaneous heparin injections since admission to the ICU. A deep vein thrombosis (DVT) was just diagnosed in her left calf, and she is noted to have a platelet count of 55,000. Which of the following is the most likely complication?

   A. Hemolytic uremic syndrome (HUS)
   B. HIT
   C. DIC
   D. ITP

5. Cryoprecipitate can be used in managing actively bleeding patients. In which of the following situations would cryoprecipitate most likely be used?

   A. Low fibrinogen level
   B. Anticoagulant overdose
   C. Thrombocytopenia
   D. Hemolytic anemia

6. A patient is admitted to the ICU following a motor vehicle collision and a complication of an abruptio placenta. She is bleeding from her IV sites and has blood in her urine. Her PT and PTT are elevated and fibrinogen levels are low. Which of the following laboratory values would indicate that she is developing microvascular occlusion?

   A. Elevated troponin
   B. Elevated lactate
   C. Elevated myoglobin
   D. Elevated thrombin time

7. A patient is suspected of developing HIT due to a sudden unexplained decrease in platelets to 55,000 while on heparin. All heparin was discontinued. Which of the following is the most appropriate intervention?

   A. Administer platelet transfusions
   B. Obtain direct Coomb's test
   C. Initiate Argatroban IV drip
   D. Restart heparin after platelets increase to 100,000

8. A patient with a low platelet count is diagnosed with ITP. Which of the following medications is most appropriate to treat ITP?

   A. Heparin
   B. Fondaparinux
   C. Decadron
   D. Acyclovir

9. Which of the following is the most common cause of mortality after transfusion therapy?

   A. Acute hemolytic transfusion reaction (AHTR)
   B. TRALI
   C. Transfusion-transmitted disease (TTD)
   D. Anaphylactic transfusion reaction (ATR)

10. Following a hemolytic blood transfusion reaction, which of the following laboratory test(s) is important to verify the transfusion reaction?

    A. Direct antiglobulin test
    B. Myoglobin
    C. Enzyme-linked immunosorbent assay (ELISA) test
    D. PT/aPTT

Neurological System Review

In this chapter, you will review:

■ Ischemic strokes
■ Hemorrhagic strokes
■ Subarachnoid hemorrhage (SAH): Aneurysms and arterial venous malformations (AVM)
■ Seizure and seizure management
■ Severe traumatic brain injuries
■ Brain death determination
■ Neurological infectious diseases
■ Neuromuscular disorders
■ Hydrocephalus
■ Intracranial pressure (ICP) monitoring and lumbar drains

ISCHEMIC STROKES

■ *What differentiates a transient ischemic attack (TIA) from a stroke?*
■ **Length of time for symptoms**

A stroke occurs following loss of blood flow to an area of the brain resulting in ischemic injuries and permanent cerebral infarction. TIAs are brief episodes of neurological dysfunction resulting from focal cerebral ischemia not associated with permanent cerebral infarction (Box 5.1).

Box 5.1 Quick Comparison of Thrombotic and Embolic Strokes

	Thrombotic	Embolic
Cause	Atherosclerotic plaque narrows lumen of the cerebral vessel; plaque ruptures and causes thrombus from obstructing blood flow distally	The clot originates typically in the heart and is thrown in to the cerebral circulation; the clot obstructs smaller vessels resulting in loss of blood flow distally; the most common location is the middle cerebral artery (MCA)
Presentation	Tends to have a progressive worsening of symptoms	Typically abrupt onset without progression of symptoms
Timing	May occur at rest or on awakening	May occur following activity or exercise

PATHOPHYSIOLOGY

■ *What is the term used in strokes to indicate the ischemic (reversible injury) zone?*
■ **Penumbra**

> **❯ HINT**
> Penumbra may be used in questions discussing the administration of thrombolytic and reversing an injury.

■ *What is hemorrhagic transformation in ischemic stroke?*

■ **Bleeding into the infarction area**

Hemorrhagic transformation is considered to be a natural evolution of an embolic stroke and is usually asymptomatic. Computed tomography (CT) scans following an acute embolic stroke and potentially after reperfusion can demonstrate hemorrhage in the infarcted area of the brain. Because the bleeding tends to occur within the infracted zone (irreversible injury), it is usually asymptomatic.

PREVENTION OF STROKES

Primary stroke prevention is to prevent a stroke from occurring. Secondary stroke prevention is to prevent a stroke patient from having a recurrent stroke.

■ *What class of medications is recommended in primary thrombotic stroke prevention?*

■ **Antiplatelet**

The recommended drug therapy is an aspirin (81 to 100 mg) a day for high-risk patients. Aspirin is not recommended for low-risk patients. An (HMG-CoA) reductase inhibitor (statin) medication is also recommended in patients with heart disease or in certain high-risk people.

■ *What class of medications is recommended in secondary thrombotic stroke prevention?*

■ **Antiplatelet**

Antiplatelet drugs are preferred to oral anticoagulation therapy. Other recommendations include antihypertensive medications to manage hypertensive patients and statin therapy. The recommendations are:

1. Aspirin (50 to 325 mg) monotherapy
2. Combination aspirin/dipyridamole (Aggrenox)
3. Clopidogrel (Plavix) monotherapy

Cardioembolic Stroke Prevention

■ *Which of the ischemic strokes is the most preventable?*

■ **Cardioembolic stroke**

Atrial fibrillation (AF) is the most common cause of embolic strokes and is also the most preventable type of stroke. Anticoagulation therapy is recommended for stroke prevention in this population. Warfarin (Coumadin) is the most commonly used drug. Direct thrombin inhibitors, such as dabigatran (Pradaxa), may also be used to prevent a secondary cardioembolic stroke.

> ❭ HINT
> Questions may include how to monitor the anticoagulation effect of these medications and recognize the side effects of a hemorrhagic stroke (intracerebral hemorrhage).

SYMPTOMS/ASSESSMENT

■ *What does F.A.S.T. stand for when teaching symptoms of a stroke?*
■ **Face, arms, speech, and timing**

Facial and arm weakness along with speech abnormalities are common symptoms of a stroke. Timing reminds them to call 911 immediately when symptoms occur (Box 5.2).

Box 5.2 Symptoms of Cardioembolic Stroke

Ataxia	Alteration behavior
Aphasia	Visual field cuts
Facial palsy	Agnosia
Neglect syndrome	Deviated gaze
Cranial nerves (CN) palsies	Dysarthria
Paresis/ paralysis	Dysphasia
Loss of sensation	Nystagmus
Changes in level of consciousness (LOC)	"Locked in" syndrome

■ *What is a nontraditional symptom of a stroke?*
■ **Shortness of breath**

Sudden pain or numbness in the face, arms, or legs, changes in mental status, generalized neurological symptoms (hiccupping, nausea, and vomiting [N&V]), sudden chest pain or palpitations, sudden tiredness, and shortness of breath are all nontraditional symptoms of a stroke. Shortness of breath is the most common.

■ *Which population is more likely to present with nontraditional symptoms?*
■ **Women**

Women are 60% more likely than men to present with nontraditional symptoms.

DIAGNOSIS

■ *Which radiographic study is considered to be the gold standard in diagnosing a stroke?*
■ **Noncontrast CT scan**

Even though the actual infarct may not be recognized on a CT scan until after 12 to 24 hours, the scan can be used to rule out hemorrhagic strokes and other causes of neurological deterioration. Some of the disorders that may mimic an ischemic stroke include: postictal state following a seizure, central nervous system (CNS) infections, intracerebral tumor, toxic–metabolic disturbances, hypoglycemia or hyperglycemia, hemorrhagic stroke, and subdural hematoma (SDH).

Newer imaging modalities are available in some comprehensive stroke centers that use diffusion-weighted imagery (DWI) and perfusion-weighted imagery (PWI), which will identify ischemic strokes earlier on and have the ability to differentiate between reversible and irreversible injuries. The newer magnetic resonance imaging (MRI) capability may be used to determine candidates for thrombolytic therapy instead of using a time window.

■ *When obtaining a recent history of symptoms, what is the single most important historical information to be obtained?*

■ **Last known normal**

The clock starts for thrombolytic therapy when the patient was at his or her previous baseline or symptom free. It is the time of onset of symptoms or when the patient was last known to be normal.

■ *Which of the following patient scenarios would be a candidate for thrombolytic therapy? Patient A woke up with facial drooping and upper extremity paresis. Patient B had facial drooping and upper extremity paresis 6 hours ago, which completely resolved, but he now presents in the emergency department (ED) within 30 minutes of onset of slurred speech and ataxia.*

■ **Patient B**

The symptoms of stroke found on awakening are called "wake-up" stroke and are *not* considered to be a candidate for thrombolytics because the actual onset of the symptoms is unclear (the patient was asleep at the time). But if a patient reports symptoms of a stroke, which resolved completely, then the time is reset (i.e., the patient is back to baseline). This is a TIA and the time starts when the symptoms of a stroke are presented.

NEUROLOGICAL EXAMINATION

■ *What is the neurological assessment tool used to determine the severity of the stroke?*

■ **National Institute of Health Stroke Scale (NIHSS)**

NIHSS is a tool used by health care providers to objectively quantify the impairment caused by a stroke. The higher the number, the greater the severity of the stroke.

MANAGEMENT

■ *In which situation would you allow a patient with ischemic stroke to remain hypertensive for the first 24 hours without treating for high blood pressure (BP)?*

■ **A patient with ischemic stroke who is *not* a candidate for thrombolytic therapy**

If the patient is not a candidate for thrombolytic therapy and a hemorrhagic stroke has been ruled out, then the recommendation is to monitor BP unless systolic is greater than 220 mmHg or diastolic is greater than 120 mmHg. If the patient is a candidate for thrombolytic therapy, then the systolic BP is kept lower than 180 mmHg.

> **HINT**
The test question may present a hypertensive stroke patient with time of onset of symptoms in the scenario and then ask how you would manage BP. First, determine whether or not the patient would be a candidate for thrombolytics.

■ *Within how many hours from onset of symptoms is it recommended to administer an intravenous (IV) thrombolytic in an ischemic stroke patient?*
■ **3 hours**

Based on the American Heart Association (AHA)/American Stroke Association (ASA) guidelines, the time can be expanded to 4.5 hours in some patients but the goal is still within 3 hours of onset.

> **HINT**
Questions are frequently asked regarding timing of interventions.

■ *What is the age when a patient is not to be considered a candidate for expanded hours (up to 4.5 hours) for administering an IV thrombolytic?*
■ **Older than 80 years of age**

The goal for administration of a thrombolytic agent remains 3 hours. There are certain patients that may be extended to 4.5 hours. Those who should not go to extended hours include patients

1. Older than 80 years of age
2. On oral anticoagulation therapy even with normal international normalized ratio (INR)
3. With a baseline NIH score more than 25
4. With a history of both stroke and diabetes

■ *What is the time frame for initiating IV thrombolytic following onset of neurological symptoms?*
■ **6 hours**

Endovascular therapy may also be used to recanalize and reperfuse the brain. The maximal time window following onset of symptoms for reperfusion with endovascular therapy is 6 and up to 8 hours for middle cerebral artery (MCA) and 12 hours for basilar artery occlusions.

■ *What is always the priority of care for any stroke patient?*
■ **Airway and breathing**

Airway and breathing is always a priority of care. Other management concerns include glucose levels, swallow evaluation, and temperature control.

COMPLICATIONS

■ *What consult needs to be obtained to prevent aspiration?*
■ **Speech therapy**

Swallowing difficulties and abnormal gag reflexes are complications of a stroke. A speech therapist can perform a swallow evaluation prior to feeding a patient who has had a stroke to prevent aspiration (Box. 5.3).

Box 5.3 Complications of Stroke

Paresis/paralysis
Speech problems
Swallowing difficulties
Cognitive abnormalities
Loss of independence
Personality and mood changes
Depression
Shortened life span

HEMORRHAGIC STROKES

- *Which type of hemorrhagic stroke is caused by an aneurysm rupture?*
- **Subarachnoid hemorrhage (SAH)**

Spontaneous intracerebral hemorrhagic stroke is caused by a ruptured cerebral blood vessel with bleeding into the brain tissue. SAH is caused by rupture of an aneurysm or arterial venous malformation (AVM) with bleeding into the subarachnoid space (Boxes 5.4 and 5.5).

Box 5.4 Quick Comparison of Intracerebral and Subarachnoid Hemorrhages

	Intracerebral	Subarachnoid
Cause	Most common causes are hypertension, oral anticoagulation therapy, coagulopathies	Most common causes are rupture of aneurysm, rupture of AVM
Location of bleed	Primarily into brain tissue (parenchyma) and ventricles (called extension)	Primarily into subarachnoid space and intraventricular space
Presentation	Headache, vomiting, hypertension, decreased level of consciousness, seizures	"Worst headache of my life," vomiting, focal neurological deficits, decreased level of consciousness (LOC)

Box 5.5 Common Locations for Spontaneous Intracerebral Hemorrhage (ICH)

Putamin (basal ganglia) 35%–50%	Cerebellar 5%–12%
Lobar 30%	Pontine 5%–12%
Thalamic 10%–15%	

PATHOPHYSIOLOGY

- *Does a hypertensive intracerebral hematoma expand in size after the initial bleed?*
- **Yes**

Rupture of the artery leads to accumulation of blood in the parenchyma of the brain with substantial increases in hematoma size for up to 12 hours post–initial bleed. This increase in clot volume has been shown to be associated with clinical neurological deterioration.

■ *What is commonly found surrounding an intracerebral hemorrhage?*
■ **Cerebral edema**

The bleeding causes disruption of the brain tissue. The resultant clot compresses the adjacent tissue followed by extracellular (vasogenic) cerebral edema developing in the periphery of the hematoma. The blood clot and the cerebral edema lead to an increase in ICP with a potential for fatal herniation syndromes.

> **❯ HINT**
> Vasogenic cerebral edema is interstitial edema while cytotoxic cerebral edema is intracellular (Box. 5.6).

Box 5.6 Causes of Injury Following ICH

Cerebral edema
Disruption of brain tissue
Elevation of ICP
Fatal herniation syndromes

■ *What is the most common cause of a spontaneous ICH?*
■ **Hypertension**

Other causes include vasculitis, venous thrombosis, vascular tumors, coagulopathies, anticoagulation/antiplatelet therapy, sympathomimetic drugs (cocaine, amphetamines), hemorrhagic transformation in ischemic strokes, arteriopathy, and trauma.

RISK FACTORS

■ *Who has the highest risk for an ischemic stroke, an African American male or a White female?*
■ **African American male**

Nonmodifiable risks include gender and race. Men have a greater risk than women for strokes. African Americans have a higher risk for stroke than Caucasians (Box 5.7).

Box 5.7 Risk Factors for Hemorrhagic Stroke

Race	Higher in African Americans
Gender	Higher in men
Age	Risk increases after 55 years of age
Hypertension	
Cigarette smoking	
Alcohol ingestion	Dose related
Genetics	

SYMPTOMS/ASSESSMENT

Case: A patient presents with sudden-onset headache and associated nausea and vomiting. Symptoms began when the patient was mowing the yard. On further assessment, it was noted that the patient was confused and had a decreasing level of consciousness (LOC).

■ **Which of the above symptoms would be a red flag that this patient is experiencing an ICH?**

■ **Sudden-onset headache associated with nausea and vomiting**

The classic clinical presentation includes the onset of a sudden focal neurological deficit, commonly a headache or altered LOC, which progresses over minutes to hours. Other symptoms include nausea and vomiting, seizures, and focal neurological deficits. Onset usually occurs with activity and rarely occurs at night.

> **❯ HINT**
> Vomiting is more common with ICH than with either ischemic stroke or SAH. Symptoms rarely occur at night, whereas patients with ischemic strokes frequently awaken with symptoms.

DIAGNOSIS

■ **What diagnostic test would you expect the managing clinician to order on the above patient?**

■ **Noncontrast CT scan**

A noncontrast CT scan will locate the hemorrhage and determine the size and possible etiology. CT scans are considered superior to MRIs for the diagnosis of acute ICH. The volume of the hemorrhage can be estimated and is important for the prognosis.

■ **What associated finding on the CT scan would indicate a poor prognosis in ICH?**

■ **Intraventricular extension**

This occurs when the vessel ruptures near the ventricles and the tissue loss is through the ventricular system. Bleeding then occurs into the ventricular system, resulting in damage to the ventricles and hydrocephalus.

MEDICAL MANAGEMENT

■ **What is the priority of care following an ICH?**

■ **Airway and breathing**

The focus of caring for a stroke patient is rapid identification, diagnosis, and management, although airway and breathing should always remain a priority.

> **❯ HINT**
> Airway and breathing are always a priority of care in a patient with a decrease in LOC.

■ *Following an ICH, what is the goal for BP management?*
■ **Systolic BP less than 160 mmHg**

The amount of BP control has not been established but a decrease in systolic BP to less than 160 mmHg is reasonable. Systolic BP is frequently maintained in the range of 130 to 150 mmHg. This range may decrease the risk of hypertensive extension of the bleed but it allows for improved cerebral perfusion.

The following are suggested recommended guidelines for treating elevated BP in spontaneous ICH:

1. If systolic BP is 200 mmHg or mean arterial pressure (MAP) is 150 mmHg, then consider aggressive reduction of BP with a continuous IV infusion, with frequent BP monitoring every 5 minutes.
2. If systolic BP is 180 mmHg or MAP is 130 mmHg and there is evidence or suspicion of elevated ICP, then consider monitoring ICP and reducing BP using intermittent or continuous IV medications to keep cerebral perfusion pressure (CPP) greater than 60 to 80 mmHg.
3. If systolic BP is 180 mmHg or MAP is 130 mmHg and there is no evidence of or suspicion of elevated ICP, then consider a modest reduction of BP (e.g., MAP of 110 mmHg or target BP of 160/90 mmHg) using intermittent or continuous IV medications to control BP, and clinically reexamine the patient every 15 minutes.

BP is frequently controlled with a titratable agent to balance the risk of ischemia, hypertension-related rebleeding, and maintenance of cerebral perfusion. **Avoid hypotension** (Box 5.8).

Box 5.8 Intravenous Medications That May Be Considered for Control of Elevated Blood Pressure in Patients With ICH

Drugs	Loading Dose	Continuous Infusion Dose
Labetalol	5–20 mg every 15 min	2 mg/min (maximum 300 mg/d)
Nicardipine	NA	5 to 15 mg/hr
Esmolol	250 µ/kg intraveous push (IVP) loading dose	25 to 300 µ/kg/min
Enalapril	1.25 to 5 mg IVP every 6 hr*	NA
Hydralazine	5–20 mg IVP every 30 min	1.5 to 5 µ/kg/min
Nipride	NA	0.1 to 10 µ/kg/min
Nitroglycerin	NA	0 to 400 µ/min

*Because of the risk of precipitous blood pressure lowering, the first test dose for enalapril should be 0.625 mg.

■ *It has been determined that the cause of an ICH is anticoagulation therapy with warfarin. What would you expect the patient to receive to reverse the bleeding?*
■ **IV vitamin K and fresh frozen plasma (FFP)**

Management of anticoagulated bleeds is to correct coagulopathies with FFP, vitamin K (warfarin), protamine sulfate (heparin), or administer platelets (platelet inhibitor drugs) depending on which drug is to be reversed. For other management therapies for ICH see Box 5.9.

Box 5.9 Other Management Therapies for ICH

Treat an increased ICP
Administer antiepileptic medications
Manage hyperglycemia (>185 mg/dL and possibly >140 mg/dL) with insulin
Treat fever with antipyretic medications

SURGICAL MANAGEMENT

■ *What is the location in the brain for a hemorrhage that is considered the most amenable by surgery?*

■ **Cerebellum**

Surgical approaches include craniotomy with clot evacuation, stereotactic aspiration with the use of thrombolytic agents, and endoscopic evacuation. Overall, most patients with ICH will not benefit from surgery. The routine evacuation of supratentorial ICH by standard craniotomy within 96 hours of bleed is not recommended. Surgical options depend on the location and size of the hematoma. The following are situations that may be amendable by early surgery:

1. Patients with hematoma less than 1 cm from the cortical surface
2. Cerebellar hemorrhage more than 3 cm or a rapidly deteriorating clinical status

SUBARACHNOID HEMORRHAGE: ANEURYSMS AND ARTERIAL VENOUS MALFORMATIONS

PATHOPHYSIOLOGY

■ *What is an aneurysm called that is round with a neck and typically located at a bifurcation?*

■ **Sacular aneurysm**

Aneurysms are classified by their shape and size. A sacular or "berry" aneurysm is round, has a neck, and is frequently found in a bifurcation or branching vessel. A fusiform aneurysm has an outpouching of the arterial wall without a neck and can occur anywhere along the vessel.

> ❯ HINT
> A giant aneurysm measures 2.5 cm or larger and produces symptoms of a space lesion.

■ *What is the type of intracranial aneurysm caused by septic emboli commonly associated with bacterial endocarditis?*

■ **Mycotic aneurysm**

A mycotic aneurysm is due to an infectious source. The most common source is a bacterial endocarditis.

■ **What is a system of dilated vessels that shunts arterial blood directly into the venous system without the capillary network?**

■ **AVM**

AVMs are composed of the nidus, which is a fairly well-circumscribed center, as well as the feeding arteries and draining veins. Rupture of the aneurysm or AVM is frequently associated with an activity causing an increase in BP. The rupture results in bleeding, primarily into subarachnoid space, but also bleeding into the subdural or intracerebral tissue.

> ❯ **HINT**
> Aneurysms more commonly cause an SAH than an AVM.

■ **What is the most common site of an aneurysm?**

■ **Circle of Willis**

This is because of all of the bifurcations and branches in the Circle of Willis. The anterior circulation accounts for 85% of the aneurysm and the posterior circulation (vertebral and basilar arteries) account for 15%.

SYMPTOMS/ASSESSMENT

■ **What is the most common sign of an SAH?**

■ **Headache**

Headache in SAH is frequently described as "the worst headache of my life" (Box 5.10). Warning signs are present in about 50% of the bleeds (Box 5.11). The SAH is graded on the severity of the presenting signs and symptoms.

Box 5.10 Other Symptoms of SAH

Loss of consciousness or change in level of consciousness	Pupillary changes
	Stiff and painful neck
Cranial nerve deficits (especially CN III)	Positive Kernig's and Brudzinski's signs
Visual disturbance	Photophobia
Hemiparesis or hemiplegia	Possible temperature elevation
Vomiting	

Box 5.11 Warning Signs of SAH

Lethargy	Cranial nerve dysfunction
Localized headache	Audible bruits
Neck pain	

■ **What is the grading system most commonly used following an SAH?**

■ **Hunt and Hess**

Hunt and Hess grading is based upon clinical presentation. Grade I is minimal symptoms and grade V is the worst presentation (Box 5.12).

Box 5.12 Hunt and Hess Grading System

Grade I	Asymptomatic, mild headache, slight nuchal rigidity
Grade II	Moderate to severe headache, nuchal rigidity, no neurologic deficit other than cranial nerve palsy
Grade III	Drowsiness/confusion, mild focal neurologic deficit
Grade IV	Stupor, moderate to severe hemiparesis
Grade V	Coma, decerebrate posturing

DIAGNOSIS

- *What is the diagnostic test for SAH?*
- **Noncontrast CT scan and cerebral angiogram**

A noncontrast CT scan is the initial diagnostic test used to screen patients presenting with headache and neurological deficits. A CT scan demonstrating an SAH indicates the need for follow-up angiography.

- *What is the most life-threatening complication within the first 24 hours following an aneurysm rupture?*
- **Rebleeding**

The peak incidence of a rebleed occurs within the first 24 to 48 hours (Box 5.13).

Box 5.13 Interventions to Prevent Rebleeding

Prevent hypertension
Avoid straining
Manage anxiety or pain
Bed rest
Quiet room
Decrease physical stimulation

- *Your patient is 7 days post-SAH. During the day, he has a sudden decrease in LOC. Which complication is the most likely cause?*
- **Vasospasms (VS)**

A VS is defined as the focal narrowing of the cerebral arteries. It most commonly occurs within 7 to 10 days following an SAH. Symptoms of VS can be any neurological deficit. Diagnosis is confirmed with angiography and/or transcranial Doppler studies.

> **HINT**
> Questions frequently use the number of days after an SAH to determine the cause of a neurological change.

■ *The treatment of VS includes "triple H therapy." What is triple H therapy?*

■ **Hypervolemia, hypertension, and hemodilution**

Triple H therapy is used to attempt to open the vessel in VS and perfuse the brain distally. The calcium channel blocker nimodipine (Nimotop) is administered from the time of admission for 14 to 21 days. It has been found to improve neurological outcomes. An interventional neurologist may use angioplasty and intra-arterial antihypertensives to open the vessels and reperfuse the brain. Other complications of SAH include hydrocephalus, cerebral edema, and hyponatremia.

SURGICAL MANAGEMENT

■ *What is the surgical management of an intracerebral aneurysm?*

■ **Surgical clipping**

Surgical clipping of the neck of the aneurysm has been the primary treatment of intracerebral aneurysms. Interventional therapy may also be used to manage aneurysms and includes coiling the aneurysm.

SEIZURES

TERMINOLOGY

■ *What is an abnormal excessive neuronal discharge in the brain called?*

■ **Seizure**

Epileptic seizure is a transient symptom due to an abnormal excessive neuronal discharge. This definition allows for differentiation of epileptic seizures from other seizures that may not be epileptic in nature and may be accompanied by convulsions. Epilepsy is a disorder of the brain characterized by an enduring predisposition to generate epileptic seizures. Definitions of epilepsy typically include the occurrence of more than one epileptic seizure. Status epilepticus (SE) is a condition of recurrent seizures or continuous seizure activity without return to normal function (a seizure lasting > 5 minutes). Refractory SE occurs when the seizure does not respond to two different antiepileptic medications within 20 minutes.

■ *What is it called when the electroencephalogram (EEG) findings indicate*
  seizure activity without the motor movements of a convulsive seizure?

■ **Nonconvulsive status epilepticus (NCSE)**

NCSE is a type of status epilepticus in which the patient does not exhibit any motor movements, but the brain could be experiencing abnormal excessive neuronal activities of an epileptic seizure. It is suspected in patients with altered mental status and can be diagnosed with a continuous EEG monitor. NCSE is frequently found in patients after a generalized seizure. Any patient who is slow to awaken or remains unresponsive after a convulsive generalized seizure should have an EEG taken.

CAUSES OF SEIZURES

All neurological disorders can increase the risk of a seizure (Box 5.14). Other causes of epilepsy include genetic defects or metabolic disorders of the brain.

Box 5.14 List of Common Neurological Risk Factors of Seizures

Traumatic brain injury	Infectious CNS disorders
Subdural hematomas	Hypoxic or anoxic brain injuries
Brain tumors	Subarachnoid hemorrhage
Ischemic strokes	Neurodegenerative disorders
Hemorrhagic strokes	Antiepileptic medication or alcohol withdrawal

■ *What are three electrolyte abnormalities that can cause a seizure?*
■ **Hyponatremia, hypocalcemia, hypoglycemia**

Electrolyte abnormalities can result in a seizure and need to be monitored closely. Sodium abnormalities, especially hyponatremia, hypocalcemia, and hypoglycemia, are the three most electrolyte abnormalities commonly found to cause seizures. Hypomagesium and hypernatremia may also cause seizures.

> ❯ HINT
> The question may start with a scenario about a patient with an electrolyte abnormality, such as hyponatremia, and lead to questions on seizures.

CLASSIFICATION OF SEIZURES

■ *What is the name of the classification of a seizure in which the neuronal discharge is localized to an area of the brain?*
■ **Partial seizure**

Seizures are classified as partial (focal) or generalized seizures. Generalized seizures have a neuronal discharge occurring within and rapidly engaging bilateral hemispheres. Partial seizures have a neuronal discharge that initiates in one focal site and is limited to one hemisphere. Partial seizures are further divided into simple partial or complex partial seizures. The difference between a simple and a complex partial seizure is the awareness and recall of the seizures. It is important to note the patient's awareness during the seizure and whether the patient has any recall of the seizure afterward (Box 5.15).

Box 5.15 Types of Seizures

Focal Seizure	Generalized Seizure
Focal motor	Tonic–clonic (in any combination)
Jacksonian march	Absence
Somatosensory	Myoclonic
Fencer's position	Clonic

(continued)

Box 5.15 Types of Seizures (*continued*)

Focal Seizure	Generalized Seizure
Affective	Tonic
Automatisms	Atonic
Psychic	
Postural	

■ *A patient may have an aura before a seizure. What classification is an aura?*
■ **Simple partial seizure**

An aura is a distinct sensory or motor event that precedes a generalized seizure. It is frequently a somatosensory focal seizure. Focal seizures can progress to generalized seizures.

■ *What is the period immediately following a seizure called?*
■ **Postictal**

Following a seizure, the patient is usually postictal. This time usually requires prolonged sleep or rest. He or she may experience severe headache; muscle aches are also common after muscle contractions. The assessment of airway and breathing are important. Placing the patient in a lateral position can prevent aspiration if vomiting occurs during or after a seizure.

■ *After a seizure, your patient experiences temporary blindness. What is this called?*
■ **Todd's paralysis**

Todd's paralysis is a temporary neurological deficit, commonly a paralysis or blindness, which resolves itself spontaneously. It may last from minutes to hours after the motor seizure.

SYMPTOMS/ASSESSMENT

■ *Following a seizure, what complication should be closely assessed?*
■ **Potential injury**

Convulsive seizures can frequently result in injury from falls, repetitive impacting solid surfaces, and oral trauma (Box 5.16).

Box 5.16 Obtaining History of Patient's Seizures

Description of past seizures
Frequency of seizures
Seizure patterns
Precipitant of seizure
Current antiepileptic drug (AED)
Compliance status

MANAGEMENT

- *What should be done with the side rails on a bed for patients with seizure precautions?*
- Pad the side rails

Padding side rails can potentially help limit injuries that may occur during a seizure (Box 5.17).

Box 5.17 Seizure Precautions

Set bed in the lowest position
Bed should be locked
Side rails are in the upright position
Pad side rails
Place oral airway at bedside
Suction and oxygen equipment should be available

- *What is the preferred first-line AED used to stop a seizure?*
- Lorazepam (Ativan)

The side effect of lorazepam is respiratory depression but this should not deter from administering the medication to stop the seizure. It is better to secure the airway and adequately treat the seizure. This is important because the longer the seizure lasts, the greater the potential for irreversible brain damage. This is due to an increase in metabolic demands of the brain during a seizure.

The preferred second-line medication is phenytoin sodium (Dilantin) or fosphenytoin (Cerebyx). The full antiepileptic effect of these drugs is not immediate, so the initial drug is still a benzodiazepine. The dose and infusion rate of IV Cerebyx is expressed as phenytoin sodium equivalents (PSE) to avoid the need to perform molecular weight-based adjustments when converting between fosphenytoin and phenytoin sodium dosages (Box 5.18).

> ❯ HINT
>
> Phenytoin should not be administered faster than 50 mg/min and fosphenytoin's maximal administration is no faster than 150 mg PSE/min because of hypotension.

Box 5.18 AEDs Used During Seizure

First line:
Benzodiazepines
Ativan or Valium
Second line:
Dilantin
Cerebyx
Third line:
Versed
Propofol
Keppra
Depacon
Vimpat
Fourth line:
Pentobarbital

> **HINT**
>
> Pentobarbital is reserved as a fourth-line drug because of significant side effects of hypotension, cardiac depression, respiratory depression, and immunosuppression.

- **What is the recommended bedside monitoring for refractory status epilepticus (RSE)?**
- **Continuous EEG monitoring**

Titration of IV infusions of AEDs is best through burst suppression on a continuous EEG. Continuous EEG is also used to recognize a nonconvulsive seizure and is recommended in cases of abnormal mental status, a comatose patient, and in survivors of cardiac arrest.

SEVERE TRAUMATIC BRAIN INJURIES

PATHOPHYSIOLOGY

- **Following a blunt mechanism, what is a brain injury occurring on the opposite side of impact called?**
- **Contracoup injury**

A coup injury occurs on the side of the impact and a contracoup injury is on the opposite side of impact. The most common site for a coup–contracoup injury is an impact to the temporal area of the skull, causing a side-to-side impact of the brain in the skull.

> **HINT**
>
> A contracoup injury is caused by brain impacting the skull and bony protrusions.

- **What is a nondisplaced fracture of the skull called?**
- **Linear skull fracture**

A linear skull fracture is a nondisplaced skull fracture and may be recognized on a lateral skull fracture. A basilar skull fracture cannot be identified with a lateral x-ray but is typically identified with CT scan or clinical presentation (Box 5.19).

Box 5.19 Types of Skull Fractures

Linear skull fracture	Nondisplaced fracture
Comminuted skull fracture	Fragmented disruption of skull with multiple linear fractures
Depressed skull fracture	Displaced comminuted fracture with depression
Basilar skull fracture	Fracture of the basilar skull through anterior or middle fossa

- **Which two secondary injuries are the most predictive for a worsened neurological outcome following a traumatic brain injury (TBI)?**
- **Hypotension and hypoxia**

Brain injury is classified as either primary and secondary injury. Interventions to improve outcomes are aimed at secondary injuries. Of all the secondary injuries, hypotension and hypoxia are the two most significant in worsening neurological outcomes. Immediate goals for managing TBIs are airway protection, adequate oxygenation, and improved brain perfusion. Following a TBI, there is loss of autoregulation in the area of injury resulting in focal edema and an ischemia of uninjured tissue because of a "steal" phenomenon (Box 5.20).

Box 5.20 Primary and Secondary Injuries

Primary Injuries	Secondary Injuries
Concussion (mild traumatic brain injury [TBI])	Hypoxia/anoxia
Contusions	Hypotension
Diffuse axonal injury (DAI)	Anemia
Lacerations	Hyperthermia
Subarachnoid hematoma (SAH)	Hypercapnia/hypocapnia
Subdural hematoma (SDH)	Electrolyte imbalances (e.g., hyperglycemia)
Epidural hematoma (EDH)	Cerebral edema
	Hydrocephalus

> **HINT**
> Diffuse axonal injury may be used in the scenario of a TBI patient in test questions.

■ *What is cerebral edema caused by injury to the blood–brain barrier and increased interstitial fluid called?*
■ **Vasogenic cerebral edema**

Vasogenic cerebral edema is a result of injury to the brain tissue, such as trauma, brain tumors, and strokes. Cytotoxic cerebral edema is intracellular fluid in the brain caused by hypoxic or anoxic brain injuries. Both vasogenic and cytotoxic cerebral edema are commonly found in severe TBI patients.

> **HINT**
> Mannitol is most effective with vasogenic cerebral edema.

■ *What population is more likely to present with a chronic SDH?*
■ **The elderly**

SDH is bleeding into the subdural space. It often occurs as a result of an injury to the bridging veins and can result in rapid neurological changes (acute), delayed symptoms (subacute), and chronic presentations. Elderly people, alcoholics, and patients with dementia have some brain atrophy and a higher risk of falls and head trauma, which allows for more room to bleed into the cranial vault before ICP increases. It can be managed with burr holes and evacuation of the hematoma or by surgical craniotomy.

DIAGNOSIS

■ *What is the preferred method for testing fluid from the nose or ears for cerebrospinal fluid (CSF) following a trauma?*

■ Halo test

The halo test involves placing the fluid from the nose or ears on gauze dressing; the blood separates from the CSF with the CSF forming a ring or halo. Glucose testing can be used to differentiate nasal drainage from CSF, but if the drainage is bloody, a halo test is not recommended because of false positives.

> ❯ HINT
> Most questions regarding skull fractures will focus more on basilar skull fractures.

SYMPTOMS/ASSESSMENT

■ *What are the clinical signs of a basilar skull fracture?*

■ Raccoon eyes and battle signs

Clinical signs of a basilar skull fracture include bilateral periorbital ecchymosis (raccoon eyes) and/or bruising on mastoid process (battle signs). They may exhibit CSF fluid drainage from the nose (rhinorrhea) or from the ears (otorrhea). Do not use intranasal packing. Basilar skull fractures have a higher incidence of CNS infections.

> ❯ HINT
> All tubes (e.g., gastric tubes, endotracheal tubes, suction catheters) should be placed orally, not nasally. Nasal tubes can enter the brain through the cribiform fracture.

■ *A rapidly expanding epidural hematoma (EDH) results in a dilated, nonreactive pupil. Which pupil is affected?*

■ Ipsilateral pupil

Cranial nerve III (oculomotor) is responsible for pupil size and reaction to light. Cranial nerves remain ipsilateral (except for cranial nerve IV) so injury to cranial nerve III causes a dilated, nonreactive pupil on the ipsilateral side. This is a result of uncal herniation, in which the unilateral mass pushes the temporal lobe downward through the tentorial opening.

> ❯ HINT
> EDH is an arterial bleed, frequently caused by injury to the middle meningeal artery following a blunt trauma. It causes rapid deterioration of neurological status, typically following a period of being lucid.

MANAGEMENT

- ■ *What affect does CO_2 have on the cerebral vasculature?*
- ■ **Cerebral vasodilation**

Hyperventilation, which reduces $PaCO_2$, has been used to lower ICP through cerebral vasoconstriction. This lowers the blood volume, thus lowering the ICP. It is not recommended to routinely hyperventilate because even though hyperventilation can lower ICP, it also decreases cerebral blood flow. Hyperventilation, with a goal of $PaCO_2$ at 32 to 34, can be used in situations of increased ICP refractory to other treatments.

> ❭ HINT
> Avoid an increase in $PaCO_2$, which elevates the ICP.

- ■ *When administering mannitol (Osmitrol), what laboratory values should be monitored closely?*
- ■ **Serum osmolality and serum sodium**

Mannitol is the most commonly used osmotic diuretic in the treatment of increased ICP. It increases serum osmolality, creating a gradient between the plasma and the brain tissue. Serum osmolality and serum sodium levels can increase during repeated administration of mannitol and should be closely monitored. Mannitol should not be administered if serum osmolality becomes higher than 320 mOsm. The patient may need to be rehydrated if he or she becomes too hyperosmolar.

> ❭ HINT
> Arterial hypotension should be avoided because of the adverse effect
> on cerebral blood flow.

Another hyperosmolar treatment currently used to manage increased ICP caused by cerebral edema is hypertonic saline (HS). It does not have the diuretic effect of mannitol. HS administration can have the complication of central pontine myelinolysis (CPM) in a hyponatremic patient. (Box 5.21).

> ❭ HINT
> Hypernatremia should be excluded before the administration of HS.

Box 5.21 Treatment of TBI

Craniectomy	Bone flaps and hemicraniectomy	Allows room for swelling Lowers risk herniation
Fluid resuscitation	Normal saline recommended Avoid hypotonic solutions	Prevent hypovolemia and hypotension
Steroids	Not recommended for TBI May be used in other neurological disorders	Stabilizes cell membranes to decrease cerebral edema

(continued)

Box 5.21 Treatment of TBI (*continued*)

Blood pressure management	Maintain cerebral perfusion pressure (CPP) > 60 Do not aggressively attempt to keep CPP > 70	Adequate pressure to increase cerebral blood flow (CBF) Avoid complications of fluid overload (e.g., acute respiratory distress syndrome [ARDS])
Hypnotics and sedatives	Short-acting or reversible	Lowers cerebral demand Lowers intracranial pressure (ICP) May also decrease CBF
Barbiturate coma	Pentobarbital, thiopental	Lowers cerebral metabolism Lowers ICP May also decrease CBF
Temperature control	Avoid hyperthermia (fever) May or may not induce hypothermia	Lowers cerebral metabolism Neuroprotectant Decreases ICP
Glucose control	Avoid hyperglycemia Avoid hypoglycemia	Prevents furthering of cellular injury

- *Which two monitoring techniques are recommended for a barbiturate coma?*
- **ICP and continuous EEG with burst suppression**

ICP is monitored to determine the effectiveness of the therapy. The induced barbiturate coma results in loss of the ability to assess a patient's neurological status. Continuous EEG monitoring is used to guide the dosing of the barbiturate. Dosing is guided by the extent of burst suppression. Beyond the point of burst suppression, it may increase the risk of complications without offering further therapeutic benefit. Other monitoring may include arterial line and pulmonary artery catheter due to the cardiovascular complications (myocardial depression) of the barbiturate (Box 5.22).

Box 5.22 Nursing Interventions to Lower ICP

Maintaining head-of-bed elevation to facilitate venous drainage
Maintaining good head alignment to facilitate venous drainage
Providing good pulmonary toiletry for oxygenation and avoiding hypercarbia
Spacing activities to limit the response of ICP

BRAIN DEATH DETERMINATION

- *What type of death involves an irreversible cessation of brain function?*
- **Brain death**

The Uniform Determination of Death Act (UDDA) defines death as follows: "An individual who has sustained either (a) irreversible cessation of circulatory and respiratory functions, or (b) irreversible cessation of all functions of the entire brainstem, is dead" (Wijdicks et al., 2010). The UDDA does not define how to determine brain death.

Most states in the United States have adopted the UDDA, but some states have added amendments stating certain criteria are needed to determine brain death. There are published practice guidelines for brain death determination but the actual process remains variable throughout the country.

> **HINT**

For the exam, brain death determination may be different from your hospital practice. Be familiar with the national standards.

- *What is a clinical examination performed at the bedside?*
- **Brainstem reflexes**

There are three clinical findings required to confirm irreversible cessation of all functions of the entire brain, including the brainstem. This includes determining the coma is irreversible and has a known cause; there is an absence of brainstem reflexes and the patient is determined to be apneic.

- *What has to be normalized before the determination of brain death?*
- **Body temperature**

The patient must have a body temperature above 36°C. A drug and alcohol screen is also frequently recommended to ensure the coma is not the effect of a CNS-depressant drug. If the patient has received a neuromuscular blocking (NMB) agent, the effects must be reversed totally. This can be determined by the presence of train-of-four twitches with maximal ulnar nerve stimulation. There should be no severe electrolyte or acid–base imbalance. Achieve normal systolic pressure (> 100 mmHg) to assure a reliable neurological examination.

- *How do you define a "coma"?*
- **Absence of all responses to any noxious stimuli**

No motor response, eye opening, or eye movement with application of a noxious stimulation, other than spinal reflexes. Some patients who are brain dead may still have nonbrain-mediated spontaneous movements and spinal reflexes.

- *What are the commonly tested brainstem reflexes?*
- **Pupillary response to light, ocular movements, corneal reflex, cough (tracheal reflex), and gag (pharyngeal reflex)**

Bilateral pupils are frequently midsize to dilated and fixed, with no reaction to light. If the pupils are pinpoints, drug overdose should be suspected. Ocular movement is tested using the oculocephalic test (doll's eyes) and the oculovestibular test (cold calorics).

> **HINT**

Doll's eyes and cold calorics tests are done when testing for a reflex. If the reflex is there (positive), then the patient is not brain dead. If the reflex is absent (negative), it is one step toward the determination of brain death. Doll's eyes test: The eyes should move in the opposite direction of head movement. Barbie dolls have their eyes painted on the head, so when you move their heads side to side, the eyes go in the same direction. Remember Barbie dolls are brain dead!

■ *Which blood gas abnormality is required for an apnea test to be positive?*
■ **Hypercarbia**

The absence of a breathing drive (apnea test) is tested with a CO_2 challenge. Documentation of an increase in $PaCO_2$ above normal levels is typical practice. Prerequisites include eucapnia and no prior evidence of CO_2 retention (e.g., chronic obstructive pulmonary disease [COPD]). Abort the test if systolic BP is less than 90 mmHg or oxygen saturation is less than 85% for longer than 30 seconds. If respiratory movements are absent and $PaCO_2$ is greater than 60 mmHg, the apnea test is positive.

Other ancillary tests include EEG, cerebral angiography, nuclear scan, transcranial Doppler, CT angiography, and MRI/magnetic resonance angiography (MRA).

NEUROLOGICAL INFECTIOUS DISEASE

BACTERIAL MENINGITIS

Pathophysiology

■ *Where is the primary location of the infection in meningitis?*
■ **Meninges**

Bacterial meningitis is an inflammation or an infection in the meninges, particularly involving the pia and arachnoid layer (subarachnoid space). The routes of entry for the bacteria into the meninges are listed in Box 5.23.

Box 5.23   Routes of Entry Bacterial Meningitis

Bloodstream
Middle ear infection
Sinusitis
Direct route
Mouth/nose droplets

Symptoms/Assessment

■ *What is the triad of symptoms in meningitis?*
■ **Nuchal rigidity, headache, and fever**

Meningitis typically presents with headache, fever, and nuchal rigidity. This is considered the classic triad of symptoms (Box 5.24).

Box 5.24 Other Symptoms of Meningitis

Headache
Photophobia
Seizure
Cranial nerve palsy (e.g., CN II, III, IV, VI, VIII)
Petechiae and cutaneous hemorrhage
Brudzinski's sign
Kernig's sign

■ *What is it called when the hips or knees flex in response to passive neck flexion?*

■ **Brudzinski's sign**

Brudzinski's sign and Kernig's sign are indications of meningeal irritation. Kernig's sign is severe stiffness or pain in the hamstring causing an inability to straighten the leg when hip is flexed at a 90-degree angle.

Diagnosis

■ *Is the CSF glucose high or low in bacterial meningitis?*

■ **Low**

CSF analysis is used to diagnose meningitis and determine the underlying causative microorganism. The normal glucose level in the CSF is two-thirds of the glucose in the blood. So if the serum glucose is within normal range than the CSF glucose normal is 45 mg/dL. A ratio of CSF glucose to serum glucose less than 0.4 is a predictor of bacterial meningitis. Viral meningitis has a normal CSF glucose (Box 5.25).

> ❯ HINT
>
> Think of a bacteria as an animal; an animal has to eat. It eats glucose, whereas a virus is not an animal, and does not need to eat and will have a normal CSF glucose level.

Box 5.25 CSF Analysis of Bacterial Meningitis

Opening pressure is in the range of 200 to 500 mm H_2O
Elevated protein levels
Elevated lactate levels
Positive Gram stain

■ *Which white blood cells (WBC) are expected to be elevated in bacterial meningitis?*

■ **Neutrophils**

Neutrophils are typically elevated in a bacterial infection. Lymphocytes are typically elevated in viral infections.

> ❯ HINT
>
> Gram stains provide an accurate, rapid identification of the causative bacterium.

■ *What would be an indication for a head CT scan before performing a lumbar puncture?*

■ **Abnormal LOC, focal neurological deficit, or presence of papilledema**

The presence of an abnormal neurological evaluation may indicate an increase in ICP. Performing a lumbar puncture on a patient with an increased ICP can result in brain herniation; thus, a head CT scan is needed first to identify any space-occupying lesions. The lumbar puncture results in a temporary decrease in CSF pressure due to removal of CSF.

Treatment

■ *What is the priority of care in managing bacterial meningitis?*
■ **Administration of antibiotics**

Management includes early administration of an antimicrobial agent. Any delay in treatment might be associated with an adverse outcome. The use of dexamethasone is controversial in adults and may be initiated with the first dose of the antimicrobial agent.

Complications

■ *What is a common complication following bacterial meningitis related to a cranial nerve abnormality?*
■ **Hearing loss**

Complications of bacterial meningitis include hearing loss, visual acuity deficits, and post-meningitis sequelae.

> ❯ HINT
>
> Following a meningeal coccal meningitis, a complication may include amputations due to the vasculitis and thrombophlebitis.

NEUROMUSCULAR DISORDERS

MYASTHENIA GRAVIS

Pathophysiology

■ *In myasthenia gravis (MG), what do the antibodies destroy resulting in fatigable muscle weakness?*
■ **Acetylcholine receptors**

MG is a chronic autoimmune disease that affects the neuromuscular junction causing a fatigable muscle weakness, which worsens with repeated use of the muscles and improves with rest. Antibodies destroy the acetylcholine (ACh) receptors on the postsynaptic muscle end plate, thus decreasing the effect of acetylcholine. This reduces the number of receptor sites at the neuromuscular junction and the voltage to elicit action.

Symptoms/Assessment

■ *What is the hallmark sign of MG?*
■ **Muscle weakness with repetitive movement**

The first time the movement is performed there are receptor sites available for acetylcholine and the contraction is strong. Further attempts of the movement become weaker until a person is unable to preform the movement. This is due to the loss of receptor sites on the muscle end plate.

> ❯ HINT
> Examples of repetitive movements include chewing, talking, swallowing, and movement of the extremities.

■ *What is the primary concern when a patient with MG is admitted in a crisis?*
■ **Pulmonary compromise**

Assessment of the patient's ventilatory capability is very important. In a crisis, a patient with MG may develop significant weakness in the diaphragm and intercostal muscles and progress rapidly to respiratory failure. Assess the quality of the voice and the ability to talk. Assess the ability to cough and suction as needed. Administer oxygen as needed and obtain arterial blood gases to monitor ventilation ($PaCO_2$).

> ❯ HINT
> Other areas of concern include difficulty swallowing and choking caused by weakness of the laryngeal and oropharyngeal muscles.

■ *Which two pulmonary function tests are used most often to evaluate ventilatory effort of patients with MG?*
■ **Forced vital capacity (FVC) and negative inspiratory force (NIF)**

Pulmonary function tests are monitored frequently, and significant changes from baseline are an indication of respiratory failure. An FVC less than 15 mL/kg or an NIF less than 20 cm H_2O are indications of the need for mechanical ventilation.

Treatment

■ *During crisis, what are two therapies that may be used to rapidly reverse the crisis in MG?*
■ **IV immunoglobulin (IVIG) or apheresis**

IVIG or plasmapheresis is indicated during an MG crisis. IVIG therapy may be preferred in patients with hemodynamic instability, in which apheresis (plasma exchange) may be contraindicated. Steroids may also be initiated but can result in an exacerbation in muscle weakness within 5 to 10 days of initiation of the steroid and may still require the above therapies concomitantly. The cholinesterase inhibitors may actually be held initially during the crisis.

> **HINT**
Corticosteroids (prednisone) and immunomodulatory drugs
(azathioprine, cyclosporine, mycophenolate) may also be used to
manage MG during a crisis. Remember, this is an autoimmune disease.

■ *What is the name of the crisis induced by an overdose of cholinesterase-inhibitor drugs used to manage MG?*

■ **Cholinergic crisis**

A cholinergic crisis can also present with an increase in weakening of muscles and respiratory failure. Determining the time of the last dose is helpful in differentiating a cholinergic crisis from a myasthenia crisis. If the onset of weakness is 3 to 4 hours after the dose, the probable cause is an acute worsening of the disease process itself. If it is within 15 to 60 minutes of the last dose, it is more likely a cholinergic crisis (Box 5.26). The treatment is typically to hold the cholinesterase inhibitor medications until symptoms are resolved. Intense monitoring for signs of respiratory failure and increased weakness is necessary.

Box 5.26 Symptoms of Cholinergic Crisis

Slurred speech
Dyspnea
Increased diplopia
Increased salivation
Muscle cramping
Fasciculations
Bradycardia
Abdominal symptoms

GUILLAIN-BARRÉ

Pathophysiology

■ *What is the hallmark presentation of a patient with Guillain-Barré?*

■ **Ascending, bilateral paralysis**

Guillain-Barré (GB) syndrome is an acute inflammatory, autoimmune polyradiculoneuropathy frequently presenting as an ascending, bilateral paralysis. The process causes demyelination of the peripheral nerves, including the cranial nerves, ventral and dorsal nerve roots, entire length of the peripheral nerves, and the autonomic nervous system (ANS). When the pathological process is completed, regeneration of the myelin sheath occurs and function is restored. Reinnervation of the muscle occurs due to new growth from the cone of the axon.

Symptoms/Assessment

■ *Which of the cranial nerves are more important to assess during an acute process of GB?*

■ **CN IX, X, XII**

Cranial nerves IX, X, and XII are responsible for the gag and swallow reflexes. As the paralysis ascends, the patient may have weakened reflexes or loss of the gag and swallow reflexes. This puts the patient at high risk for aspiration.

> ❭ HINT
> The other cranial nerves commonly involved are CN III, IV, and VI for extraocular eye movement and should be assessed on a regular basis.

■ *What are the signs of involvement of the autonomic nervous system?*
■ **Alteration in heart rate**

The autonomic nervous system (ANS) includes the sympathetic and parasympathetic nervous system. The ANS may also be affected by the demyelination of the peripheral portion of the nerves (Box 5.27).

Box 5.27 Signs of ANS Abnormalities in GB

Heart rate abnormalities (tachycardia or bradycardia)
Inverted T waves
Alteration in BP (hypo- or hypertensive)
Facial flushing
Loss of sweating ability

■ *Is the resolution of paralysis ascending or descending?*
■ **Descending**

The resolution of muscle weakness or paralysis is in the opposite direction of the onset of GB. The muscle weakness begins with gait and paralysis in the lower extremities. Muscle strength is regained in a descending fashion, with the resolution of spontaneous ventilation before the ability to ambulate.

Treatment

■ *What is the acute medical treatment for GB?*
■ **IVIG and/or apheresis**

The treatment of GB is similar to that of MG. Apheresis (plasma exchange) involves the removal of antibodies, which decreases the autoimmune response in the peripheral nerves (Box 5.28).

> ❭ HINT
> Nursing assessment and care for both MG and GB should focus on ventilatory efforts and the presence of respiratory failure.

Box 5.28 Complications of Apheresis

Clotting disorders	Hypotension
Hypocalcemia	Autonomic dysfunction
Infections	Phlebitis
Decreased serum proteins	

HYDROCEPHALUS

PATHOPHYSIOLOGY

- *What is hydrocephalus called when it occurs because of an obstruction within the ventricular system?*
- **Noncommunicating hydrocephalus**

When there is an obstruction within the ventricular system, the flow of CSF from the ventricles to the subarachnoid space is impaired. The most common form is a mass lesion, intraventricular or extraventricular, disrupting the ventricular system. Tumors can cause blockage anywhere along the CSF flow.

A communicating hydrocephalus occurs because of overproduction of CSF, interference with reabsorption of CSF, or venous drainage insufficiency. The ventricular system communicates with the subarachnoid space. The most common cause is damage to the arachnoid villi, which interferes with the reabsorption of CSF. This commonly occurs in SAH and bacterial meningitis.

SYMPTOMS/ASSESSMENT

- *What are two common signs of hydrocephalus?*
- **Headache and nausea/vomiting**

Hydrocephalus is an increase in CSF volume and typically presents with headache and nausea/vomiting (Box 5.29).

Box 5.29 Symptoms of Hydrocephalus

Decreased LOC	Diplopia
Headache	Seizures
Nausea and vomiting	

TREATMENT

- *What is the primary surgical treatment for the management of hydrocephalus?*
- **Shunt placement**

A shunt provides an open communication between the ventricular system and a drainage cavity, most often the peritoneum. Other cavities to drain include the right atrium and pleura. Complications of a shunt include obstruction, overdrainage of CSF, and shunt infection.

ICP MONITORING AND LUMBAR DRAINS

▪ *Where is an intraventricular catheter placed for ICP monitoring?*
▪ **Anterior horn of lateral ventricle**

ICP monitoring is commonly used when managing a patient with a neurological disorder resulting in an increase in ICP. In combination with BP, it is currently the best way to continuously monitor cerebral perfusion. ICP monitors can be placed in several areas of the brain, including the epidural space, subarachnoid space, intraparenchymal, and intraventricular. Intraventricular catheters are considered the gold standard because they are placed directly into the ventricles, typically the anterior horn of the lateral ventricle.

> ❯ **HINT**
> The intraventricular catheters can also be used to manage increased ICP by draining CSF.

INDICATIONS FOR ICP MONITORING

▪ *What is the most common reason for placement of an ICP monitor?*
▪ **Decrease in LOC**

There are many different neurological scenarios that warrant the placement of an ICP monitor. The most common indications include a TBI with a Glasgow Coma Scale (GCS) score of 8 or less and a significantly abnormal CT scan (Box 5.30).

Box 5.30 General Indications for ICP Monitoring

Hydrocephalus: communicating and noncommunicating	Infections: meningitis, encephalitis
	Brain relaxation in the operating room (OR)
Subarachnoid hemorrhage (SAH): acute hydrocephalus or Hunt and Hess Grade ≥ III	Space-occupying lesions
Cerebral edema	
Surgical mass lesions	

> ❯ **HINT**
> ICP monitoring not only provides information regarding pressure and perfusion, but it also shows compliance of the brain. ICP waveform analysis is used to determine compliance.

▪ *What ICP waveform abnormality would indicate a decrease in brain compliance?*
▪ **P2 component greater than the P1 component**

The normal ICP waveform is a three-peaked wave, similar in shape to the arterial waveform. The peaks are labeled P1, P2, and P3. The P1 component is the highest in amplitude, followed by P2 and P3 in a descending manner. As the ICP increases, the amplitude of all the peaks also increases. When the P2 component becomes greater than the P1, it is an indication of noncompliance in the cranium and may require intervention at this time.

■ **What is the external landmark used to level the transducer of the ICP monitor?**
■ **Tragus of the ear or outer canthus of the eye**

Either landmark is acceptable. It is recommended though that the same external landmark be used consistently. These external landmarks approximate the transducer level to the foramen of Monro, which is the zero reference level.

■ **How do you control the amount of CSF drainage from an external ventricular drain (EVD)?**
■ **Raise or lower the drainage system**

Drainage of CSF is based on hydrostatic pressure. Leveling the fluid-filled EVD at or above the zero reference level controls the amount of drainage. When the ICP is higher than the set pressure level, CSF will drain. The lower the pressure level, the greater the amount of CSF drainage.

■ **How do you calculate CPP?**
■ **CPP = MAP − ICP**

MAP is the driving force and ICP is the opposing force. The difference between the two is the pressure needed to perfuse the brain. A decrease in MAP or an increase in ICP can cause hypoperfusion. A normal CPP is greater than 60 mmHg. A CPP between 40 and 60 mmHg is hypoperfusion and a CPP less than 40 mmHg indicates anoxic brain injury. The goal is typically to maintain CPP greater than 60 or 70 mmHg, depending on the neurological disorder.

■ **What is a complication of overdrainage of CSF?**
■ **Hemispheric shift**

If the CSF is drained too rapidly or an overdrainage occurs, it can cause a shift of the brain laterally and an uncal herniation (Box 5.31).

Box 5.31 EVD Complications and Management

Complication	Prevention	Management
Infection	Antibiotic-impregnated ventricular catheters Aseptic technique of placement of catheter Aseptic technique of flushing the EVD tubing with initial setup Strict sterile dressing change	Cerebrospinal fluid (CSF) analysis if infection is suspected Antimicrobial therapy Remove infected catheters, if possible
CSF leak	Assess catheter site and dressing for CSF drainage	Inform physician immediately if intracranial pressure (ICP) dressing is wet May place a suture or remove the catheter

(continued)

Box 5.31 EVD Complications and Management (*continued*)

Complication	Prevention	Management
Aneurysm rebleed	Monitor ICP and ICP drainage carefully Prevent CSF overdrainage	Rapid recognition and notification of the physician Control blood pressure
Hemispheric shifts	Monitor ICP and ICP drainage carefully Prevent CSF overdrainage	Rapid recognition and notification of the physician Clamp the EVD
CSF overdrainage Subdural hematoma formation Herniation	Maintain the EVD drip chamber at the prescribed level Inform patient/family not to change level of bed without assistance Ensure zero reference is maintained Clamp EVD any time there is a procedure that may cause CSF overdrainage	Rapid recognition and notification of the physician Clamp the EVD
Hemorrhage	Assure international normalized ratio (INR) is within normal range prior to catheter placement	May require surgical management
Misplacement of catheter	Ensure postprocedural CT scan, if ordered, is performed in a timely manner Perform ICP waveform assessment Assure catheter drainage is CSF by performing a halo test	Removal and replacement of catheter

LUMBAR DRAINS

Lumbar drainage devices (LDDs) are systems that are placed in the subarachnoid space at the lumbar level (L_2–L_3 level or below) and are used to obtain CSF samples or drain CSF. LDDs are commonly used in the treatment of dural fistulae, shunt infections, and in the diagnostic evaluation of idiopathic normal-pressure hydrocephalus (Box 5.32).

Box 5.32 Relative and Absolute Contraindications for LDDs

Relative Contraindications	Absolute Contraindications
Coagulopathy	Increased intracranial pressure (ICP)
Brain abscess	Unequal pressures between supratentorial and infratentorial compartments
History prior to lumbar spine surgery	Infected skin over needle-entry site
History of prior lumbar vertebral fracture	Spinal epidural abscess
	Intracranial mass
	Obstructive noncommunicating hydrocephalus
	Spinal arteriovenous malformation

■ *What is a common complication following placement of a lumbar drain?*
■ **Postprocedural puncture headache**

A common complication of a lumbar puncture or drain is a headache following the procedure. This may be managed by keeping the head of the bed flat and administering analgesics. If this does not alleviate headache, a blood patch may be performed (Box 5.33).

Box 5.33 Complications of Lumbar Drain

Radicular nerve pain
CSF leak
CNS infection (e.g., meningitis)
EDH
Catheter fracture
Herniation
Cerebral venous thrombosis
Overdrainage of CSF
Occlusion of tubing

> **HINT**
> A patient with an epidural catheter for pain management could have similar potential complications to those needing lumbar drains.

■ **What should you do with the LDD when making changes in the patient's position?**

■ **Clamp the drainage system**

A position change can affect the amount of drainage. Clamping the catheter's drainage system while making changes in the patient's position will prevent overdrainage from occurring. Overdrainage can result in SDH and tension pneumocranium. After repositioning, the LDD should be leveled and the drainage assessed.

BIBLIOGRAPHY

Broderick, J., et al. (2009). AHA/ASA guidelines for the management of spontaneous intracerebral hemorrhage in adults. *Stroke, 38*, 2001–2023.

del Zoppo, G. J., Saver, J. L., Jauch, E. C., & Adams, H. P. Jr. (2009). Expansion of the time window for treatment of acute ischemic stroke with intravenous tissue plasminogen activator. *Stroke, 40,* 2945–2948.

Easton, J. D., Saver, J. L., Albers, G. W., Alberts, M. J., Chaturvedi, S., Feldmann, E., Sacco, R. L., American Heart Association, American Stroke Association Stroke Council, Council on Cardiovascular Surgery and Anesthesia, Council on Cardiovascular Radiology and Intervention, Council on Cardiovascular Nursing, & Interdisciplinary Council on Peripheral Vascular Disease. (2009). Definition and evaluation of transient ischemic attack. *Stroke, 40*, 2276–2293.

Fisher, R. S., Van Emde Boas, W., Blume, W., Elger, C., Genton, P., Lee, P., & Engel, J. Jr. (2005). Epileptic seizures and epilepsy definitions proposed by the International League Against Epilepsy (ILAE) and the International Bureau for Epilepsy (IBE). *Epilepsia, 46*, 470–472.

Goldstein, B., et al. (2011). Guidelines for primary prevention of stroke. *Stroke, 42*, 517–584.

Tunkel, A. R., Hartman, B. J., Kaplan, S. L., Kaufman, B. A., Roos, K. L., Scheld, W. M., & Whitley, R. J. (2004). Practice guidelines for the management of bacterial meningitis. *Clinical Infectious Diseases, 34*, 1267–1284.

Wijdicks, E., Varelas, P. N., Gronseth, G. S., & Greer, D. M. (2010). Evidence-based guideline update: Determining brain death in adults. *Neurology, 74*, 1911–1918.

Questions

1. A postcraniotomy patient suddenly stops responding and begins to have a tonic–clonic seizure. Which of the following drugs is considered the preferred first-line antiepileptic agent to give during a seizure?

   A. Diazepam
   B. Lorazepam
   C. Phenytoin
   D. Phenobarbital

2. A family member of a patient in the ICU, who recently experienced a TBI, asks the nurse how long the patient will have to be on seizure medications as the patient has not had a seizure. Which of the following would be the nurse's best answer?

   A. The patient will have to be on seizure medications for the rest of her life.
   B. Ask the neurologist that question.
   C. Typically, following trauma, seizure medications are given for 7 days if no seizures occur.
   D. The neurologist will reevaluate her during the 3-month follow-up clinic visit.

3. A patient is diagnosed with an ischemic stroke but is 4.0 hours out from the initial onset of stroke symptoms. Which of the following is an additional exclusion if considering using the 4.5-hour window to administer IV tPA?

   A. If taking oral anticoagulants, INR must be < 2.5
   B. Has a baseline National Institutes of Health (NIH) Stroke Scale < 20
   C. History of both stroke and diabetes
   D. Patient is younger than 50 years old

4. When is it recommended to administer antihypertensive agents to a patient with acute ischemic stroke who is not a candidate for tPA?

   A. Systolic > 220 mmHg
   B. Diastolic > 105 mmHg
   C. Systolic > 180 mmHg
   D. Diastolic > 90 mmHg

5. Which of the following should be treated to prevent infarct expansion and worsening of cerebral edema in acute ischemic stroke patients?

   A. Hypernatremia
   B. Fever
   C. Hyperkalemia
   D. Metabolic alkalosis

6. When administering hyperosmolar therapy to manage an increased ICP, when would the nurse hold the dose of mannitol?

   A. ICP > 20 mmHg
   B. Urine output > 200 mL/hr

C. Serum osmolality > 320 mOsm/kg

D. Sodium levels < 125 mEq/L

7. During the first 24 to 48 hours after an SAH due to a ruptured aneurysm, which of the following is the most appropriate medical intervention?

A. Administer PRBCs

B. Administer albumin

C. Administer antihypertensives

D. Administer vasoconstrictors

8. Which of the following diagnostic procedures is considered the gold standard for the diagnosis of VS following SAH?

A. NIH Stroke Scale

B. Cerebral angiography

C. Transcranial Doppler

D. MRI

9. Mr. C was admitted 7 days ago for an SAH. An MCA aneurysm was coiled and the patient has been monitored in the ICU. He has suddenly developed a decrease in LOC. It is suspected that he has cerebral VS. Which of the following interventions is considered to be a part of the "triple H therapy"?

A. Hypertension

B. Hypovolemia

C. Hypothermia

D. Hyponatremia

10. A postcraniotomy patient develops respiratory failure and requires emergency intubation. Rapid sequence intubation (RSI) is proposed for the intubation process. Which of the following drugs would be the preferred induction drug in neurological patients?

A. Succinylcholine

B. Propofol

C. Vecuronium

D. Midazolam

11. A patient is admitted to the ICU with an intracerebral hemorrhage from chronic hypertension. His BP is currently 210/108 mmHg. The physician has ordered BP parameters of 130 to 150 mmHg. Which of the following antihypertensives would more likely exacerbate cerebral edema and increase ICP?

A. Labetalol

B. Nicardipine

C. Esmolol

D. Nipride

12. Following an SAH, a patient has been noted to have a sodium level of 124 mEq/L. He was found to have cerebral salt wasting syndrome and 3% hypertonic NaCl was ordered to correct the sodium level. Which of the following can be a complication of administering the hypertonic solution too rapidly?

    A. Cerebral herniation
    B. Coma
    C. CPM
    D. Cerebral edema

13. A patient with a history of MG is admitted because of increased weakness. His vital capacity and negative inspiratory force were evaluated by the respiratory therapist and impending respiratory failure was predicted. He stated he had been feeling bad lately and had been doubling his dose of pyridostigmine. Which of the following is the most likely cause for the respiratory failure?

    A. Cushing's syndrome
    B. Steroid overdose
    C. Myasthenia crisis
    D. Cholinergic crisis

14. A myasthenia crisis can be a clinical emergency with a need for rapid intervention. Which of the following is considered the initial intervention of choice for a hemodynamically unstable patient in a myasthenia crisis?

    A. IV immunoglobulin
    B. IV steroids
    C. Plasmaphoresis
    D. Anticholinesterase inhibitors

15. Following a gunshot wound to the head, an MRI was ordered by the physician. Which of the following is the most appropriate response by the nurse?

    A. Take the patient to get an MRI as ordered
    B. Inform the physician a CT scan is a better radiographic study for TBIs
    C. Remind the physician of the concern of metal fragments remaining within the cranium
    D. Discuss with the physician the need for immediate surgery

16. Ms. K is a 22-year-old female who was thrown from a vehicle and admitted for a TBI. The report from the previous nurse states she is localizing to pain and pupils are equal and reactive to light. During your assessment, you note her left pupil is dilated and unresponsive. Which of the following would be the most likely cause for the change in neurological status?

    A. Left-sided EDH
    B. Bilateral cerebral edema
    C. Right-sided acute SDH
    D. Right-sided EDH

17. Following a blunt TBI, Ms. G is in the ICU with a ventriculostomy, mechanically ventilated, and receiving propofol for sedation. The family asks the nurse how long Mrs. G

will be in the ICU and on sedation. Which of the following would be the best answer by the ICU nurse?

A. Most patients only have to have ICP monitoring for 24 hours after their injury
B. She will typically be sedated and monitored for at least 2 to 3 days until the peak period of cerebral edema is reached
C. You will have to ask the neurosurgeon when he plans to take her to surgery
D. Sedation is required in managing her brain injury and may continue indefinitely

18. Which of the following ventilator techniques used to manage acute respiratory distress syndrome (ARDS) should be avoided in a TBI patient with an increased ICP?

A. Positive end-expiratory pressure (PEEP)
B. Pressure release ventilation (PRV)
C. Pressure control ventilation (PC)
D. Permissive hypercapnia

19. A patient has been in the ICU for 5 days following a craniotomy for a tumor resection. He has been on decadron, propofol, and fentanyl to manage an elevated ICP and cerebral edema. He is now developing metabolic acidosis and hyperkalemia. Which of the following would be the most likely cause?

A. Cushing's disease
B. Long-term neurological and cognitive dysfunction (LNCD)
C. Sepsis
D. Propofol infusion syndrome

20. During testing for brain death, which two complications may occur during the apnea testing and should be closely monitored?

A. Hypercapnia and metabolic acidosis
B. Hypotension and cardiac arrhythmias
C. Bradycardia and hypertension
D. Aspiration and hypoxia

21. Which CNs should be assessed prior to allowing patients with neurological injury to drink liquids?

A. III, IV, and VI
B. V, VII, and VIII
C. IX, X, and XII
D. I, II, and III

22. During ICP monitoring, a patient's ICP is noted to be 15 mmHg and his ICP waveform has changed. The P2 component is now greater than the P1 component. What does this most likely represent?

A. Noncompliance of the brain
B. Increased ICP
C. Onset of A waves
D. It is not a significant finding

23. Potential organ donors can develop hemodynamic instability that may have an adverse effect on the donor organs. Typically, thyroxine T4 is administered with a goal to decrease vasopressor requirements. Which of the following is the most correct statement regarding the mechanism of improving hemodynamics with thyroxine?

A. Increases the release of catecholamines to improve BP
B. Reverses the diabetes insipidus (DI) and volume loss
C. Replaces the deficient hormone due to pituitary dysfunction
D. Improves sympathetic tone by stimulating the ANS

24. Where is the most common site for an obstructive hydrocephalus (noncommunicating) to occur?

A. Aqueduct of Sylvius
B. Foramen of Magnum
C. Posterior horn of the lateral ventricle
D. Foramen of Monro

25. Which of the following is the most effective management of anoxic brain-injured patients?

A. Mannitol
B. Steroids
C. Hypertonic 3% NaCl
D. Therapeutic hypothermia

Gastrointestinal System Review

In this chapter, you will review:

- Pancreatitis
- Gastrointestinal hemorrhage
- Acute liver failure
- Abdominal trauma
- Bowel infarctions/obstructions/perforations
- Malabsorption and malnutrition
- Abdominal compartment syndrome
- Enteral and parenteral nutrition

PANCREATITIS

- *Which of the types of pancreatitis has the greatest morbidity and mortality?*
- **Hemorrhagic (necrotizing) pancreatitis**

Pancreatitis is an inflammatory response with potential necrosis of pancreatic cells, resulting from premature activation of pancreatic digestive enzymes. It is caused by the escape of enzymes into surrounding pancreatic tissue, producing interstitial edema. Interstitial (edematous) pancreatitis is more self-limiting with lower acuity and better outcomes. Hemorrhagic (necrotizing) pancreatitis involves fat necrosis and hemorrhage within the pancreatic parenchyma. It is more severe and has a higher mortality.

> ❯ HINT
> On initial presentation it may be difficult to determine the severity of pancreatitis.

PATHOPHYSIOLOGY

- *Does the stimulation of the pancreas to release digestive enzymes occur with activation of the sympathetic or parasympathetic autonomic nervous system?*
- **Parasympathetic nervous system (PNS)**

PNS is responsible for stimulation of the gastrointestinal (GI) system, including the pancreas, via the vagal nerve. The pancreas produces approximately 1,500 to 2,500 mL of fluid in 24 hours. Limiting pancreatic stimulation to decrease the production of digestive enzymes during periods of pancreatitis is a mainstay of treatment (Box 6.1).

> **HINT**
PNS is the "rest and feed" portion of the autonomic nervous system.

Box 6.1 Pancreatic Stimulation

Parasympathetic nervous system stimulation	Small bowel stimulation
Gastric distention	Release secretin and cholecystokinin

■ *Which of the digestive enzymes produced from the pancreas breaks down protein?*

■ **Trypsin**

Trypsinogen is the precursor to trypsin, which is a proteolytic enzyme produced to break-down or digest proteins. Normally, digestive enzymes remain inactivated until they are within the duodenum. Pancreatic injury can lead to the cleavage of trypsinogen to trypsin, causing autodigestion of the pancreas. The activated trypsin may also activate other digestive enzymes such as amylase and lipase, furthering pancreatic injury (Box 6.2).

> **HINT**
This activates the neutrophils and macrophages, causing a local inflammation within the pancreas.

Box 6.2 Digestive Enzymes

Digestive Enzymes	Role
Trypsin	Protein to amino acids
Amylase	Carbohydrate to glucose
Lipase	Lipids to free fatty acids
Elastase	Elastin

■ *What is the primary reason for injury to the pancreatic parenchyma in pancreatitis?*

■ **Activation of digestive enzymes within the pancreas**

Initial injury of the acinar cells causes the activation of the digestive enzymes, especially trypsin, within the pancreas, resulting in autodigestion of the pancreas. Hemorrhagic pancreatitis is characterized by a cycle in which release and activation of more digestive enzymes leads to further pancreatic necrosis.

> **HINT**
The continual cycle of activation and necrosis in the pancreas is the reason for serial surgeries to debride the pancreas in hemorrhagic pancreatitis (Box 6.3).

Box 6.3 Three Stages of Hemorrhagic Pancreatitis

Stage I: Activation of digestive enzymes	Premature activation of trypsin within pancreatic acinar cells Once activated, activates other digestive enzymes Begin autodigestion of pancreas

(continued)

Box 6.3 Three Phases of Hemorrhagic Pancreatitis *(continued)*

Stage II: Intrapancreatic inflammation	Activates neutrophils and macrophages Releases proinflammatory cytokines Increases vascular permeability Promotes thrombosis and hemorrhage Leads to ischemia and necrosis
Stage III: Extrapancreatic inflammation	Systemic inflammatory response Acute respiratory distress syndrome (ARDS) Multisystem organ failure

> **❯ HINT**
> Requires abdominal computed tomography (CT) scan to differentiate
> sterile and infected pancreatic necrotic tissue (Box 6.4).

Box 6.4 Necrotic Pancreatic Tissue

Sterile Pancreatic Necrosis	Infected Pancreatic Necrosis
Aseptic necrotic tissue	Presence of bacteria within necrotic tissue
Less severe	Greater severity and mortality
May involve organ failure but is less frequent	Greater incidence of multisystem organ failure

■ *What are the two most common causes of pancreatitis in the United States?*
■ **Alcoholism and gallstones**

Chronic alcoholism may cause pancreatitis through several mechanisms. Alcohol increases pressure in the pancreatic ductal system, resulting in atony and edema of the sphincter of Oddi, permitting reflux of duodenal contents with activated enzymes. Alcohol-induced ductal hypertension is also associated with permeability changes in the duct, allowing enzymes to leak out to the surrounding tissues. Excessive alcohol use may lead to activation of proteolytic enzymes within the pancreas. Gallstones cause pancreatitis by obstruction of the ampulla of Vater (common bile duct) causing pressure to back up into the pancreatic duct (Boxes 6.5 and 6.6).

Box 6.5 Causes of Pancreatitis

Chronic alcoholism	Vasculitis
Binge drinking	Iatrogenic
Pancreatic tumors	Endoscopic retrograde cholangiopancreatography
Allergies	Liver biopsy
Metal toxicities	Cardiopulmonary bypass
Pancreatic trauma	Congenital
Drug induced Salicylates Thiazide diuretics Corticosteroids Estrogen contraceptive	Autoimmune response Hypercalcemia

Box 6.6 Mechanism of Drug-Induced Pancreatitis

Pancreatic duct constriction	Accumulation of a toxic metabolite
Cytotoxic and metabolic effects	Hypersensitivity reactions

SYMPTOMS/ASSESSMENT

■ *What is the symptom considered to be the hallmark of pancreatitis?*
■ **Epigastric pain**

Severe onset of acute epigastric pain accompanied by nausea and vomiting is the hallmark of pancreatitis. Pain is frequently described as severe, relentless, knife-like, and twisting deep in the midepigastrium region or periumbilical region. It may radiate to the back. The patient will take a knee-to-chest position to relieve the pain. Supine positions typically exacerbate the pain (Box 6.7).

> ❯ **HINT**
> Onset of pain may be associated with heavy fatty meals (biliary) or binge drinking (alcohol related).

Box 6.7 Symptoms of Pancreatitis

Epigastric pain	Grey Turner' sign
Low-grade fever	Cullen's sign
Nausea and vomiting	Fox's sign
Abdominal tenderness and guarding	Jaundice (biliary)
Hypotension	Steatorrhea (biliary)
Hypoactive or absent bowel sounds	

■ *What is the presence of ecchymosis along the flank in hemorrhagic pancreatitis called?*
■ **Grey Turner's sign**

Hemorrhagic pancreatitis can cause tissue ecchymosis. When present along the flank area, the ecchymosis is in the retroperitoneal space and is called Grey Turner's sign. Cullen's sign is bruising in the periumbilical area due to ecchymosis in the intraperitoneal and Fox's sign is bruising at the inguinal ligament.

> ❯ **HINT**
> Ecchymosis signs are not usually present on initial presentation.

DIAGNOSIS

■ *Which two laboratory values are most frequently used to assist with the diagnosis of pancreatitis?*
■ **Amylase and lipase**

Damaged acinar cells release digestive enzymes systemically. Among those frequently measured are amylase and lipase. Both amylase and lipase elevate rapidly (within 3–6 hours) following the onset of pancreatitis; lipase has a longer half-life, therefore it remains elevated longer (8–14 days). Neither is specific for pancreatitis and can be elevated in other disorders.

> **HINT**
Degree of amylase or lipase elevation has no prognostic significance (Box 6.8).

Box 6.8 Other Causes of Elevated Amylase and Lipase

Perforated ulcer	Cholecystitis
Small bowel obstruction	Peritonitis
Acute kidney injury	Stomach tumors
Salivary glandular disease	

■ *Diagnosis of pancreatitis requires two of three signs. What are the three diagnostic evaluations used to diagnose pancreatitis?*

■ **Pain, amylase, and CT scan**

Diagnosis requires two of the three signs:

1. Abdominal pain characteristic of pancreatitis
2. Serum amylase and/or lipase more than three times the upper limit of normal
3. Characteristic findings of acute pancreatitis on CT scan

> **HINT**
Elevation of amylase by three times or greater than normal is almost always the result of pancreatitis.

■ *Which radiographic test is the gold standard for diagnosing pancreatitis?*

■ **Abdominal CT scan with IV contrast**

Abdominal CT scans can differentiate between interstitial and necrotizing pancreatitis reliably with IV contrast after 2 to 3 days; the degree of necrosis is also prognostic. Abdominal CT scans are used to estimate size of the pancreas, evaluate cystic lesions, and identify fluid collections. MRI is not as widely used but may have some advantages, including lack of nephrotoxicity of gadolinium and greater ability to differentiate necrosis from fluid. The use of MR cholangiopancreatography is increasingly used in evaluating pancreatitis.

> **HINT**
Early CT scan (within 24 hours of illness onset) might underestimate the amount of necrosis but is an indicator that rules out other causes of abdominal pain.

■ *Which radiographic study is the diagnostic test of choice to evaluate for gallstones?*

■ **Abdominal ultrasound**

The main role of abdominal ultrasound is to identify the presence of gallstones. It is not accurate for determining necrosis or inflammation of the pancreas. Endoscopic retrograde cholangiopancreatography (ERCP) is used to identify anomalies and evaluate the biliary tract for strictures or stones. It may be considered in recurrent episodes of pancreatitis.

■ *Which laboratory value, when elevated, may be used to assist in determining the prognosis of pancreatitis?*

■ **Hematocrit (hct)**

A concentrated hct predicts the potential for complications of pancreatitis. It is an early marker for organ failure and pancreatic necrosis when elevated within 24 hours. Leaking of exudate (third spacing) results in the increase in hct and is defined as hct greater than 44% on admission (Box 6.9).

> ❯ HINT
> A significant decrease in hct following volume replacement indicates that elevated hct was concentrated.

Box 6.9 Abnormal Laboratory Findings in Pancreatitis

Concentrated hematocrit	Hypocalcemia
Hyperamylasemia	Hyponatremia
Hyperlipasemia	Elevated liver enzymes
Leukocytosis	Hyperglycemia
Hypokalemia	Hyperlipidemia

■ *What does the Ranson criteria determine in pancreatitis patients?*

■ **Severity of pancreatitis**

Ranson criteria are frequently used to determine the severity of pancreatitis and correlate to mortality. Ranson criteria comprise a total of 11 criteria, 5 of which are determined on admission and the remaining 6 during the first 48 hours. The Apache II score and CT-based severity index can also be used to determine severity.

> ❯ HINT
> Presence of three of five Ranson criteria on admission is considered severe pancreatitis (Box 6.10).

Box 6.10 Ranson Criteria

On Admission	During Initial 48 Hours
Age older than 55 years	Hematocrit decreases > 10%
White blood cells (WBC) > 16,000/mL	Blood urea nitrogen increases of > 5 mg/dL
Lactate dehydrogenase (LDH) > 350 IU/L	Ca^{++} < 8 mg/dL
Aspirate aminotransferase > 250 IU/L	P_aO_2 < 60 mmHg
Glucose > 200 mg/dL	Base deficit > 4 mg/dL
	Fluid sequestration > 6 L

MEDICAL MANAGEMENT

■ *What is considered the most important component in the management of hemorrhagic pancreatitis?*

■ **Fluid resuscitation**

Adequate fluid replacement is required to correct the severe fluid losses due to third spacing. Inadequate fluid replacement can cause intestinal ischemia with translocation of bacteria into the pancreas (infected necrosis) as well as distal organ hypoperfusion. Early resuscitation reduces the incidence of systemic inflammatory response syndrome (SIRS) and multisystem organ failure (MSOF). The target for fluid resuscitation is to correct concentrated hct and maintain adequate urine output. Administration of supplemental oxygen or intubation with mechanical ventilation in patients with compromised respiration is necessary. Pain control is also an important aspect of medically managing pancreatitis.

> **❯ HINT**
> Lactated Ringer's solution may be recommended to prevent hyperchloremic acidosis, which occurs with large volumes of 0.9% NaCl administration.

■ **What is the purpose of nothing by mouth (NPO) status in the patient with pancreatitis?**

■ **"Rest" pancreas**

Allowing the pancreas to "rest" and not release digestive enzymes will interrupt the progression of the pancreatic injury from autodigestion. The use of octreotide (Somatostatin, Sandostatin) has been used to decrease production of gastrin and cholecystokinin and to reduce secretions of the pancreas (Box 6.11).

> **❯ HINT**
> Distal feeding through a nasojejunal tube may have less complications than parenteral nutrition.

Box 6.11 Interventions to Decrease Pancreatic Stimulation

Nasogastric (NG) tube to low wall suction	Octreotide
NPO	Total parenteral nutrition or distal enteral feeding in jejunum
Proton pump inhibitors	

SURGICAL MANAGEMENT

■ **What is the primary surgical treatment for an infected necrosis of the pancreas?**

■ **Surgical debridement**

Infected necrosis of the pancreas typically requires some route of surgical debridement and may require multiple surgeries to completely debride the necrotic areas of the pancreas. Sterile necrosis usually does not require surgical debridement and may be managed medically for 2 to 3 weeks (Box 6.12).

> **❯ HINT**
> Debridement of sterile necrosis commonly results in development of infected necrosis.

Box 6.12 Types of Surgical Debridement

Necrosectomy with closed continuous irrigation via indwelling catheter	Percutaneous placement of drainage catheter
Necrosectomy and open packing	Minimally invasive retroperitoneal necrosectomy
Necrosectomy with closed drainage without irrigation	Laparoscopic necrosectomy
CT-guided needle aspiration	

> ❯ HINT
>
> Postoperative bleeding can be a life-threatening complication of pancreatic debridement procedures.

COMPLICATIONS

■ *What is a fluid collection walled off by a rim of fibrous granulation tissue called?*

■ **Pseudocyst**

A pseudocyst is a collection of "sterile" fluid that is lined or walled off by a fibrous layer. If the fluid is infected and walled off by well-defined granulated tissue, it is called a pancreatic abscess. Pseudocysts can resolve spontaneously but they also have the potential of becoming infected, bleeding, or rupturing (Box 6.13).

> ❯ HINT
>
> Pain management is a high priority in patients who develop pseudocysts.

Box 6.13 Complications of Pancreatitis

Pancreatic Complications	Systemic Complications
Pancreatic necrosis	ARDS
Pseudocyst	Sepsis/systemic inflammatory response syndrome
Pancreatic abscess	Abdominal compartment syndrome
Fistula or pancreatic duct leak	Multisystem organ failure
	Disseminated intravascular coagulation

GASTROINTESTINAL HEMORRHAGE

■ *What is the landmark that divides the intestines between an upper and lower gastrointestinal bleed (GIB)?*

■ **Ligament of Treitz**

An upper GIB (UGIB) is defined as bleeding occurring proximal to the ligament of Treitz. The ligament of Treitz is the suspensory muscle of the duodenum that connects the duodenum to the diaphragm. This is the anatomical landmark of the duodenojejunal junction.

PATHOPHYSIOLOGY

■ *What is it called when a UGIB is caused by retching and vomiting?*
■ **Mallory–Weiss tear**

A Mallory–Weiss tear is a tear in the mucosa at the esophageal gastric junction caused by forceful vomiting or retching. The vomiting can be due to the flu, food poisoning, or eating disorders, but becomes bloody once the mucosa tears (Box 6.14).

Box 6.14 Causes of UGIB

Esophageal varices	Esophagitis
Peptic ulcer disease	Mallory–Weiss tear
Stress-related mucosal disease	Gastric/duodenal tumors
Diffuse gastritis	Angiodysplasia

■ *Critically ill patients are at a greater risk for UGIB due to the development of what GI complication?*
■ **Stress-related mucosal disease (SRMD)**

Ulcerations in the upper GI tract (stomach and duodenum) can occur within hours of a severe injury or major surgery. GI ulcerations caused by critical illness have several different names but are commonly called SRMD. The ulcerations range from superficial to deep ulcerations at risk for perforation. The most common complication of SRMD is UGIB.

> ❭ **HINT**
> Brain-injured patients and patients with burns are the two patient populations with the highest incidence of SRMD (Box 6.15).

Box 6.15 Risk Factors of SRMD

Mechanical ventilation	Hypotension and shock states
Coagulopathy	Hepatic failure
Major or multiple trauma	Renal failure
Sepsis and multisystem organ failure	Administration of steroids

■ *What causes the loss of secretion of protective mucus that shields the GI mucosa from the acids?*
■ **Hypoperfusion**

The development of SRMD is caused by multiple factors. The stomach is normally protected from the gastric acids by secretion of glycoprotein mucus that protects the mucosa and secretes bicarbonate to neutralize some of the acids. Hypotension or shock states cause vasoconstriction and shunts blood away from nonessential organs, such as the GI tract. Decreased gastric blood flow diminishes the amount of protective mucus secretions allowing acids to flow back into the mucosal layer, causing tissue injury.

> ❭ HINT
> There is also an increase in acid production during stress periods lowering the gastric pH.

■ *Which bacteria are frequently found colonizing the stomach and are associated with peptic ulcer disease?*

■ Helicobacter pylori

Colonization of the stomach by helicobacter pylori can result in chronic gastritis at the site of infection. Ulcers in the stomach and duodenum result when the consequences of inflammation allow stomach acid and the digestive enzyme pepsin to overwhelm the mechanisms that protect the stomach and duodenal mucous membrane.

■ *What is the underlying physiology that causes esophageal varices?*

■ Portal hypertension

Portal hypertension is caused by fibrotic changes in the liver that collapse and distort the hepatic vasculature; therefore, blood backs up and increases portal venous pressure. Portal hypertension results in the development of collateral circulation that redirects the portal venous blood flow through vessels of lower resistance in the esophagus and stomach (varices). Collateral blood flow also occurs in the rectum, resulting in hemorrhoids and lower GI bleeding (Box 6.16).

Box 6.16 Causes of Lower Gastrointestinal Bleed

Ulcerative colitis	Neoplasm
Mesenteric vascular ischemia	Hemorrhoids
Vascular ectasias	Angiodysplasia
Diverticulosis	

SYMPTOMS/ASSESSMENT

■ *What laboratory value is elevated in a UGIB but not in a lower gastrointestinal bleed (LGIB)?*

■ Blood urea nitrogen (BUN)

The BUN is elevated in UGIB because of greater absorption of protein in the stomach and duodenum (Box 6.17).

Box 6.17 Signs of Upper and Lower Gastrointestinal Bleeds

Upper Gastrointestinal Bleed	Lower Gastrointestinal Bleed
Hematemesis (coffee grounds or bloody)	No hematemesis
Melena stools (dark, tarry, odorous)	Bloody stools
Elevated blood urea nitrogen (normal creatinine)	Normal BUN
Decreased hemoglobin and hematocrit	Decreased hemoglobin and hematocrit

■ *What assessment tool can be used to determine the need for an intervention for a UGIB?*

■ **Blatchford score**

The Blatchford score is a tool used to assess UGIB patients to determine the likelihood that the patient will require an intervention. The higher score is more likely to require endoscopy and transfusions (Box 6.18).

Box 6.18 Blatchford Score

Admission Risk Marker	Score Component Value
BUN	
≥ 6·5 and <8·0	2
≥ 8·0 and <10·0	3
≥ 10·0 and < 25·0	4
≥ 25	6
Hemoglobin (g/L) for men	
≥12.0 and <13.0	1
≥10.0 <12.0	3
<10.0	6
Hemoglobin (g/L) for women	
≥10.0 <12.0	1
<10.0	6
Systolic blood pressure (mmHg)	
100–109	1
90–99	2
< 90	3
Other markers	
Pulse ≥100 (per minute)	1
Presentation with melena	1
Presentation with syncope	2
Hepatic disease	2
Cardiac failure	2

Scores of 6 or more are associated with a greater than 50% risk of needing an intervention.

DIAGNOSIS

■ *What is the most common diagnostic intervention for a UGIB?*

■ **Endoscopy**

An endoscopy is used to localize site of bleeding, determine the cause of the bleed, and allow the estimation of blood loss.

■ *What is the recommended diagnostic procedure to diagnose a LGIB?*

■ **Colonoscopy**

A colonoscopy is the recommended diagnostic procedure to identify a LGIB. Blood in the terminal ileocecal valve indicates the bleeding source is the small bowel. The small bowel can be visualized with push enteroscopy, double-balloon enteroscopy, and video capsule endoscopy. A more rapid bleed may use mesenteric angiography or CT angiography to localize the source. A slow bleed may be found with nuclear scintigraphy that involves nuclear tagging of the red blood cells (RBCs).

> **HINT**
> A full colonoscopy is recommended because of potential bleeding in the right colon.

MEDICAL MANAGEMENT

■ *Which two risk factors have the greatest incidence for SRMD and require prophylactic interventions?*
■ **Mechanical ventilation and coagulopathy**

Respiratory failure requiring mechanical ventilation and coagulopathy are the two risk factors for SRMD that are commonly documented as requiring GI prophylaxis. Mechanical ventilation may decrease splanchnic blood flow by lowering mean arterial pressure (MAP) and increasing vascular resistance of the GI tract. It can also initiate a proinflammatory response.

> **HINT**
> The greater the number of risk factors, the higher the risk of GI bleeding and, therefore, the greater the need for prophylaxis.

■ *Of the drugs used for GI prophylaxis, which class of drug has a greater risk for development of thrombocytopenia?*
■ **H_2-receptor antagonists**

GI prophylaxis can include antacids, H_2-receptor antagonists, sucralfate, and proton pump inhibitors. Of these drugs, H_2-receptor antagonists can cause thrombocytopenia as a side effect. Another proposed complication of H_2-receptor antagonists and antacids is a higher incidence of nosocomial pneumonias. The change of the pH from acidic to alkaline causes an overgrowth of bacteria in the stomach that can be aspirated into the lungs.

> **HINT**
> Proton pump inhibitors have been associated with a higher incidence of diarrhea and may have an association with *Clostridium difficile*.

■ *What is a potential contraindication for placement of a gastric tube following onset of vomiting blood?*
■ **Esophageal varices**

Placement of a gastric tube can damage the enlarged, tortuous varices in the esophagus, resulting in greater blood loss. Endoscopy prior to placement of a gastric tube is recommended to identify the source of bleeding and rule out esophageal varices. Gastric tubes have been used to lavage the stomach with saline or water to cause cooling. Cooling decreases peptic acid activity in the stomach, decreases gastric mucosal blood flow, and GI motility.

> ❯ HINT
>
> If a clot was present on ulcer bed, lavaging the gastric tube may dislodge the clot and worsen blood loss.

■ **What drug therapy is used to manage UGIB caused by varices?**
■ **Octreotide or terlipressin**

Octreotide administered as a continuous infusion in patients with variceal bleeds can lower the rate of hemorrhage. The effects of octreotide may include a decrease in portal hypertension and splanchnic blood flow. Terlipressin is an analog of vasopressin and produces vasoconstriction, thus reducing pressure in the portal vein. Terlipressin has minimal coronary vasoconstriction compared to vasopressin with reduced risks of causing coronary artery syndrome.

> ❯ HINT
>
> Vasopressin (Pitressin), administered as an IV infusion to manage UGIB, requires administration of nitroglycerin to protect form coronary vasoconstriction.

■ **What is the role of lactulose in managing a UGIB patient?**
■ **Prevents absorption of ammonia**

Lactulose and magnesium citrate are frequently given to patients with UGIB to prevent absorption of ammonia that is released in the bowel with blood degradation. Lactulose is metabolized by the enteric bacteria in the colon, resulting in the acidification of the stool, thus preventing ammonia from converting to an absorbable form. So, less ammonia is absorbed into the bloodstream, lowering the risk of encephalopathy. Magnesium citrate is used to purge the bowel of blood and fecal matter.

SURGICAL MANAGEMENT

■ **What would be an indication for surgical management of a UGIB caused by SRMD?**
■ **Active bleeding in a hemodynamically unstable patient**

Endoscopy therapy is the intervention of choice initially, but if the patient has ongoing bleeding and is hemodynamically unstable or required more than 6 units of packed red blood cells (PRBCs) in the past 48 hours, surgical management may be required.

> ❯ HINT
>
> A second endoscopy may be performed before surgical options are considered, because endoscopy is associated with fewer complications.

■ *What is the endoscopic treatment of varices?*

■ **Sclerotherapy or band ligation**

Sclerotherapy involves the injection of a sclerosing agent in and around the varices causing localized constrictive edema, induced thrombosis, and sclerosis of the vein, with minimal damage to the esophageal mucosa and muscle. This may be accomplished with vasoconstrictors, sclerosing agents, tissue adhesives, or saline. Band ligation can also be performed on the varice and in some studies has been shown to improve outcomes. Endoscopic band ligation is varices that are ligated and strangulated with small rubber bands. Ischemic necrosis of the mucosa within 24 hours, displacement of the bands in 3 to 7 days, and complete healing in 21 days are seen. If endoscopic therapy fails to control bleeding, a second attempt is recommended before surgical management of varices.

> **HINT**
> Indications for endoscopy intervention include actively bleeding ulcers and visible vessels in ulcer beds or varices.

■ *What is the most common surgical procedure to treat bleeding gastric ulcers not amendable by endoscopic interventions?*

■ **Antrectomy**

The removal of the antrum portion of the stomach that has the ulcer and produces acids will control hemorrhage and decrease risk of future development of gastric ulcers. The remaining portion of the stomach is anastomosed either to the duodenum (called Bilroth I) or to the jejunum (called Bilroth II). Truncal, selective, or highly selective vagotomy are other surgical options for treatment of peptic ulcer disease for acid suppression (Box 6.19).

> **HINT**
> Acid-reduction surgeries are less common because of the use of acid-suppressing proton pump inhibitors.

Box 6.19 Types of Gastric Ulcer Surgeries

Type of Gastric Ulcer	Location of Ulcer	Surgical Management
Type I	Lesser curvature of stomach	Wedge resection
Type II	Lesser curvature of stomach and duodenum	Truncal vagotomy or antrectomy
Type III	Prepyloric	Truncal vagotomy or antrectomy
Type IV	Lesser curve near cardiac and esophagogastric junction	Distal gastrectomy and Roux-en-Y reconstruction
Type V	Diffuse ulcers	Removal of the area of ulcer

■ *What is a less invasive procedure used to control hemorrhage of a gastric ulcer?*

■ **Angiography with embolization**

Angiography with embolization of bleeding vessels is another option to control hemorrhage of an actively bleeding ulcer. This involves embolization of the vessel within the ulcer bed with coils, gel foam, or polyvinyl alcohol.

> **HINT**
> Patient may remain on proton pump inhibitor therapy for continual acid suppression.

■ *What is a less invasive option for management of varices if endoscopy and variceal ligation are ineffective?*

■ **Transjugular intrahepatic portosystemic shunts (TIPS)**

In a TIPS procedure a shunt is placed between the portal and hepatic veins through a catheter in a nonsurgical procedure. The stent redirects some of the portal blood directly into the hepatic vein, thus decreasing portal pressure and decompression of varices.

> **HINT**
> Postprocedure management includes assessing for hemorrhage and management of pain (Box 6.20).

Box 6.20 Complications of TIPS Procedure

Pain	Inadvertent puncture of bile ducts, hepatic arteries, and hepatic capsule
Hemorrhage	
Infection at site or stent	New-onset encephalopathy
Allergic reaction to dye	Shunt occlusion or stenosis
Airway and respiratory compromise (conscious sedation)	Recurrent UGIB

■ *A splenorenal shunt placed for variceal bleeding reroutes which vein away from the portal vein to bypass the liver?*

■ **Splenic vein**

The splenic vein flows into the portal vein providing a portion of the blood that goes through the liver. A shunt is used to surgically manage portal hypertension by decreasing the volume of blood in the portal vein and diverting it around the liver. Splenorenal shunt involves the splenic vein shunt anastomoses to the left renal vein. Other shunts include portacaval shunt (portal vein anastomoses to inferior vena cava) and mesocaval shunt (superior mesenteric vein anastomoses to inferior vena cava). Patients who are transplant candidates are best treated with orthotopic liver transplantation.

> **HINT**
> Look at the name of the shunt to determine which vein is removed from the portal vein and where it is reconnected. The first part of the word indicates the vein that is being removed (splenic) and the second part of the word indicates where it has been anastomosed (renal vein).

■ *What is the nonshunt surgery to prevent recurrent variceal hemorrhaging?*
■ **Esophagogastric devascularization**

Esophagogastric devascularization is an effective nonshunt surgery to prevent recurrent bleeding from esophageal varices. This procedure may also be used in patients with ascites or splenic thrombosis, who are contraindicated for a shunt procedure. This involves ligation of venous branches entering the distal esophagus and proximal stomach. It combines this with highly selective vagotomy and pyloroplasty.

■ *What procedure is used to control LGIBs with hemodynamic instability?*
■ **Angiography**

Angiography is used to determine the location of the hemorrhaging in LGIB patients who are hemodynamically unstable and unable to undergo colonoscopy. It may also be used if the colonoscopy has been unable to localize the bleeding source. Embolization and intra-arterial vasopressin may be used to control hemorrhage. Surgery for an LGIB is not performed often because of complications and higher risk of mortality. Surgical management includes subtotal colectomy.

> ❯ HINT
> Patients who have undergone visceral embolization should be monitored for bowel ischemia for several days.

COMPLICATIONS

■ *A patient suddenly develops hypotension and complains of severe midsternal to midabdominal pain following an endoscopy. What potential endoscopy complications would be the most likely cause?*
■ **Esophageal perforation**

Iatrogenic perforation accounts for more than half of all esophageal perforations. Prompt recognition and treatment are required to prevent contamination of visceral spaces. Esophageal perforation is life threatening (Box 6.21).

> ❯ HINT
> Treatment of perforation of the esophagus during endoscopy is the placement of clips.

Box 6.21 Complications of Endoscopy

Esophageal perforation	Esophageal strictures
Esophageal hemorrhage	Bacteremia/sepsis
Aspiration	Myocardial infarction

■ *Following a splenorenal shunt, what is the neurological complication that may occur?*
■ **Hepatic encephalopathy**

The splenic vein is removed from the portal circulation and anastomosed to the renal artery that directly flows into the inferior vena cava. The amount of blood shunted around the liver correlates to the incidence of encephalopathy. The liver detoxifies the blood and makes ammonia water soluble to be removed by the kidneys. When blood is shunted around the liver, it results in the accumulation of ammonia and development of hepatic encephalopathy. Another complication of selective distal splenorenal shunt is ascites formation due to extensive retroperitoneal dissection.

> **HINT**
The greater amount of blood being bypassed around the liver, the greater the risk of encephalopathy.

ACUTE LIVER FAILURE

■ *How is acute liver failure (ALF) differentiated from chronic liver failure?*
■ **Length of time for onset of signs**

ALF is defined as the onset of hepatic encephalopathy and coagulopathy within 26 weeks of jaundice in a patient without preexisting liver disease. ALF can be a result of primary liver failure or secondary failure due to multisystem organ failure (MSOF).

> **HINT**
Patients with chronic liver failure typically have one or more complications.

PATHOPHYSIOLOGY

■ *What is the most common cause of ALF?*
■ **Acetaminophen**

Acetaminophen is a substance-induced ALF and is currently the most common cause of ALF. It can be due to intentional overdose or unintentional overdose. Accumulation of high levels of acetaminophen unintentionally occurs as a result of consuming multiple products containing acetaminophen. Unintended overdoses typically are not recognized until symptoms of liver failure develop (Box 6.22).

> **HINT**
The recommended dosing should not exceed 4,000 mg in a 24-hour period. The 24-hour dose may be lower (3,000 mg) in geriatric and alcohol-abuse patients.

Box 6.22 Causes of ALF

Infectious	Substance Induced	Other Disease Processes
Viral hepatitis (A to G)	Acetaminophen	Wilson disease
Coxsackie viruses	Alcohol	Fatty liver in pregnancy
Echoviruses	Carbon tetrachloride	Reye's syndrome
Adenoviruses	Wild mushrooms	Autoimmune hepatitis
	Parenteral hyperalimentation	Budd–Chiari syndrome
	Blood transfusion reaction	

■ *What is the physiological change that occurs with viral hepatitis resulting in liver failure?*

■ **Hepatocyte necrosis**

There are three major pathological changes that can occur within the liver that result in liver failure. These include necrosis of the hepatocytes, cirrhosis (widespread replacement of hepatocytes with fibrous tissue), and lesions within hepatocytes without necrosis (Box 6.23).

Box 6.23 Major Physiological Changes in Liver Failure

Hepatocyte Necrosis	Cirrhosis	Non-necrotic Lesions
Viral hepatitis	Cardiac (right heart failure)	Starvation
Drug-induced hepatitis	Biliary	Obesity
Hyperthermia	Alcohol ingestion	Alcohol ingestion
Blood transfusion reaction		Diabetes mellitus
Alcohol ingestion		Reye's syndrome
		Hyperalimentation

SYMPTOMS/ASSESSMENT

■ *What is the primary cause of the development of hepatic encephalopathy?*

■ **Elevated ammonia levels**

Liver failure patients are unable to convert ammonia (byproduct of protein) to urea for renal excretion. Hepatic encephalopathy is a clinical disorder characterized by impaired mentation, neuromuscular disturbances, and altered level of consciousness. It is due to elevated ammonia levels, which interfere with normal cerebral metabolism and the amount of energy produced by brain cells.

> **❯ HINT**
> The quantitative level of ammonia does not correlate with the grade of hepatic encephalopathy or prognosis (Box 6.24).

Box 6.24 Grades of Hepatic Encephalopathy

Grade of Encephalopathy	Symptoms
Grade I	Slight personality and behavioral changes Impaired mentation Reversal of sleep/wake patterns
Grade II	Mental confusion Asterixis (liver flap) Deterioration of handwriting
Grade III	Progressive confusion Decreased level of consciousness (LOC) but arousable Combative
Grade IV	Unresponsive

■ *What is the presence of spider angiomas across the face and chest in liver failure patients caused by?*

■ **Elevated estrogen**

The liver detoxifies substances by converting substances from a fat-soluble to a water-soluble state, which allows the kidneys to excrete the substance. Substances include sex hormones, ammonia, mineralcorticoids (aldosterone), glucocorticoids (cortisol), and numerous drugs.

> **〉 HINT**
> Drugs are typically metabolized (made water soluble) in the liver and excreted by the kidneys (Box 6.25).

Box 6.25 Symptoms of Liver Failure

Normal Liver Function	Symptoms of Liver Failure
Liver produces bile composed of bile salts to emulsify fats	Steatorrhea (fatty, clay-colored stools) Malnutrition (inability to absorb fats) Decreased absorption of fat-soluble vitamins
Synthesizes proteins (albumin)	Hypoalbuminemia Third-spacing Ascites
Stores Vitamin B	Vitamin B deficiency Anemia (folic acid deficiency) Peripheral nerve degeneration Nystagmus Paresthesia of feet
Absorption of Vitamin K	Coagulopathy
Produces coagulation factors	Thrombocytopenia
Removes activated clotting factors from blood	Elevated prothrombin time (PT)
Conjugates bilirubin (makes it water soluble for kidneys to remove)	Jaundice Dark, foamy urine Elevated bilirubin levels Pruritus (elevated bile salts deposited in skin)

(continued)

Box 6.25 Symptoms of Liver Failure *(continued)*

Normal Liver Function	Symptoms of Liver Failure

Detoxifies substances	Elevated estrogen
	  Spider angiomas
	  Gynecomastia
	  Testicular atrophy
	  Impotence in males
	Elevated ammonia
	  Hepatic encephalopathy
	Elevated aldosterone and antidiuretic
	  hormone (ADH)
	  Increased circulating blood volume
	  Palmar erythema
	  Sodium and water retention
	  Loss of potassium through kidneys
	  Increased ascites and edema
	Elevated cortisol
	  Moon face
	  Striae
	  Truncal obesity

> **HINT**
Liver function tests (LFTs) may elevate before clinical signs of liver dysfunction occur.

DIAGNOSIS

- *Which of the liver enzymes is the most specific for liver injury?*
- **Alanine aminotransferase (ALT)**

Enzymes are present within the liver cells (hepatocytes), when damaged, are released in serum. The aminotransferase enzymes are the most sensitive and widely used. ALT is also known as serum glutamic pyruvic transaminase (SGPT). It is typically found only with liver injury and is the most specific for liver damage. Aspirate aminotransferase (AST), also known as serum glutamic oxaloacetic transaminase (SGOT), is also used in diagnosing liver injury but is less specific. AST can elevate with myocardial injury and sepsis. The ratio of AST to ALT is sometimes used to differentiate between causes of liver diseases.

> **HINT**
ALT = SGPT and AST = SGOT

- *Which liver enzyme will increase with biliary duct obstructions?*
- **Alkaline phosphatase (ALP)**

ALP is the enzyme that lines the biliary ducts of the liver. Elevation of ALP occurs with biliary duct obstructions as well as intrahepatic cholestasis and infiltrative disease of the liver (Box 6.26).

Box 6.26 Liver Enzymes

Liver Enzyme	Normal Levels
Aspirate aminotransferase	5–60 U/L
Alanine aminotransferase	10–40 U/L
Alkaline phosphate	44–147 IU/L
Albumin	3.9–5.0 g/dL
Total bilirubin	0.2–1.2 mg/dL

Normal levels vary based on source or laboratory.

〉 HINT

Level of liver enzymes does not always correlate to the actual extent of liver damage or prognosis. For example, acute viral hepatitis A may develop really high AST/ALT but has full recovery, whereas chronic hepatitis C frequently has only a slight elevation of liver enzymes but has advanced damage and scarring of liver (Boxes 6.27 and 6.28).

Box 6.27 Liver Enzyme Elevation With Hepatic Injury

Highest Level Elevations of LFTs	Mild to Moderate Elevations of LFTs
Hepatitis B and C	Normal variation
Acetaminophen overdose	Chronic hepatitis C
Alcohol–acetaminophen syndrome	Fatty liver due to: Obesity Diabetes mellitus
Prolonged hypoperfusion	Biliary obstruction
Active cirrhosis	
Primary or metastatic cancer	
Alcoholic induced	
Reye's syndrome	

Box 6.28 Specific LFT Findings

Acute Viral Hepatitis	Complete Biliary Obstruction	Cirrhosis	Liver Metastasis
Aspartate aminotransferase (AST) 14 × nml	AST 3 × nml	AST 2 × nml	AST 1–2 × nml
Alanine aminotransferase (ALT) 17 × nml	ALT 4 × nml	ALT 1–2 × nml	ALT 1–2 × nml
Alkaline phosphate (ALP) 1–2 × nml	ALP 4–14 × nml	ALP 1–2 × nml	ALP 10–20 × nml

nml, normal.

■ *If the patient's total bilirubin is elevated but the direct bilirubin is normal, is the abnormality in the liver or bile ducts?*

■ Liver

If the total bilirubin is elevated, then looking at the direct and indirect bilirubin can assist with determining where the injury is located. If direct bilirubin (conjugated bilirubin) is normal, then the problem is excess of unconjugated bilirubin (indirect bilirubin). The problem is within the liver, such as the effects of viral hepatitis or due to hemolysis. If direct bilirubin is elevated, the liver is conjugating the bilirubin normally but is not able to excrete it. Bile duct obstruction by gallstones or cancer should be suspected.

> HINT
Conjugated bilirubin is water soluble and goes "directly" to the kidneys for excretion. So the laboratory value of direct bilirubin measures conjugated bilirubin (or after the liver).

MEDICAL MANAGEMENT

■ *A patient presents with an acute overdose of acetaminophen. What is the antidote used to reverse the hepatic involvement?*

■ **N-acetylcysteine (NAC)**

If a known toxin causes the ALF, acute management should include known antidotes to the toxin. For acetaminophen overdoses, intravenous NAC is the antidote recommended. In managing symptoms of ALF, including encephalopathy and coagulopathy, NAC is administered until reversal of symptoms (resolution of encephalopathy, international normalized ratio [INR] is less than 1.5, and liver enzymes are declining).

> HINT
Treat the underlying cause if possible. For example, steroids are used to treat autoimmune hepatitis, lamivudine is used for hepatitis B patients, and acyclovir is used for herpes simplex.

SURGICAL MANAGEMENT

■ *What set of criteria is commonly used to determine the prognosis of ALF and potential candidate for liver transplant?*

■ **King's College Criteria**

This is a prognostic tool that is used for patients who present with ALF and is used to determine potential candidates for liver transplantation in ALF (Box 6.29).

Box 6.29 King's College Criteria Predicting Poor Outcome in ALF

Acetaminophen Induced	Non–acetaminophen Induced
pH < 7.3 after fluid resuscitation or arterial lactate > 3.5 at 4 hours or arterial lactate > 3 at 12 hours or all of the following: INR > 6.5 Serum creatinine > 3.4 mg/dL Grade 3 or 4 hepatic encephalopathy	INR > 6.5 or any three of the following: Age younger than 10 or older than 40 years Time from onset of jaundice to the development of coma of more than 7 days PT > 50 seconds (INR > 3.5) Serum bilirubin > 17.5 g/dL

COMPLICATIONS

■ *What role does the liver play in preventing infections and bacteremia?*
■ **Filters blood**

The normal function of the liver is to filter the blood. Kupfer cells line the sinusoids to remove bacteria from the blood, especially from the GI tract. Virtually no bacteria reach systemic circulation, but in liver failure, Kupfer cells have limited ability for phagocytosis and bacteria reach systemic circulation. This causes the patient to be prone to infection, bacteremia, and overwhelming sepsis.

> **❯ HINT**
> Minimize invasive lines and administer antibiotics with signs of sepsis or SIRS.

■ *What is the most common cause of death in liver failure?*
■ **Hepatorenal syndrome**

Hepatorenal syndrome is progressive renal failure that is associated with acute or chronic liver disease. It is the leading cause of death in hepatic failure. There are no anatomical or histological changes and the syndrome is thought to be caused by decreased renal perfusion. Management includes the treatment of the underlying hepatic failure and fluid resuscitation (Box 6.30).

Box 6.30 Symptoms of Hepatorenal Syndrome

Oliguria	Increased urine osmolality
Hyponatremia	Elevated blood urea nitrogen and creatinine

■ *What is the acute complication of hepatic encephalopathy and elevated ammonia levels?*
■ **Increased intracranial pressure (ICP)**

An ICP can lead to long-term neurological deficits and is a cause of death in ALF. The mechanism of cerebral edema is not totally understood but may be due to the conversion of ammonia to glutamine by the astrocytes in the brain. Management includes treating the cerebral edema and managing ammonia levels with lactulose.

> **❯ HINT**
> Highest incidence is a rapid presentation of ALF from jaundice to encephalopathy in fewer than 4 weeks.

■ *Which drug is primarily used in the management of the coagulopathy in ALF?*
■ **Vitamin K**

The coagulopathy of ALF is caused by a combination of vitamin K deficiency, abnormal clotting cascades, and platelet dysfunction. Clinically significant bleeding is relatively uncommon and management typically includes empirical administration of vitamin K. Fresh frozen plasma (FFP) should only be used to reverse coagulopathy in a patient with clinically significant bleeding. Cryoprecipitate may be used in a patient with low fibrinogen levels.

> **HINT**
> To prevent complication of GI bleeding, GI prophylaxis is important with either H_2-receptor antagonists or proton pump inhibitors.

ABDOMINAL TRAUMA

■ *What type of abdominal organs are more likely to be injured in a blunt mechanism?*

■ **Solid organs**

Common organs injured by blunt mechanism include the solid organs such as the spleen, liver, and pancreas. Hollow organs, like the stomach, collapse with blunt mechanism. Other abdominal organs frequently injured include the small bowel, especially the duodenum. The duodenal injury occurs with a sudden deceleration mechanism due to ligament of Treitz securing the duodenum, while the small bowel is relatively mobile, resulting in a tear (Box 6.31).

Box 6.31 Mechanism of Injury of Blunt Abdominal Trauma

Entrapment of organ between vertebral column and impacting force	Change in organ position
Sudden increase in uniform pressure	Puncture from bone fractures

■ *Which two abdominal organs are most commonly injured in penetrating injuries to the abdomen?*

■ **Bowel and liver**

Bowel is at a greater risk of injury with penetrating injury because of the quantity of bowel present in the abdomen. The liver is one of the most commonly injured organs in the abdomen because of the liver's size and location. The spleen and liver are commonly injured in blunt mechanism.

■ *Which abdominal organs are commonly damaged by a lap belt?*

■ **Colon and bladder**

Mechanism of injury includes crush injury or sudden decompression of an air-filled bowel or urine-filled bladder with the lap belt. Colon and bladder injuries are commonly associated with pelvic fractures.

PATHOPHYSIOLOGY

■ *Are the kidneys located in the peritoneal or retroperitoneal space?*

■ **Retroperitoneal space**

The abdominal cavity is divided into peritoneal and retroperitoneal space. Certain diagnostic tests are able to locate injuries in the peritoneal cavity better than the retroperitoneal space. Organs in the retroperitoneal space that sustain an injury are more likely to be missed due to the greater difficulty in diagnosis (Box 6.32).

Box 6.32 Peritoneal and Retroperitoneal Organs

Peritoneal Space	Retroperitoneal Space
Stomach	Duodenum
Small bowel	Ascending colon
Liver	Descending colon
Spleen	Kidneys
Gallbladder	Part of the bladder
Transverse colon	Pancreas
Sigmoid colon	Major vessels
Upper one-third of rectum	
Part of bladder	
Uterus	

■ *What is the most common cause of death following liver injury in abdominal trauma?*

■ **Hemorrhage**

The liver is very vascular as both the portal vein and hepatic artery bring blood into the liver. It is the most common cause of hemorrhagic shock in abdominal trauma (both penetrating and blunt) followed by the spleen and kidneys.

> **HINT**
> Initially "damage" control is frequently performed intraoperatively to control bleeding, followed by a return trip to the operating room later to actually repair the liver injury.

■ *Which part of the bladder, when ruptured, would result in intraabdominal injury (peritonitis)?*

■ **Dome of the bladder**

Bladder rupture results from a blunt trauma to the lower abdomen when the bladder is full. The dome is the weakest point of the bladder and is the most common site of rupture. The dome of the bladder is covered by the peritoneum, so rupture of the dome causes urine to enter the intraperitoneal space.

> **HINT**
> Extraperitoneal bladder ruptures are usually associated with pelvic fractures.

SYMPTOMS/ASSESSMENT

■ *What is the most common finding for stomach injuries following penetrating trauma to the abdomen?*

■ **Bloody gastric aspirate**

The most common sign of stomach injury is blood in the gastric aspirate. Other findings include rapid-onset epigastric pain, tenderness and signs of peritonitis due to release of gastric contents, and free air on abdominal x-ray.

> **HINT**
> Blunt trauma may result in blood in gastric aspirate without stomach injuries, if facial trauma or oral-cavity injury resulted in swallowing of blood.

- *Why does a duodenal tear not cause immediate peritonitis, as seen often with gastric injuries?*
- **Alkaline fluid in duodenum**

The fluid in the stomach is acidic and when spilled into the peritoneal cavity causes a rapid, severe peritonitis. Gastric injuries typically present with abdominal pain, abdominal tenderness, or a "board-like" abdomen. Duodenal tears, however, may have minimal signs of peritonitis with mild irritation or tenderness of the abdomen initially. This is because the fluid in the duodenum and small bowel is alkaline, which causes less irritation. Symptoms of peritonitis occur later as a result of infection in the peritoneum.

> **HINT**
> Duodenal injuries may be missed due to the delayed presentation of peritonitis because it is a retroperitoneal organ (Box 6.33).

Box 6.33 Symptoms of Delayed Peritonitis With Duodenal Injuries

Fever	Increased bilirubin and amylase
Leukocytosis	High intestinal obstruction
Third spacing with hypovolemia	Jaundice

- *What is pain in the neck area because of irritation of the phrenic nerve following splenic injury called?*
- **Saegesser's sign**

Following splenic injury, pain occurs as generalized abdominal pain that is localized in the left upper quadrant and can refer to the neck region (Saegesser's sign) or to the left shoulder or scapula (Kehr's sign). Splenic injuries can cause life-threatening hemorrhage with signs of shock.

DIAGNOSIS

- *What may be found on a chest x-ray (CXR) or kidneys, uterers, and bladder (KUB) x-ray that would be an indication for surgery?*
- **Free air or foreign bodies**

An upright CXR and left lateral decubitus are used to identify free air (ruptured hollow organ) or presence of foreign bodies. Supine abdominal x-ray can identify retroperitoneal free air, gross organ injury, presence of blood, or foreign objects in the abdominal cavity.

■ **What is the diagnostic focused abdominal sonography trauma (FAST) test that is used to evaluate blunt abdominal trauma?**

■ **Ultrasonography of the abdomen**

FAST is ultrasonography that can be used to evaluate the abdomen following blunt trauma. It can detect the presence of free intraperitoneal or pericardial fluid. Ultrasound can estimate the amount of blood in the abdomen, thus preventing unnecessary laparotomies and can identify candidates for observation. It is not as reliable for the retroperitoneal space.

> **HINT**
> Greater than 1,000 mL of fluid (blood) in the peritoneum needs immediate surgical intervention.

■ **Which diagnostic test is the gold standard to evaluate the abdomen following a blunt trauma?**

■ **Abdominal CT scan**

Abdominal CT scans are able to view both the retroperitoneal cavity as well as intra-abdominal injuries. Abdominal CT scans able to identify the organs involved and grade the severity of injury. This allows for the ability to observe some patients with less-severe injuries instead of performing an exploratory laparotomy (Box 6.36).

> **HINT**
> Unstable patients require evaluation in the emergency department and may not be able to be transported to CT scan (Box 6.34).

Box 6.34 Diagnostic Evaluation of Blunt Abdominal Trauma

Diagnostic Test	Advantages	Disadvantages
KUB or CXR	Performed in the ED Free air indicates hollow organ rupture without having to perform further workup	Unable to identify severity of organ injuries or fluid in the abdomen
Ultrasound	Performed in the ED High sensitivity to detect intra-abdominal fluid	Not accurate in obese patients, ileus, emphysema Unable to differentiate blood, bile, urine, or ascites Decreased accuracy of retroperitoneal injuries

(continued)

Box 6.34 Diagnostic Evaluation of Blunt Abdominal Trauma *(continued)*

Diagnostic Test	Advantages	Disadvantages
CT scan	View retroperitoneal space Identify organs injured Grade severity of organ injury Determine patients for observation instead of surgery	Transport patient out of the ED May miss mesenteric, bowel, or diaphragm injuries More expensive
Diagnostic peritoneal lavage (DPL)	Performed in the emergency department	Unable to identify retroperitoneal injuries Inability to determine type or severity of injury False-negative results False-positive results Potential bowel or bladder perforation

■ *Would a patient with pelvic injuries more likely have a false-positive or a false-negative result with a diagnostic peritoneal lavage (DPL)?*

■ **False-positive result**

Patients with pelvic injuries may receive a positive DPL due to blood from the pelvic region being found in the peritoneum. False-positive and false-negative results can occur with a DPL. For example, multiple previous abdominal surgeries resulting in adhesions can sequester the blood and cause a false-negative result.

> ❯ **HINT**
>
> A false-positive result occurs when a DPL is positive, indicating surgery, when an injury was not present, whereas a false-negative result means the DPL was negative but an injury was present.

■ *What should be placed prior to performing a DPL?*

■ **Foley catheter**

Bladder or bowel perforation can occur with the placement of the peritoneal catheter to perform the DPL. A Foley catheter should be inserted prior to placement of the catheter to empty the bladder and lower the risk of unintentional perforation (Boxes 6.35 and 6.36).

Box 6.35 Relative Contraindications for DPL

Advanced pregnancy	Morbid obesity
Pelvic injuries	Advanced cirrhosis
History of previous abdominal surgeries	Coagulopathy

Box 6.36 Positive Findings in DPL

Aspiration > 10 mL of blood	Hematocrit > 2%
> 100,000 RBCs	Presence of bile, bacteria, or fecal material
> 500 WBCs	Elevated amylase

MEDICAL MANAGEMENT

■ *What is a medical option for a hemodynamically stable blunt abdominal trauma patient with a splenic injury Grade II?*

■ **Observation**

The American Association for the Surgery of Trauma (AAST) developed a grading system for organ injury based on the CT scan to determine potential success for a nonoperative approach. Hemodynamically stable patients with low-grade injuries of the spleen or liver without any other evidence of intraabdominal injuries may be observed without initial surgery. Another nonsurgical method is embolization of the spleen or liver (Boxes 6.37 and 6.38).

Box 6.37 Grading Liver Injuries

Grade	Description of Injuries
Grade I	Subcapsular hematoma < 10% surface area Capsular tear < 1-cm depth
Grade II	Subcapsular hematoma with 10%–50% surface area Intraparenchymal hematoma < 10-cm diameter Capsular tear 1- to 3-cm depth, < 10-cm length
Grade III	Subcapsular hematoma > 50% surface area, or ruptured with active bleeding Intraparenchymal hematoma > 10-cm diameter Capsular tear > 3-cm depth
Grade IV	Ruptured intraparenchymal with active bleeding Parenchymal disruption involving 25%–75% of hepatic lobes
Grade V	Parenchymal disruption involving >75% of hepatic lobes Vascular: Juxtahepatic venous injuries (inferior vena cava [IVC], major hepatic vein)
Grade VI	Vascular: Hepatic avulsion

Reprinted with permission, *The Journal of Trauma*, 1995; 38(3), 323–334.

Box 6.38 Grading Spleen Injuries

Grade I	Capsular tear, < 1 cm parenchymal
Grade II	Capsular tear, 1- to 3-cm depth, which does not involve a trebecular vessel
Grade III	Laceration > 3-cm parenchymal depth involving trabecular vessels Ruptured subcapsular or parenchymal hematoma Intraparenchymal hematoma > 5 cm or expanding
Grade IV	Laceration involving segmental or hilar vessels producing major devascularization (>25% of spleen)
Grade V	Shattered spleen or hilar vascular injury, which devascularizes spleen

Reprinted with permission, *The Journal of Trauma*, 1995; 38(3), 323–334.

SURGICAL MANAGEMENT

■ *What surgical procedure would a patient with ongoing blood loss from an unknown source following a blunt trauma require?*

■ **Exploratory laparotomy**

Following a blunt trauma, the most common site to cause hemorrhagic shock is the abdomen. If a patient remains unstable and an immediate source of blood loss is unable to be located, the patient should undergo an exploratory laparotomy (Box 6.39).

Box 6.39 Indications for Exploratory Laparotomy

Penetrating trauma to abdomen	Ongoing blood loss from unknown source
Presence of free air on x-ray	Known significant injuries found with diagnostic studies
Eviscerated bowel or omentum	Positive peritoneal signs
Significant bleeding from NG tube or rectum	

■ *What is the priority in an emergency exploratory laparotomy performed on an abdominal trauma patient?*

■ **Control blood loss**

The immediate priority in an exploratory laparotomy in a trauma patient is to find the source of blood loss and control the bleeding. The most common organs involved in significant blood loss are the liver, spleen, and kidneys. Typically, an unstable patient may require control of bleeding by either removing the organ (spleen or kidneys) or packing to tamponade the bleeding liver (Box 6.40).

Box 6.40 Exploratory Laparotomy Priority

First priority	Find source of blood loss and control bleeding
Second priority	Locate any colonic injuries to control fecal contamination
Third priority	Identify injured organs
Fourth priority	Repair injured organs

■ *What is "damage control" when managing a bleeding liver intraoperatively?*

■ **Temporary control of blood loss**

Control of blood loss from the liver is frequently obtained by a technique called "damage control." If hemorrhage is severe, the liver may be packed with lap pads to tamponade the bleeding. Other techniques used in "damage control" include use of fibrin glue (sealant made from concentrated fibrinogen and thrombin) and/or selective hepatic artery or portal vein ligation. Following packing of the liver, a temporary closure is used to cover the abdomen and a planned reoperation to control bleeding and repair the liver is performed. The packing may be kept in place for 48 to 72 hours while the patient is being maintained in the intensive care unit (ICU) (Box 6.41).

> **❯ HINT**
> Assess for uncontrolled hemorrhage, monitor coagulation studies, administer FFP, and warm the patient to reverse the coagulopathy.

Box 6.41 Surgical Interventions of Abdominal Organ Injuries

Stomach	Debridement of devitalized tissue
	Closure with sutures
	Partial gastrectomy
	NG tube postoperative for decompression

(continued)

Box 6.41 Surgical Interventions of Abdominal Organ Injuries *(continued)*

Duodenum and small bowel	Debridement of devitalized tissue Bowel resection and anastomosis NG tube and/or duodenal tube for decompression
Pancreas	Suture and drain if minor injury Debridement of pancreas if major injury Occurs over several days Placement of drains around pancreatic bed
Liver	Control bleeding ("damage control") Debridement of devitalized tissue Minor injuries may be sutured, topical agents applied or electrocautery performed Placement of drains around hepatic bed Drain bile ducts
Spleen	Minor injury repaired Major injury may require splenectomy Surgery if separated from blood supply or macerated
Colon	Primary closure Resection with primary anastomosis Primary closure with proximal colostomy Delayed closure Colostomy (double-barrel loop colostomy)

> **HINT**
Postoperative management and complications of stomach injuries are the same as for postoperative gastrectomy patients.

■ *What is a common laboratory finding following a splenectomy?*
■ **Elevated platelets and WBCs**

Following a splenectomy, the platelet count typically is elevated (thrombocytosis) and can cause thrombotic evens such as an acute myocardial infarction, mesenteric vein thrombosis, and venous thromboembolism (VTE). The incidence of thrombocytosis will peak between 9 and 10 days postoperatively. Platelet counts typically return to normal within weeks to several months post splenectomy. Leukocytosis can also be seen following splenectomy.

> **HINT**
Prophylaxis for VTE is recommended post splenectomy.

COMPLICATIONS

■ *Which combination of organs injured following abdominal trauma will have the highest rate of postoperative sepsis?*
■ **Liver and colon**

When injured the colon will leak or spill fecal material into the peritoneum. The liver is very vascular and susceptible to bleeding. Abscess formation is due to foreign body fragments, necrotic tissue, blood, or bile remaining at the site of injury. The combination of blood and fluid with fecal contamination in the peritoneum increases the risk of peritonitis and sepsis.

> ❯ HINT
>
> Postop fluid collections or abscesses can be drained by CT-guided placement of a catheter.

■ *Following a splenectomy to control hemorrhaging, what needs to be given to the patient prior to discharge?*

■ **Pneumococcal vaccination**

A complication of a splenectomy is overwhelming postsplenectomy sepsis (OPSS), which can occur as a result of the loss of some immune responses that will increase the mortality rate. The majority of OPSS occurs within 1 year post-splenectomy but can occur several years later. *Streptococcus pneumoniae* (pneumococcus), *Haemophilus influenzae* type B, and *Neisseria meningitidis* are organisms that cause OPSS. Infections are associated with mortality as high as 50% to 80% following a splenectomy. Pneumovax vaccination is required before discharge (Box 6.42).

Box 6.42 Complications of Abdominal Organ Injuries

Stomach	Breakdown of anastomosis
	Abscesses
	Fistulas
	Alkalosis
	Hypokalemia
	Peritonitis
Duodenum and small bowel	Breakdown of anastomosis
	Peritonitis
	Abscess
	Wound dehiscence
	Bowel ischemia
	Fistula formation
	Bowel obstruction
	Abdominal compartment syndrome
Pancreas	Hemorrhage
	Signs of peritonitis
	Fluid and electrolyte imbalance
	Pseudocyst
	Abscess
	Fistulas
	Sepsis
	ARDS
	Necrosis due to autodigestion

(continued)

Box 6.42 Complications of Abdominal Organ Injuries *(continued)*

Liver	Hemorrhage
	Sepsis
	ARDS
	DIC
	Abdominal abscess
	Hematobilia (free communication between biliary tree and vascular system)
	Hepatorenal syndrome
	Jaundice
	Bile peritonitis
Spleen	Hemorrhage
	Overwhelming postsplenectomy sepsis
Colon	Fistulas
	Abscesses
	Peritonitis
	Sepsis
	Bowel obstruction
	Incisional infection

> ❯ HINT
>
> Duodenal fistulas cause acidosis secondary to loss of bicarbonate from pancreatic juices, whereas jejunal fistulas produce low volumes of neutral pH fluid with little change in acid–base balance (Box 6.43).

Box 6.43 Late Complications From Abdominal Trauma

Peptic ulcers	Fistulas
Intestinal obstruction from adhesions	Chronic abscess
Hernia	Cholelithiasis and cholecystitis

BOWEL INFARCTIONS/OBSTRUCTIONS/PERFORATIONS

- *Is bowel ischemia related to venous obstruction a result of thrombosis or embolism?*
- **Thrombosis**

Acute mesenteric ischemia is a syndrome of inadequate blood flow through the mesenteric vessels resulting in infarction, necrosis, and death. Bowel ischemia can be caused by either arterial or venous system abnormalities. Occlusive venous disease is due to thrombosis, whereas arterial disease may be caused by thrombosis or embolism. Arterial disease that is not caused by occlusion of blood flow that results in hypoperfusion is also possible (Box 6.44).

Box 6.44 Acute Mesenteric Ischemia

Nonocclusive mesenteric ischemia (NOMI)
Occlusive mesenteric arterial ischemia (OMAI)
Acute mesenteric arterial embolism
Acute mesenteric arterial thrombosis
Mesenteric venous thrombosis (MVT)

■ *What is a complication following abdominal surgery that can cause a bowel obstruction?*

■ **Adhesions**

Acute bowel obstruction occurs when the forward flow of intestinal contents is interrupted and can occur anywhere in the intestines. The obstruction is classified as either small- or large-bowel obstructions. The three most common causes of bowel obstruction are intra-abdominal adhesions, malignancy, and abdominal hernias.

> ❯ HINT
> Bowel obstructions may be complete or partial.

PATHOPHYSIOLOGY

■ *What artery supplies blood to the jejunum?*

■ **Superior mesenteric artery**

The arteries that supply the GI viscera branch off the anterior portion of the descending aorta. The most clinically important is the territory of the superior mesenteric artery, which affects the small and large intestines. The esophagus and stomach are not commonly affected by local ischemia versus a global ischemia (Box 6.45).

Box 6.45 Arterial Supply of the Gastrointestinal System

Celiac Artery	Superior Mesenteric Artery	Inferior Mesenteric Artery
Esophagus	Inferior portion duodenum	Left one-third of transverse colon
Stomach	Jejunum	Descending colon
Superior portion duodenum	Ileum	Sigmoid colon
Liver	Cecum	Rectum
Spleen	Appendix	Upper portion anal canal
	Ascending colon	
	Right two-thirds of transverse colon	

■ *What is a common cause in an ICU patient for nonocclusive arterial bowel infarction?*

■ **Hypotension**

Arterial disease is divided into occlusive and nonocclusive ischemia. Occlusive bowel ischemia is typically caused by an obstruction to flow due to either an embolism or thrombosis, whereas nonocclusive ischemia is decreased blood flow through the mesenteric vessels. Critically ill patients frequently experience periods of shock and hypotension. Blood may be shunted away from the GI system, causing hypoperfusion to the bowel.

> ❯ HINT
> Vasoactive drugs may also cause nonocclusive bowel infarctions (Box 6.46).

Box 6.46 Causes of Acute Arterial Mesenteric Ischemia

Nonocclusive Arterial Mesenteric Ischemia	Occlusive Arterial Mesenteric Thrombosis	Occlusive Arterial Mesenteric Embolism
Hypotension	Atherosclerotic disease	Cardiac emboli Atrial fibrillation Septic emboli
Vasopressor drugs	Aortic aneurysm	Fragments of atheromatous plaque
Ergotamine	Aortic dissection	
Sympathomimetic drugs cocaine	Arteritis	
Digitalis	Dehydration	

■ *What disease state most commonly causes mesenteric venous ischemia due to venous congestion?*

■ **Hepatic failure**

Venous congestion occurs in portal hypertension from hepatic failure. Portal hypertension can cause venous blood to back up into mesenteric vessels, causing venous stasis and thrombosis (Box 6.47).

Box 6.47 Causes of Mesenteric Venous Ischemia

Hypercoagulable state	Abdominal compartment syndrome
Tumor causing venous obstruction	Venous trauma
Intraabdominal infection	Decompression sickness
Venous congestion	

■ *What happens proximal to bowel obstruction?*

■ **Dilation of bowel**

Proximal to the bowel obstruction, the intestinal lumen dilates due to accumulation of secretions, ingested food and fluid, bowel contents, and gas. There is little to no movement of bowel contents or flatus distal. This results in an increased intraluminal pressure. Distal bowel collapses and alters the normal secretory or absorptive function of the bowel.

> **❯ HINT**
> Fluid and electrolyte abnormalities commonly occur with bowel obstruction.

■ *What is a major concern in bowel obstructions that affects management and mortality?*

■ **Vascular compromise**

Bowel dilation and obstruction increase intraluminal pressures. When pressures exceed venous pressures, the bowel becomes edematous and swollen. This leads to compromised arterial flow and bowel ischemia. Bowel obstruction can occur with or without vascular compromise.

> **HINT**
Presence of vascular compromise to the bowel determines the need for surgery instead of medical management (Box 6.48).

Box 6.48 Causes of Bowel Obstruction

Intraabdominal adhesions	Intraabdominal abscess
Malignancy	Foreign bodies
Abdominal hernia	Diverticulosis
Inflammatory bowel disease	Fecal impaction
Intestinal intussusception	Crohn's disease
Volvulus	Parasitic infestation

- *What is it called when there is a complete twist of the intestine?*
- **Volvulus**

Volvulus is the complete twisting of a loop of intestine around the mesenteric attachment. It is a malposition or malrotation of the intestines. It can cause bowel obstruction and bowel ischemia. In the elderly population, it most commonly occurs at the sigmoid colon.

> **HINT**
Intussusception occurs when the intestine is invaginated into another section of the intestines, resulting in obstruction.

SYMPTOMS/ASSESSMENT

- *Bloody diarrhea is most likely to be the presentation of bowel infarction, bowel obstruction, or bowel perforation?*
- **Bowel infarction**

All of the above can present with severe abdominal pain, nausea and vomiting, and diarrhea. Infarctions are more likely to develop bloody diarrhea than obstructions or perforation. In small-bowel infarctions, bleeding from the rectum may be seen as a late sign caused by tissue necrosis. Colonic infarctions may involve bloody diarrhea but not necessarily to the point of significant blood loss. Bowel obstructions, if complete, will not allow passing of stool but partial obstructions may present with diarrhea.

> **HINT**
Colonic infarctions have more severe abdominal pain than small-bowel infarctions. Small-bowel ischemia may be very nonspecific until signs of peritonitis appear (Box 6.49).

Box 6.49 Symptoms of Bowel Infarctions

Small-Bowel Infarction	Colonic Infarction
Abdominal pain	Severe abdominal cramping
Increased peristalsis	Diarrhea
Vomiting	Bloody diarrhea
Diarrhea	Ileus
Blood from rectum	Signs of sepsis
Signs of peritonitis	
Signs of sepsis	

> **HINT**
> Abdominal pain is frequently described as a constant, diffuse, nonlocalized, colicky type of pain.

- *During abdominal auscultation in early bowel obstruction, what would you expect to occur with bowel sounds?*
- **Bowel sounds should be hyperactive and high pitched**

Early obstruction typically results in hyperactive, high-pitched bowel sounds. The colon may develop loud borborygmi due to increased peristalsis. Late obstruction may present with minimal bowel sounds due to hypotonia.

> **HINT**
> Emesis may be odorous and frequently has a feculent odor due to intestinal stasis and the effect of bacteria on abdominal contents (Box 6.50).

Box 6.50 Symptoms of Bowel Obstruction

Colicky abdominal pain	Cessation of flatus and stool
Nausea and vomiting	Signs of dehydration
Abdominal distention	High-pitched bowel sounds
Palpable abdominal mass	

DIAGNOSIS

- *What is the most confirmative diagnosis for small-bowel infarction?*
- **Exploratory laparotomy**

Plain radiographs are not useful in the diagnosis of acute mesenteric ischemia. A diagnostic finding is intramural or intravascular air but this is a late sign of intestinal infarction. A CT scan may identify a thickening of the bowel wall, characteristic "thumb printing" caused by submucosa necrosis, and intramural or intravascular air may also be seen. Other diagnostics include MRI, MRA, and ultrasonography. Frequently, the confirmation of the diagnosis is an exploratory laparotomy.

> ⟩ HINT
>
> Angiography is beneficial for occlusive arterial disease but has been shown to be less effective with nonobstructive or venous thrombosis disease.

■ **What electrolyte is typically found elevated in patients with mesenteric ischemia?**

■ **Phosphate**

Phosphate is somewhat sensitive to mesenteric ischemia and infarctions and will increase in the first 4 hours. Hematocrit initially is elevated due to third spacing and hemoconcentration but will decrease with GI bleeding. Amylase levels may be elevated but are nonspecific (Box 6.51).

Box 6.51 Laboratory Findings of Mesenteric Ischemia

Hyperphosphatemia	Moderately elevated amylase
Elevated hematocrit initially	Elevated lactase
Leukocytosis	Metabolic acidosis
Elevated D-dimer	

■ **Does bowel obstruction with emesis result in metabolic acidosis or metabolic alkalosis?**

■ **Metabolic alkalosis**

Obstruction in the bowel leads to high intraluminal pressures and commonly presents with emesis. Gastric acids, potassium, chloride, and hydrogen ions are lost with emesis. The kidneys reabsorb bicarbonate and further lose chloride, contributing to metabolic alkalosis. The loss of fluids from the stomach and kidneys also contribute to hypovolemia and dehydration. Hypochloremic metabolic alkalosis is a combination of a loss of acids and reabsorption of bicarbonate.

> ⟩ HINT
>
> If a patient with a bowel obstruction presents with metabolic acidosis, suspect bowel ischemia. Lactate levels will be elevated due to anaerobic metabolism (Box 6.52).

Box 6.52 Abnormal Laboratory Findings in Bowel Obstruction

Hypokalemia	Increase in bicarbonate
Hypochloremia	Elevated blood urea nitrogen
Metabolic alkalosis	Elevated hemoglobin (hgb) and hematocrit

■ **Which radiographic diagnostic test is used most frequently to diagnose bowel obstruction?**

■ **Plain abdominal radiograph**

A plain abdominal radiograph is used to determine the presence of dilated loops of small bowel or dilated colon with decompressed small bowel. Early obstruction or high duodenal or jejunal obstruction may not appear on a plain radiograph and require abdominal CT scan. An advantage of abdominal CT scan over plain radiograph is the ability to identify the location of a cause of the obstruction. Other diagnostic examinations include ultrasonography, MRI, and contrast fluoroscopy.

> **HINT**
> CT scans are not as valuable for partial obstructions and the patient may require fluoroscopy.

MEDICAL MANAGEMENT

■ *What is the initial treatment of patients with bowel ischemia and bowel obstruction?*
■ **Fluids and antibiotics**

The initial management includes fluid resuscitation, correction of electrolyte and other metabolic abnormalities, and initiation of antibiotic therapy. Antibiotics are administered to prevent or treat infections caused by bowel infarction and necrosis. Antibiotics used for bowel obstruction prevent bacterial overgrowth and translocation of bacteria causing septicemia.

> **HINT**
> Antibiotics should cover gram-negative organisms and anaerobes.

■ *What other treatment may be used to conservatively manage a high-grade bowel obstruction?*
■ **Decompression of the intestines**

Conservative management includes fluid and electrolyte management as well as a nasogastric tube to suction for decompression. Other drugs may include probiotics, oral magnesium hydroxide, and simethicone.

> **HINT**
> Patient will have NPO status to "rest" bowel while aggressively replacing fluid intravenously.

■ *What is the treatment for patients with acute mesenteric venous thrombosis?*
■ **Anticoagulation therapy**

Heparin may be used in the acute care setting as an anticoagulant to treat the venous thrombosis. If no bowel necrosis exists, anticoagulation therapy is used to treat without surgical intervention. Warfarin is commonly used for long-term management of mesenteric venous thrombosis.

> **HINT**
> Venous thrombosis anywhere in the vasculature is managed with anticoagulation therapy.

SURGICAL MANAGEMENT

▪ *Nonocclusive arterial mesenteric ischemia is initially managed with which minimally invasive procedure?*

▪ **Angiography with papaverine infusion**

Angiography with papaverine infusion may be used in all forms of arterial mesenteric ischemia but in nonocclusive ischemia it is the only treatment except bowel resection. Papaverine infusion through a catheter placed in an angiogram will relieve vasospasms in the occluded arterial vessel. Thrombolytic infusion may be used for embolic mesenteric ischemia in patients without peritonitis or bowel infarction.

> ❯ **HINT**
> Signs of peritonitis indicate the need to stop infusion of thrombolytics
> for embolic mesenteric ischemia and prepare patient for surgery.

▪ *What complication indicates the need for surgery in all types of mesenteric ischemic disease?*

▪ **Bowel necrosis**

Bowel necrosis presents as peritonitis and is an indication for surgery and bowel resection in all types of mesenteric ischemia. Signs of peritonitis include fever, leukocytosis, abdominal pain, and a "board-like" abdomen. Thrombotic mesenteric occlusion may undergo emergency revascularization surgery if the gut is not gangrenous. Transthoracic endarterectomy is an alternative when no vein is available for bypass.

▪ *Which two complications of bowel obstruction would indicate the need for immediate abdominal surgery?*

▪ **Bowel ischemia and perforation**

Onset of peritonitis or unexplained sepsis with abdominal signs would indicate a complication of bowel obstruction and need for surgical management. Another indication for abdominal surgery is to manage the underlying cause of obstruction such as hernia or adhesion.

> ❯ **HINT**
> Abdominal tumors will need to be evaluated to determine whether
> surgery or palliative care is indicated.

COMPLICATIONS

▪ *Bowel obstruction and the resulting ischemia can cause what complication?*

▪ **Bowel perforation**

Following bowel obstruction, perforation can occur. Vascular compromise leads to ischemia and is the most common site of perforation. This typically occurs in the small bowel but can also occur in the colon or cecum with large dilation.

> **HINT**
Free air found in an upright KUB is diagnostic of bowel perforation.

MALABSORPTION AND MALNUTRITION

■ *What is the malabsorption syndrome commonly associated with the ICU?*
■ **Sepsis**

Malabsorption is defined as intestinal absorption capacity of 85% or less. It is commonly associated with sepsis and multiple organ dysfunction or failure (such as acute renal failure). Malabsorption is the clinical sign of intestinal dysfunction or failure.

> **HINT**
Malabsorption can contribute to translocation of bacteria.

■ *Hypercatabolism in critically ill patients can result in loss of what?*
■ **Muscle mass**

Hypercatabolism is recognized in critically ill patients to cause a cachectic state in which the person's muscle is used as an energy source. This results in a loss of muscle mass, including the respiratory muscles. Critically ill patients have a high metabolism rate and require an increase in caloric and nutrient requirements (Box 6.53).

Box 6.53 Risk for Malnutrition

Obese	Increased nutrient loses
Underweight	Malabsorption
Recent weight loss	Short bowel syndrome
Inadequate digestion	Fistula
Recent gastrointestinal surgeries	Draining wounds
Alcohol or substance abuse	Renal dialysis, peritoneal dialysis
NPO status	Severe diarrhea
Increased nutrient requirements	Corticosteroid therapy
Burns	
Trauma	
Sepsis	
Fever	
Surgery	
End-stage renal disease (ESRD)	

PATHOPHYSIOLOGY

■ *What function of the intestines, when altered in critical illness, can result in an ileus?*
■ **Motility**

A function of the intestine is coordinated intestinal transport or motility. A decreased motility results in an ileus, malnutrition, and increased risk of translocation of bacteria.

Critically ill patients are at risk for altered intestinal activity due to a decrease in splanchnic blood flow (Box 6.54).

> **HINT**
Adequate absorption in the intestines is important in critically ill patients for improvement.

Box 6.54 Functions of the Intestines

Motility	Mucosal immunological response
Coordinate exocrine digestive functions (pancreas, jejunum, liver)	Intestinal barrier function

■ *What is a common cause of intestinal disruption in the ICU?*
■ **Bowel rest**

Complete bowel rest causes progressive atrophy, disruption, and degenerative changes of the intestinal mucosa. These changes can occur within a few days of assigning NPO status. Parenteral nutrition does not prevent intestinal disruption. Translocation of bacteria can occur during bowel rest. Enteral nutrition can help prevent sepsis from bowel origin (gram-negative bacteria).

> **HINT**
Early feeding can lower the incidence of bacteremia from translocation of bacteria.

■ *What is the amino acid required to replace the intestinal mucosa?*
■ **Glutamine**

The bowel mucosa relies on nutrients from the bowel lumen. One important nutrient is an amino acid called glutamine. Glutamine is a principle metabolic fuel for the intestinal epithelial cells. The entire lining of the GI tract mucosa is replaced every 2 to 8 days. The replacement of these cells is dependent on the nutrition of the patient. Food has a trophic effect on the GI mucosa.

> **HINT**
Glutamine is the major fuel of the cells of the small intestine.

SYMPTOMS/ASSESSMENT

■ *What is a symptom of protein malnutrition and cachectic state?*
■ **Muscle wasting**

Wasting of muscle and subcutaneous fat are signs of protein malnutrition. The body begins to break down its own supply of protein and fat to meet the high caloric demands of critically ill patients.

> HINT

The diaphragm is a muscle, so critically ill patients in cachectic states may have increased difficulty weaning from ventilators.

DIAGNOSIS

- *What hepatic protein is considered the best predictor of nutrition in critically ill patients?*
- **Prealbumin**

Prealbumin levels are used in assessing nutritional status in critically ill patients. They have been shown to predict outcomes and correlate to patient recovery. Prealbumin is the earliest indicator of protein malnutrition and is not as affected by liver disease as other proteins.

> HINT

Prealbumin may allow earlier recognition and intervention for malnutrition. A prealbumin less than 15 mg/L requires nutritional consult (Box 6.55).

Box 6.55 Plasma Proteins

Plasma Proteins	Half-Life	Range
Albumin	20 days	3.30–4.8 g/L
Prealbumin	2 days	16–35 mg/L
Transferrin	10 days	0.16–0.36 g/L

> HINT

These are called negative acute phase proteins.

MEDICAL MANAGEMENT

- *Which two drugs are commonly used as prokinetics to improve tolerance to feeding?*
- **Erythromycin and metoclopramide**

Prokinetic therapy is used in patients with feed intolerance and gastroparesis. The two drugs used as first-line therapy as a prokinetic include erythromycin and metoclopramide. Erythromycin is a dopamine agonist and metoclopramide is a promotility agent. Metoclopramide has been found most effective in improving gastric emptying. Erythromycin has been found effective in both gastric emptying and improving tolerance to feeding but may cause an increase in bacterial resistance. A combination of both erythromycin and metoclopramide may be more effective with less tachyphylaxis.

> ❯ HINT
> Prolongation of QT interval is a potential complication of erythromycin and metoclopramide administration.

COMPLICATIONS

- ■ *What is the pulmonary complication of total parenteral nutrition (TPN) with overfeeding?*
- ■ **Elevated PaCO$_2$**

Overfeeding can impair pulmonary function. Too much caloric intake from lipids or carbohydrates alone can result in an increased production of carbon dioxide (CO_2). This can cause a difficulty in weaning patients from ventilators due to hyperventilation. Avoid overfeeding by monitoring caloric intake and using balanced lipids and carbohydrates to supply the calories (Box 6.56).

Box 6.56 Complications of Total Parenteral Nutrition

Catheter-related sepsis
Central-line complications
Air embolus
Pneumothorax
Central venous thrombosis
Catheter occlusion
Hypoglycemia or hyperglycemia
Gram-negative sepsis
Elevated PaCO$_2$

TESTABLE NURSING INTERVENTIONS

ABDOMINAL COMPARTMENT SYNDROME

- ■ *When pressure within an anatomical compartment increases to the point of compression and tissue perfusion compromise, what is it called?*
- ■ **Compartment syndrome**

Compartment syndrome can occur in the extremities, as well as in intracranial, thoracic, and abdominal areas. Compression results in altered cellular oxygenation and initiates a cycle of progressive cellular injury, with edema and hypoperfusion leading to anaerobic metabolism, metabolic acidosis, and cellular death.

- ■ *When the pressure increases in the abdominal cavity to the extent of causing organ dysfunction/failure, what is it now known as?*
- ■ **Abdominal compartment syndrome (ACS)**

This syndrome was initially recognized and managed in abdominal trauma patients but it is now known to occur in any critically ill patient (also medical patients without abdominal conditions). ACS results in multiple complications, including acute respiratory distress; acute renal failure; dehiscence of abdominal wound and evisceration of bowel, bowel ischemia, sepsis, and MSOF. Intraabdominal pressure (IAP) is a compartment pressure that is monitored and measured and is defined as a steady-state pressure concealed within the abdominal cavity (Box 6.57).

Box 6.57 Factors That Influence IAP

Abdominal organ volume	Grossly swollen bowel (occupies several times original volume)
	Excessive crystalloid resuscitation
Presence of space-occupying substances (blood, ascites, tumor, free air)	Bleeding, leakage of abdominal contents, bowel edema
	Blood or blood clots
Abdominal wall compliance	Mechanical ventilation
	Positive end expiratory pressure (PEEP)
	Increased body mass index (BMI)

■ *What is the primary injury that occurs in ACS?*
■ **Trauma or ischemic insult**

The "primary" injury occurs due to the direct trauma or ischemic insult. The "secondary" injury occurs due to cytokine release and systemic inflammatory response. The inflammatory response results in an increase in capillary permeability and edema. The goal of treatment is to manage or prevent the secondary injuries. Recurrent ACS is a "second hit" phenomenon in which ACS redevelops following initial medical or surgical treatment of either primary or secondary ACS.

> ❯ **HINT**
> Chronic ACS occurs in the presence of cirrhosis and ascites, often end-stage disease.

■ *How does ACS cause respiratory distress and pulmonary complications?*
■ **Upward displacement of the diaphragm**

When the IAP increases, the abdominal organs displace the diaphragm upward, resulting in respiratory distress and pulmonary complications. The abdominal pressure is also displaced on the bladder and kidneys, resulting in renal dysfunction and elevation of bladder pressures. The elevated IAP can also cause elevation in thoracic and cerebral pressures. An increase in thoracic pressures affects the venous return and cardiac output.

> ❯ **HINT**
> The increase in ACS causes a decrease in venous return from the cerebral circulation. This can cause an increased ICP (Box 6.58).

Box 6.58 Organ Involvement in ACS

Acute kidney injury	Gastrointestinal
Cardiovascular	Altered blood flow to gut, liver, pancreas
Decreased venous return	Bowel ischemia/infarction
Increased afterload	Eyes
Pulmonary	Rupture of retinal capillaries
Decreased lung compliance	Decreased central vision (Valsalva retinopathy)
Increased peak inspiratory pressure	Surgical wound
Decreased tidal volume	Abdominal wound dehiscence
Neurological	
Increased intracranial pressure	

■ *Which patient population is at the greatest risk for development of ACS?*

■ **Abdominal trauma**

Abdominal trauma and abdominal surgeries are the most common causes of ACS and patients with abdominal injury were the first who were recognized to have complications from increased IAP. Since there is an increased awareness of ACS, multiple patient populations, including medical patients, have been found to have ACS (Box 6.59).

Box 6.59 Causes of ACS

Abdominal trauma	Liver failure with ascites/liver transplant
Abdominal surgery	Multiple blood transfusions (>10 U blood/24-hour period)
Damage-control laparotomy	Pneumonia/pneumonitis
Ischemic bowel	Mechanical ventilation/PEEP
Abdominal infections/abscesses/masses	Hypothermia (core temperature < 33°C)
Gastroparesis/gastric distention/ileus	Coagulopathy (platelets < 55,000, or PT > 15 sed. Or
Major burns (with or without abdominal	PTT > 2× normal or INR > 1.5
eschar)/trauma	Kidney transplant
Bacteremia/sepsis	Rupture of aortic aneurysms
Massive fluid resuscitation (> 5 L/24 hrs)	Pelvic fracture
Acute hemorrhagic pancreatitis	

■ *What is frequently monitored to determine elevated IAP and ACS?*

■ **Bladder pressure**

Aggressive monitoring of IAP and assessing for the development of ACS is important to prevent complications and mortality. Monitoring is performed with bladder pressure readings to determine IAP. Clinical examination and assessment of abdominal girth have been found to be poor indicators of ACS. The frequency of monitoring depends on the patient. Some resources recommend monitoring every 4 to 6 hours until IAP remains less than 12 mmHg for at least 24 hours in the absence of organ dysfunction in high-risk patients.

> **HINT**
>
> Obtain readings at end-expiration with the zero reference level at the iliac crest midaxillary line.

■ *What pressure is considered elevated in ACS?*

■ **Greater than 12 mmHg**

An elevated IAP is defined as greater than or equal to 12 mmHg. End-organ damage is observed with IAP as low as 10-cm H_2O pressure. It is graded based on the degree of elevation of pressures (Box 6.60).

> **HINT**
>
> Morbidly obese patients often also range from 9 to 14 mmHg.

Box 6.60 Grading of IAP

Grade	Intraabdominal Pressure
I	12–15 mmHg
II	16–20 mmHg
III	21–25 mmHg
IV	>25 mmHg

■ *What is the equation for calculating abdominal perfusion pressure (APP)?*

■ **MAP – IAP = APP**

The MAP minus the IAP is used to calculate the perfusion pressure of the abdomen. Resuscitative therapy is titrated to maintain an adequate APP and has been found to correlate better with survival than maintenance of any particular IAP. Normotensive or hypertensive patients may have outcomes better than patients who are hypotensive.

> **HINT**
>
> APP is similar to cerebral perfusion pressure (CPP). The MAP is the "driving force" and the IAP is the "opposing force."

■ *A patient "fighting" the ventilator can demonstrate elevated IAP. What drugs can be used to lower IAP in this particular patient?*

■ **Sedation and neuromuscular blocking agents**

Medical management can assist with lowering IAP. The goal of the medical intervention is to reduce IAP and optimize APP, maintaining APPs higher than 60. Increased resistance during ventilation caused by a patient "fighting" the ventilator can increase IAP. Providing sedation and neuromuscular blocking agents if sedation is not adequate can lower the resistance and the IAP (Box 6.61).

Box 6.61 Medical Interventions for ACS

Avoid excessive fluid resuscitation	Administer albumin or hypertonic solutions
Administer diuretics	NG tube to low-wall suction to decompress stomach
Perform continuous venovenous ultrafiltration	Rectal tube to decompress colon

(continued)

Box 6.61 Medical Interventions for ACS (*continued*)

Administer prokinetic agents (i.e., Metoclopramide)	Remove constrictive abdominal dressings
	Maintain head-of-bed elevation > 30° (reverse
Minimize or discontinue enteral feeding	Trendelenburg position to "unfold the abdomen")
Provide adequate sedation and analgesics	Avoid prone position
Administer neuromuscular blocking agents	Vasopressors to increase mean arterial pressure

> ❯ **HINT**
>
> A goal in managing ACS is a negative fluid balance within 3 days of injury.

- ■ *What is the most common surgical procedure used to manage ACS?*
- ■ **Decompressive laparotomy**

An excessively high IAP or progressive ACS or refractory ACS typically requires a decompressive laparotomy. Many surgeons now leave high-risk patients' abdomens open following surgery to prevent elevated IAP and ACS. After the patient's abdominal pressure decreases and the visceral edema recedes, the abdomen can be closed.

> ❯ **HINT**
>
> Open abdomens commonly require sedation and even neuromuscular blocking agents to prevent injury (Box 6.62).

Box 6.62 Complications of an Open Abdomen

Serous fluid losses	Bowel perforation
Infection/peritonitis	Bleeding
Enterocutaneous fistulas	Inability to close wound edges later
Ventral hernia	Hypothermia
Increased abdominal scarring	Ileus

- ■ *What type of dressing can be used on an open abdomen that draws fluid away from the abdominal cavity?*
- ■ **Negative pressure wound dressing**

Negative pressure systems control the abdominal contents with an open abdomen, manage third-space fluids, and facilitate wound closure. Vacuum-assisted fascial closure (VAFC) systems provide constant tension on the abdominal wound edges, facilitating the ability to successfully perform a late fascial closure. The open abdomen can also be covered with a temporary closure to maintain and protect the viscera.

ENTERAL AND PARENTERAL NUTRITION

- ■ *Does enteral or parenteral nutrition have a greater incidence of gram-negative septicemia?*
- ■ **Parenteral**

Prolonged exclusive use of TPN can cause intestinal atrophy, loss of small-bowel integrity that results in increased permeability and a decrease in absorptive capacity. Enteral feeding enhances cell renewal, decreases epithelial cell death, and increases expression of collagen. Enteral nutrition (EN) also has a trophic effect on the GI mucosa and is recommended over parenteral nutrition.

> **HINT**
> Even "trickle" enteral feeding has a lower incidence of septicemia than NPO or parenteral nutrition (Box 6.63).

Box 6.63 Prevention of Infections With Total Parenteral Nutrition

Maintain sterile set up
Change tubing every 24 hours
Use dedicated line total parenteral nutrition
No medication administration in this line
Exception: lipid infusions
IV site care sterile technique
Treat hyperglycemia

> **HINT**
> Monitor blood glucose levels every 6 hours and if lipids are administered, measure serum triglyceride levels.

■ *What is the goal for initiating enteral feeding in an ICU patient?*
■ **Within 24 to 48 hours of injury**

Timing of enteral feeding is critical in an ICU patient. If the patient is adequately resuscitated, then EN is started within 24 to 48 hours following injury or admission to the ICU. Early EN has been found to reduce infectious complications and decreased length of stay (LOS). It may blunt the hypermetabolic response and modulate the inflammatory reaction of critically ill patients. EN has been found to preserve gut mucosa.

> **HINT**
> A contraindication to early enteral feeding is complete bowel obstruction.

■ *When signs of enteral feeding intolerance occur, what alternative nutrition may be recommended?*
■ **Combination of enteral and parenteral**

Patients with enteral feeding can develop signs of enteral feeding intolerance. When this occurs, an alternative treatment is to decrease the enteral feeding rate and add parenteral nutrition to assure adequate calories and nutrition. Two common signs of enteral feeding intolerance include high gastric residuals and severe diarrhea.

■ *What is the recommended method for determining correct placement of an oro- or nasogastric tube for the purpose of enteral feeding?*
■ **KUB**

Routine for assessing correct placement of a gastric tube has been auscultation of air bolus. If the purpose of the gastric tube is administration of enteral nutrition, a KUB radiographic study should be performed to assure correct placement before initiation of feeding or administering medications. Dislodgment of the feeding tube with reinsertion should have the tube reverified for correct placement with radiographic KUB.

> **❯ HINT**
> Air auscultation alone may miss adverse placement of the gastric tube in the lungs. A KUB is more definitive ability in determining the location of the feeding tube.

■ What is the best method to prevent obstruction of the enteral feeding tube?
■ Frequent flushes

Frequent flushes used to irrigate the feeding tube are the best method for prevention of tube occlusion. Current recommendation is 20 to 30 mL of warm water flushed every 4 hours during continuous feeding and before and after medication administration. Tube occlusion may occur due to a stagnant enteral feeding formula and improperly crushed medications. Liquid medications or elixirs should be used if possible to avoid occlusion with pill fragments.

> **❯ HINT**
> Use pancreatic enzymes to remove the obstruction in the feeding tube.

■ What is the best method to prevent aspiration during EN?
■ Elevate the head of the bed (HOB)

Elevation of HOB 30 degrees to 45 degrees can decrease the risk of reflux (if not contraindicated). Coloring the feeding formula with dye has also been used in the past but is currently not recommended. Risks are higher using the blue dye than is the perceived benefit. The presence of blue dye in the tracheal aspirate is not a sensitive indicator of aspiration. Stop tube feedings 10 to 15 minutes prior to turning or flattening the HOB.

> **❯ HINT**
> Current studies show that the risk of aspiration with feeding in the duodenum is the same as gastric feeding. The time and effort needed to advance into the duodenum may not be justified and delays initiation of nutrition.

■ How often are gastric residuals typically recommended with continuous enteral feeding?
■ Every 4 hours

The most commonly recommended frequency required for assessing gastric residuals with enteral feeding is every 4 hours. Studies have not found a correlation between gastric residuals and feeding intolerance or risk for aspiration. Current recommendations are to hold tube feeds for residuals greater than 250 mL, recheck residuals every 2 hours, and restart tube feeds when residuals decrease below 250 mL. The North American Summit states to hold tube feeds if gastric residuals are greater than 250 mL for 2 consecutive hours.

> **HINT**
Clinical judgment may also be used when determining when to hold the tube feeds, including the rate of administration. Monitor for gradual increasing residuals or other signs of intolerance to feeding (Box 6.64).

Box 6.64 Signs of Enteral Feeding Intolerance

Absent bowel sounds	Diarrhea
Gastric distension/bloating	Constipation
Cramping	High gastric residuals
Nausea/vomiting	

■ *What type of enteral formula should be used in patients who develop noninfectious diarrhea with tube feeding?*
■ **Fiber-enriched formula**

Fiber-enriched formulas of enteral feeding or bulking agents, such as Metamucil, may be used to manage diarrhea and normalize stools. Certain medications may increase the likelihood of diarrhea and alternatives should be considered if possible. Prevent bacterial contamination of delivery sets with meticulous hand washing prior to set-up and handling of the enteral formula. Limit time of formula hanging at room temperature to 8 hours and rinse bag in between. Change administration sets every 24 hours.

> **HINT**
Send a stool sample to assess for *C. difficile* if diarrhea develops.

■ *In a malnourished patient, what should be monitored due to the risk of refeeding syndrome?*
■ **Electrolytes**

Malnourished patients are at risk for the development of refeeding syndrome, causing sudden fluid shifts and electrolyte imbalances. This can be life threatening. Glucose, sodium, chloride, potassium, magnesium, and phosphorous should be monitored routinely. Diabetics or those with risk for glucose intolerance may require insulin during enteral feeding (Box 6.65).

Box 6.65 Risk Factors of Refeeding Syndrome

Chronic alcoholism	Eating disorders
Acute weight loss post weight-loss surgery	Long-term use of antacids (binds phosphate)
Postoperative	Long-term use of diuretics
Elderly	Obesity
Chronic malnutrition	Little or no nutritional intake for 7–10 days

> **HINT**
The hallmark of refeeding syndrome is hypophosphatemia.

■ *What is the drug interaction that occurs with phenytoin and enteral feeding?*
■ **Decreases absorption of phenytoin**

Administration of phenytoin with enteral feeds lowers the absorption and peak serum levels of phenytoin. It may be necessary to increase dosing to maintain therapeutic serum concentrations. If the continuous tube feeding is discontinued, the dosage needs to be adjusted down and levels followed closely.

> **HINT**
Hold tube feeding 1 to 2 hours before and after administration of phenytoin to improve absorption.

BIBLIOGRAPHY

DeWaele, J. (2011). Intra-abdominal hypertension and abdominal compartment syndrome. *American Journal of Kidney Diseases, 57*(1), 159–169.
Moore et al. (1995). Organ injury scaling: Spleen and liver: *The Journal of Trauma: Injury, Infection and Critical Care, 38*(3), 323–334, Lippincott Williams & Wilkins.

Questions

1. A patient in the ICU begins vomiting blood and becomes hemodynamically unstable. His heart rate increased to 120 bpm, BP decreased to 90/54, and oxygen saturations decreased to 90% on 40% facemask. Which of the following is the priority of care at this time?

   A. Assist with placement of a central venous access
   B. Intubate and place on mechanical ventilation
   C. Assist with endoscopy to localize source of bleeding
   D. Initiate fluid resuscitation

2. Which of the following drugs used in managing a UGIB typically requires concurrent administration of nitroglycerin?

   A. Octreotide
   B. Terlipressin
   C. Pitressin
   D. Magnesium citrate

3. Mr. M is admitted to the ICU following a motor vehicle collison with blunt abdominal injuries. He has undergone an exploratory laparotomy. He had several small-bowel repairs, splenectomy, and a double-barrel loop colostomy. Which of the following laboratory findings would be expected following the injury he has sustained?

   A. Hyperkalemia
   B. Concentrated hematocrit
   C. Leukopenia
   D. Thrombocytosis

4. What is the most appropriate method to verify placement of a feeding tube?

   A. X-ray
   B. Air bolus auscultation
   C. Check pH of aspirate
   D. Bilirubin

5. Mr. J is at postoperative day 3 after femoral popliteal bypass surgery. His protein intake was inadequate and nutritional consult was obtained. His prealbumin level was 7.4 g/dL and he had an albumin level of 1.6 g/dL. He has lost 10 pounds and demonstrates muscle weakness. Which of the following is the best assessment of this patient's protein malnutrition?

   A. Muscle weakness
   B. Weight loss
   C. Albumin
   D. Prealbumin

6. A patient presenting with severe abdominal pain and vomiting is diagnosed with pancreatitis. Which of the following findings on admission would most predict an increased severity of pancreatitis?

   A. Hematocrit 45%
   B. Amylase > 140 U/L
   C. Lipase > 70 U/L
   D. Potassium 4.5 mEq/L

7. A 54-year-old patient with history of alcohol abuse is admitted with acute hepatic dysfunction. While in the unit, he starts to develop abnormalities with his ability to write as well as asterixis. What stage of encephalopathy is the patient in?

   A. Stage I
   B. Stage II
   C. Stage III
   D. Stage IV

8. Within 6 hours of an exploratory laparotomy for blunt abdominal trauma, the patient develops increased difficulty with ventilation. A CXR finds fluffy infiltrates and the patient's saturation is decreasing. Which of the following is the most likely cause for the early respiratory changes?

   A. Congestive heart failure (CHF)
   B. Acute respiratory distress syndrome (ARDS)
   C. ACS
   D. Dilated cardiomyopathy

9. A patient was diagnosed with a gastric tumor involving the distal esophagus and gastroesophageal junction. The surgeon performed an esophagectomy and partial gastrectomy. Postop, you note that the patient has developed subcutaneous air in the chest and neck region. Which of the following is the most probable reason for the subcutaneous air?

   A. Rupture of the anastomosis
   B. Normal finding with this surgical procedure
   C. Developed pneumothorax
   D. Ruptured bleb

10. In hemorrhagic pancreatitis, which of the following is an indication for surgical debridement of the pancreas?

    A. Edematous pancreatitis
    B. Pancreatic fistula
    C. Pseudocyst
    D. Infected necrosis

Renal System Review

In this chapter, you will review:

■ Acute kidney injury and chronic kidney disease
■ Contrast-induced nephropathy
■ Rhabdomyolysis
■ Electrolytes

ACUTE KIDNEY INJURY AND CHRONIC KIDNEY DISEASE

■ **What urine output (UO) is considered a criteria for an acute kidney injury (AKI)?**
■ **Less than 0.5 mL/kg/hr for 6 consecutive hours**

AKI is an abrupt or rapid decline in renal function and is defined by the serum creatinine (SCr) increase and decrease in UO. This definition is from the Acute Kidney Injury Network (AKIN) (Box 7.1).

Box 7.1 Criteria for AKI

Serum creatinine rises by ≥0.3 mg/dL within 48 hours *or*
Serum creatinine rises ≥ 1.5-fold from reference value (if known) *or*
Urine output is < 0.5 mL/kg/hr for more than 6 consecutive hours

> **HINT**
> Remember, a low UO is based on less than 0.5 mL/kg/hr instead of less than 30 mL/hr.

■ **AKIN devised the RIFLE staging system for AKI. What does the "R" in RIFLE mean?**
■ **Risk**

Earlier recognition of renal involvement can improve outcomes. The RIFLE criteria are used to identify early changes in renal function to allow for early interventions. RIFLE categorizes AKI into three grades of increasing severity using SCr or glomerular filtration rate (GFR) and UO criteria. Risk of AKI is considered if SCr increases by more than 1.5 or GFR decreases by more than 25% or UO is less than 0.5 mL/kg/hr for 6 hours.

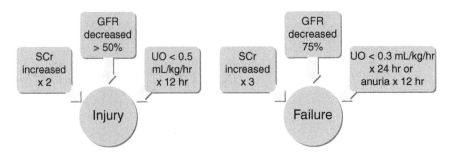

FIGURE 7.1 RIFLE staging.

> ❯ HINT
> The "I" stands for injury and the "L" in RIFLE is the "loss" that is
> persistent in complete loss of renal function for longer than 4 weeks.
> The "E" is "end stage" or complete loss of renal function for longer
> than 3 months (Figure 7.1).

■ *Chronic kidney disease (CKD) is defined as a GFR of less than what?*

■ **Less than 60 mL/minute**

CKD is defined as a GFR less than 60 mL/minute for 6 months or longer (Box 7.2).

Box 7.2 CKD Criteria

GFR > 90 but disease diagnosed
GFR 60–89, mild
GFR 30–59, moderate
GFR 15–29, severe
GFR < 15, end-stage renal disease

■ *What are the three categories of acute renal failure (ARF)?*

■ **Prerenal, intrarenal, or postrenal failure**

Prerenal, intrarenal, and postrenal failures are terms used to describe the underlying causes
of ARF. Prerenal failure is hypoperfusion without actual kidney damage. Intrarenal failure is
kidney injury that includes reversible and irreversible injury. Postrenal failure occurs "after the
kidneys" caused by obstruction to outflow. Postrenal failure results in kidney injury (Box 7.3).

Box 7.3 Causes of Prerenal, Intrarenal, and Postrenal Failure

Prerenal Failure	Intrarenal Failure	Postrenal Failure
Shock	Ischemia	Urinary tract obstructions
Sepsis	Prerenal etiology	Blood clots
Cardiogenic		Benign prostatic hypertrophy
Hypovolemic		Urethral strictures
Anaphylaxis		Tumor
		Urinary stones
Trauma	Immune/infections	Urinary tract infections

(continued)

Box 7.3 Causes of Prerenal, Intrarenal, and Postrenal Failure (*continued*)

Prerenal Failure	Intrarenal Failure	Postrenal Failure

Congestive heart failure	Nephrotoxicity
	  Aminoglycosides
	  Nonsteroidal anti-inflammatory
	   agents (NSAIDs)
	  Radiographic contrast dye
	  Antibiotics
	  Myoglobin
		Neuropathy
		  Spinal cord-injured patient

Hepatorenal syndrome	Glomerulonephritis
	  Systemic lupus erythematosus
	  Postinfections
	  Good pasture syndrome
		Trauma
		  Bilateral ureteral injuries
		  Bladder rupture
		  Urethral injury

Medication induced
  NSAIDs
  Angiotensin converting
   enzyme inhibitors/
   angiotensin receptor-
   blocking agents
  Vasoconstrictors
	Medication induced
	  NSAIDs
	  Amphotericin B
	  Radiocontrast agents
	  Antiretrovirals
		Medication induced
		  Anticholinergic drugs

Diuretics (excessive diuresis)		
Abdominal compartment syndrome		

> **HINT**
> The same mechanism can cause prerenal and intrarenal failure. In prerenal AKI, the kidneys are not injured and can still function, whereas intrarenal failure kidneys are injured and can no longer function appropriately.

PATHOPHYSIOLOGY

■ *What electrolyte is reabsorbed by the renal system in response to hypoperfusion?*

■ **Sodium**

Prerenal AKI is caused by renal hypoperfusion. Because the kidneys are not damaged, they respond appropriately to aldosterone and reabsorb sodium and water. This is a compensatory mechanism for volume depletion.

■ *Nonsteroidal anti-inflammatory drugs (NSAIDs) affect renal perfusion by blocking which substance in the body?*

■ **Prostaglandins**

Prostaglandins are partially responsible for vasodilating afferent arterioles. Prostaglandins play a role in renal perfusion during periods of hypoperfusion. NSAIDs block the prostaglandins, resulting in a decrease in GFR and renal blood flow, exacerbating hypoperfusion of kidneys during periods of decreased blood flow. Drugs that affect the vasodilation of the afferent or vasoconstriction of the efferent arterioles can result in prerenal failure.

> **HINT**
Vasodilation of afferent (toward glomerulus) and vasoconstriction of efferent (away from glomerulus) will increase GFR. There is more flow going in and less flow coming out. NSAIDs affect the inability to vasodilate afferent.

- *Do angiotensin converting enzyme (ACE) inhibitors and angiotensin receptor-blocking agents (ARBs) affect the afferent or efferent arterioles?*
- **Efferent**

ACE inhibitors and ARBs prevent efferent vasoconstriction by inhibiting angiotensin II vasoconstriction and the kidneys' ability to maintain an adequate perfusion.

> **HINT**
Angiotensin II is a potent vasoconstrictor.

- *Acute tubular necrosis (ATN) is a common problem causing intrarenal failure. This affects which part of the kidneys?*
- **Renal tubules**

Renal tubules are responsible for dilution and concentration of urine. ATN is characterized by the failure to maximally dilute or concentrate the urine. This is called isosthenuria. ATN is associated with prolonged prerenal insult or a direct nephrotoxin (Box 7.4).

Box 7.4 Five Types of Intrarenal Failure

	Tubular Injury	Interstitial Injury	Glomerular Injury	Vascular Injury	Intratubular Obstruction
Site of injury	Renal tubules	Kidney interstitium	Glomerular nephrons	Renal artery	Renal tubules
Mechanism of injury	Prolonged ischemia or nephrotoxins	Inflammatory infiltrates and edema within interstitium	Immunological mechanism triggers inflammation and proliferation	Major renal artery obstruction or severe abdominal aortic disease	Precipitation of proteins or crystals within tubule lumen causing obstruction
Clinical presentation	Failure to maximally dilute or concentrate urine	Fever, rash, eosinophila	Fever, malaise, arthralgia	Microangiopathic anemia, thrombocytopenia	
Urine characteristics	"Muddy brown" sediment (casts)		Severe proteinuria and erythrocyte casts		
Treatment	Steroid		Corticosteroids and cyclophosphamide		

■ *In postrenal failure, upper urinary tract obstruction can cause AKI. What must happen for this to occur?*
■ **Bilateral obstruction**

The upper urinary tract involves the ureters and renal pelvis. For AKI to occur, both ureters need to be involved in the obstruction, otherwise only one kidney is affected. The lower tract involves the bladder and urethra. Obstruction at any level in the lower tract can cause AKI. Obstruction of the flow of urine results in backing up into the renal parenchyma, leading to hydronephrosis. If not treated immediately, it can cause CKD due to elevated tubule pressure.

> **❯ HINT**
> The upper urinary tract has two ureters that drain to one bladder out through one urethra. For AKI to occur in the upper tract, both ureters must be obstructed (unless only one functioning kidney).

SYMPTOMS/ASSESSMENT

■ *Which of the renal failure categories is more likely to result in anuria?*
■ **Postrenal failure**

Obstruction to outflow is the most likely cause of a sudden cessation of urine rather than development of oliguria. There is an initial increase in intratubular pressure that decreases the filtration-driving force, and reabsorption of urine occurs. Once the pressure gradient equalizes, the depressed GFR depends on renal efferent vasoconstriction, which results in anuria.

> **❯ HINT**
> Postrenal failure may also present with sudden anuria with intermittent periods of polyuria.

■ *AKI causes electrolyte abnormalities. Which two electrolytes significantly elevate following renal injury?*
■ **Potassium and phosphate**

Hyperkalemia and hyperphosphatemia occur with AKI and CKD due to the inability of the kidney to remove excess potassium and phosphates. Intrarenal failure results in a loss of sodium as well as dilutional sodium (Box 7.5).

> **❯ HINT**
> Early in prerenal failure, potassium may be low because the kidney responds to aldosterone by conserving sodium and water. If the kidney reabsorbs sodium, then potassium is lost in urine.

Box 7.5 Electrolyte Abnormalities in Kidney Injury

Hyperkalemia	Hyponatremia
Hyperphosphatemia	Normal to elevate magnesium
Hypocalcemia	

> ❯ HINT
> Remember, phosphorous and calcium have an inverse relationship. As phosphate levels increase, the calcium levels decrease.

■ *In kidney injury, is there a metabolic acidosis or alkalosis?*
■ **Metabolic acidosis**

Metabolic acidosis occurs as a result of accumulation of excessive acidic substances in the blood as well as the renal tubules' inability to secrete H^+ ions and reabsorb bicarbonate.

> ❯ HINT
> Other abnormalities caused by AKI include anemia due to the decrease in production of erythtropoetin.

DIAGNOSIS

■ *A fractional excretion of sodium (FENa) less than 1% indicates which of the categories of AKI, pre-, intra-, or postrenal failure?*
■ **Prerenal failure**

A FENa measures the ratio of sodium excreted (urine sodium × volume) to sodium filtered (serum sodium × GFR). The ratio is used in determining whether the kidneys can function by conserving sodium during periods of hypoperfusion.

> ❯ HINT
> Loop diuretics can increase sodium excretion, making FENa less useful in diagnostics. Exception to prerenal cause is in myoglobinuria, which will have a FEN less than 1% but is classified as intrarenal failure.

Urine sodium levels are also used to determine the ability of the kidneys to reabsorb sodium. In prerenal failure, the renal tubules still function so they readily reabsorb Na^+. This gives a low urine sodium concentration (< 20–40 mEq/L). In intrarenal failure, the renal tubules are unable to reabsorb Na^+, so the urine concentration will be elevated (> 40 mEq/L). Elderly patients may have an obligatory loss of sodium in the urine.

> ❯ HINT
> Glomerulonephritis is an intrarenal failure that maintains the ability to reabsorb sodium, because renal tubules remain intact.

■ *A patient with AKI has a blood urea nitrogen (BUN) of 40 and a SCr of 3.8. Based on this BUN:creatinine ratio, would this be prerenal or intrarenal failure?*
■ **Intrarenal failure**

The BUN:creatinine ratio is also used to determine the category of AKI. A normal BUN:creatinine ratio is 10:1 up to a 15:1 ratio. An abnormal ratio of more than 20:1 indicates prerenal failure. The kidneys increase reabsorption of urea because of the slow renal tubular flow rates, but creatinine is not reabsorbed in the renal tubules and will increase out of proportion to the BUN. An elevated creatinine and BUN that remain within a normal ratio indicates intrarenal or postrenal failure (Box 7.6).

Box 7.6 Summary for Differentiation of Renal Failure

Lab Test	Prerenal	Intrarenal	Postrenal
Urine Na$^+$	< 10–20	> 20–40	> 20–40
Urine osmolality	> 500	< 350–400	< 350–400
Urine specific gravity	> 1.015	~1.010	~1.010
Urine sediment	No cells, casts	RBC, WBC, casts	RBC, no casts
Blood urea nitrogen:creatinine	> 20:1	10:1	10:1
Fractional excretion of sodium	< 1%	> 1%	Variable

RBC, red blood cell; WBC, white blood cell.

> **〉 HINT**
> BUN and creatinine are typically elevated in all AKI but the ratio is what is used to assist in determination of categories of AKI. Liver impairment affects BUN levels and not the SCr (Box 7.7).

Box 7.7 Factors Affecting SCr

Greater muscle mass increases SCr	Men: Greater SCr levels than women
Old age lowers SCr	Inadequate protein diet decreases SCr
African Americans: Higher SCr	Neuromuscular disease increases SCr

■ *What are the two urine tests that are used to determine the ability of the kidneys to concentrate the urine?*
■ **Urine osmolality and urine specific gravity**

One of the functions of the kidneys is to concentrate the urine. Urine osmolality and urine specific gravity are indicators of the kidneys' ability to concentrate urine. If the kidneys are hypoperfused, the renin–angiotensin system (RAS) is initiated and aldosterone is released. This causes the kidneys to reabsorb sodium and water, thus concentrating the urine. In prerenal failure the kidneys are still able to concentrate urine, but in intrarenal failure they are unable to concentrate urine.

> **〉 HINT**
> In AKI, urine laboratory tests are required to determine whether the urine is concentrated or dilute. Urine in renal failure is typically dark amber and appears to be concentrated even when dilute.

■ *What laboratory test is used to determine the GFR?*
■ **Creatinine clearance**

GFR is the volume of blood filtered by the glomerulus in 1 minute. Creatinine clearance is a calculated number that provides information about the GFR. Normal rate of clearance is 85 to 135 mL/min (normal GFR). Men have a higher normal GFR than women.

> **〉 HINT**
> Above the age of 40 years, creatinine clearance decreases by 1 mL/min per year. In postrenal failure, the urine sodium is abnormally elevated in chronic kidney injury and usually low in AKI.

■ *What is the gold standard for diagnosing upper tract obstruction in postrenal failure?*

■ **Ultrasound**

Ultrasound is the gold standard for diagnosing upper tract obstruction but can be less reliable in a volume-depleted situation. It is recommended that the ultrasound be repeated after successful fluid resuscitation. Placement of a urinary catheter or irrigation of the present catheter may assist with the diagnosis of a lower tract obstruction.

MANAGEMENT

■ *What is the primary treatment in prerenal failure?*

■ **Reestablish perfusion to the kidneys**

The primary management of prerenal failure is to treat the underlying cause of the hypoperfusion. If the patient is hypovolemic, administer volume replacement.

■ *What is the purpose of administering a loop diuretic to a patient with AKI?*

■ **Convert oliguric to nonoliguric renal failure**

Loop diuretics may be used when attempting to convert an oliguric to a nonoliguric renal failure. Nonoliguric renal failure has a better prognosis due to control of volume and some electrolytes. Overuse or high doses of diuretics do not benefit the patient and can actually worsen renal function. Other drugs that have been used to manage AKI but are not supported in the research include low-dose dopamine and fenoldopam. Currently, there is no specific pharmacological management of AKI considered to be effective.

> ❯ **HINT**
> High doses of a loop diuretic increase risk of ototoxicity.

■ *What is the complication of poor nutrition in an AKI patient that causes an increase in release of amino acids from skeletal muscle?*

■ **Protein catabolism**

Protein catabolism occurs in ARF with the excessive release of amino acids from skeletal muscle and sustained negative nitrogen balance. Energy expenditure can increase by 30% or more if AKI is associated with sepsis and multiple organ dysfunction. It is recommended that patients with AKI should receive 25 to 30 kcal/kg per day with the energy intake not to exceed 30 kcal/kg/day.

> ❯ **HINT**
> Overfeeding a critically ill patient can lead to metabolic complications such as hypertonic hydration and metabolic acidosis.

■ *What is the primary treatment in patients with severe AKI?*

■ **Renal replacement therapy (RRT)**

In severe AKI, RRT is the recommended management. There are no set guidelines on when to initiate RRT and initiation is based on individual patient risks and benefits of RRT. Recent studies indicate that early initiation of RRT may improve outcomes but this finding requires further research (Box 7.8).

Box 7.8 Indications of Renal Replacement Therapy

Metabolic acidosis	Drug overdose
Hyperkalemia	Volume overload
Symptomatic uremia	Azotemia

■ *What is the main risk of intermittent hemodialysis (IHD)?*
■ **Hypotension**

IHD is typically delivered three to six times a week and performed over a 4- to 6-hour period. The advantage is rapid removal of toxins and life-threatening electrolytes. The disadvantage is that rapid removal or shifts of fluid can result in hemodynamic instability. Another complication of rapid removal of solutes is a sudden decrease in serum osmolality, allowing fluid to shift extravascularly. This leads to cerebral edema and is called disequilibrium syndrome.

> **HINT**
> Slower removal of solutes may be required in neurological patients who are more susceptible to cerebral edema.

■ *What type of RRT is recommended in hemodynamically unstable patients?*
■ **Continuous renal replacement therapy (CRRT)**

CRRT is performed continuously 24 hours a day. This allows the water and solutes to be removed at a slower, more consistent rate, lowering the risk of hypotension. Hemodynamically unstable patients are candidates for CRRT, which has a lower incidence of hypotension and can prevent hypervolemic occurrences between hemodialysis. CRRT is performed through a venovenous access (Box 7.9).

Box 7.9 Types of Continuous Renal Replacement Therapy

Continuous venovenous hemofiltration (CVVH)	Solutes cleared by convection No dialysate is used Rate of ultrafiltration determines convective clearance Replacement fluids may be used
Continuous venovenous hemodialysis (CVVHD)	Solutes removed by diffusion Dialysate is used Ultrafiltration used for volume control
Continuous venovenous hemodiafiltration (CVVHDF)	Combination of convective solute removal and diffusion Replacement fluids may be used

■ *What is a disadvantage of CRRT for intensive care unit (ICU) patients?*
■ **Use of anticoagulation therapy**

IHD requires less anticoagulation therapy due to the rapidity of the procedure. CRRT is a slower, continuous procedure that takes place over 24 hours and is more likely to develop issues with filter clotting. Other disadvantages are the amount of nursing time and skill required to perform CRRT at the bedside, as well as its costs.

■ **Which electrolyte is most likely to become abnormally low during CRRT therapy?**

■ **Phosphate**

Hypophosphatemia (< 2 mg/dL) develops frequently with CRRT. The incidence has been found to increase with longer therapy and more intense RRT. Hypophosphatemia causes muscle weakness, including weakness of the respiratory muscles, and is associated with prolonged use of mechanical ventilation.

> ❯ **HINT**
> Phosphate is frequently added to the replacement fluids or dialysate solutions to prevent complication of hypophosphatemia.

COMPLICATIONS

■ **A renal dialysis patient presents with fever, chills, and chest pain. What is the most likely cause?**

■ **Pericarditis**

Uremic- or dialysis-related pericarditis is a complication of chronic renal failure and RRT. It is thought to be caused by accumulation of bioirritants in the pericardial sac, such as uric acid. The immune system may also play a role in development of inflammation in the pericardial space. It typically presents with chest pain (may not be as significant as other pericarditis patients), fever, chills, and pericardial friction rub. Management is typically with RRT. If large effusions or tamponade develop, it may require pericardiocentesis.

■ **What electrolyte abnormality may contribute to the arrhythmias?**

■ **Hyperkalemia**

Hyperkalemia frequently results in ventricular arrhythmias and may be seen in renal failure patients. RRT is used to manage hyperkalemia but may require administration of kayexalate in between dialysis (Box 7.10).

Box 7.10 Complications of AKI and CKD

Electrolyte imbalances	Stomatitis
Pericarditis	Drowsy, lethargy to delirium
Pericardial effusions and/or tamponade	Itching, dryness (uticaria)
Pulmonary edema	Thrombocytopenia
Dysrhythmias	Anemia
Anorexia, nausea, vomiting, diarrhea	

CONTRAST-INDUCED NEPHROPATHY

■ *What is the primary risk factor for development of contrast-induced nephropathy (CIN)?*

■ **Hypovolemia**

CIN is defined as an increase in baseline creatinine level by 25% or 0.5 mg/dL or greater within 24 to 48 hours after a procedure that requires contrast material. Almost 10% of all hospital-acquired AKI is directly related to contrast material. Hypovolemia or overall volume depletion is a primary risk for the development of CIN (Box 7.11).

> **❯ HINT**
> Recovery typically occurs 3 to 5 days after exposure unless the patient develops persistent renal failure.

Box 7.11 Risk Factors of CIN

Chronic kidney disease	Anemia
Dehydration	Cardiac disease
Diabetes mellitus	Proteinuria
Hyperglycemia	Nephrotoxic medications
Advanced age	High osmolar contrast agents
Hypertension	Greater volume of contrast agents used

■ *How long before a contrast study is it recommended to discontinue nephrotoxic agents?*

■ **24 hours prior**

It is recommended that nephrotoxic agents be discontinued 24 hours prior to performing a procedure with contrast medium. High-risk patients should be identified and preventive interventions implemented prior to the procedure.

> **❯ HINT**
> In critically ill patients, holding some of these drugs may be a risk-versus-benefit decision (Box 7.12).

Box 7.12 Nephrotoxic Agents

Nonsteroidal anti-inflammatory drugs
Angiotensin converting enzyme inhibitors/angiotensin receptor-blocking agents
Metformin
Aminoglycosides
Loop diuretics
Cyclosporine

■ *What is the primary recommended intervention to prevent CIN?*

■ **IV hydration**

Adequate IV fluid hydration before and after the procedure is beneficial and has been found to lower the incidence of CIN. The IV fluid recommended is 0.9% NaCl, with some physicians using isotonic sodium bicarbonate to alkalinize the urine in addition to fluid resuscitation. N-acetylcysteine (Mucomyst) is an antioxidant of oxygen-free radicals and vasodilator in kidneys. It can be administered prior to the study and after the study in high-risk patients.

> **HINT**
Administer fluids more cautiously in congestive heart failure (CHF) patients.

RHABDOMYOLYSIS

■ *What is the mechanism that results in rhabdomyolysis?*
■ **Skeletal muscle injury or breakdown**

Myoglobin is a protein found in skeletal and smooth muscle cells. The injury causes an alteration in the cell membrane integrity of the muscle, allowing the intracellular contents to escape into the plasma. Myoglobinuria is the presence of myoglobin in urine, which can occur if plasma levels exceed 1.5 mg/dL. Myoglobin is toxic to the kidneys, resulting in rhabdomyolysis-induced AKI.

> **HINT**
Acidity of the urine will affect the amount of damage in the renal tubules (Box 7.13).

Box 7.13 Causes of Rhabdomyolysis

Trauma	Drug induced
Crush injuries	Cocaine
Burns	Heroin
	Barbiturates
Muscle injury from overuse	Amphetamines
Status epilepticus generalized seizures	Diazepam
Fever	Alcohol
Thyroid storm	Phencyclidine (PCP)
Strenuous exercise	Lipid-lowering agents (statins)
Delirium tremors	
	Infections
Ischemic injury to muscle	Sepsis
Prolonged immobility	Infectious hepatitis
Shock states	Viral influenza
Arterial occlusion	Tetanus
Postcardiac arrest	

■ *Which two serum laboratory tests are frequently obtained to diagnose rhabdomyolysis?*
■ **Myoglobin and creatinine kinase (CK)**

Following muscle injury, the myoglobin and CK levels will increase. Muscle injury causes an alteration in the cell membrane integrity of the muscle, allowing the intracellular contents to escape into the plasma. Myoglobin and CK are found in skeletal and smooth muscle cells. Other intracellular components include potassium and phosphates and can elevate following trauma (Box 7.14).

> **HINT**
> Urine hematest will be positive for hemoglobin, but few or no RBCs are commonly found on urinalysis. The urine hematest is unable to differentiate hemoglobin from myoglobin.

Box 7.14 Laboratory Values of Rhabdomyolysis

Elevated creatinine kinase	Hyperphosphatemia
Elevated myoglobin	Hypocalcemia
Hyperkalemia	Myoglobinuria

- **What is the primary intervention used to manage rhabdomyolysis?**
- **Fluid resuscitation**

Fluid resuscitation is the primary management used to flush the myoglobin molecules through the kidneys to decrease injury to the renal tubules. NaCl is the fluid of choice, typically at a rate of 10 to 15 mL/kg/hr to achieve high urinary flow rates. Mannitol, an osmotic diuretic, can be administered if the patient becomes oliguric. It is used to increase renal perfusion, dilate renal vasculature, and "wash out" tubular debris and toxic wastes.

> **HINT**
> The goal for UO is greater than 100 mL/hr.

- **What urine pH is the goal when administering sodium bicarbonate to prevent injury in rhabdomyolysis?**
- **Higher than 6.5**

Sodium bicarbonate is used to alkalinize the urine to decrease the nephrotoxicity of myoglobin. It is administered as a continuous infusion to maintain urinary pH higher than 6.5. Bicarbonates side effects include metabolic alkalosis and hypocalcemia.

> **HINT**
> Metabolic alkalosis shifts the oxyhemoglobin dissociation curve, causing hemoglobin to hold on to oxygen, resulting in hypoperfusion of tissues.

ELECTROLYTES

See Box 7.15.

Box 7.15 Normal Values for Electrolytes

Calcium	8.5–10.5 mg/dL (2.2–2.6 mmol/L)	Magnesium	1.5–2.3 mg/dL
Ionized calcium	4.5–5.6 mg/dL (1.1–1.4 mmol/L)	Phosphate	3.0–4.5 mg/dL
Potassium	3.5–5.0 mEq/L	Sodium	135–145 mEq/L

Values will vary based on the laboratory.

PATHOPHYSIOLOGY

■ *Which hormones are responsible for regulating calcium in and out of bone?*
■ **Parathyroid hormone (PTH) and calcitonin**

Calcium is primarily stored in bone. The PTH and calcitonin controls movement of calcium in and out of bones using a negative feedback system based on serum calcium levels. PTH allows calcium to move intravascularly, and calcitonin increases the resorption of calcium in bone.

> **❯ HINT**
> Calcitonin is used to manage hypercalcemia by "pushing" calcium back into the bone.

■ *What is the most common cause of hypocalcemia in ICU patients when measuring total calcium?*
■ **Hypoalbuminemia**

A low albumin level is the most common reason for low total serum calcium levels in ICU patients. This may not require management of the calcium levels because a low albumin level does not affect ionized calcium levels. Total serum calcium should be corrected in the presence of low albumin or ionized calcium levels should be used to determine the need for treating the low calcium (Boxes 7.16 and 7.17).

Box 7.16 Causes of Hypocalcemia

Sepsis	Chelating agents (bind calcium)
Hypoalbuminemia	Citrate in packed red blood cells (PRBCs)
Pancreatitis	Ethylene glycol ingestion
Parathyroid hormone deficiency	Radiographic contrast medium
Hyperphosphatemia	Sodium bicarbonate
Alkalosis	Aminoglycosides
	Protamine sulfate
	Hypothyroidism

Box 7.17 Forms of Total Serum Calcium

Ionized	Bound to Proteins	Complexed
45% total serum calcium	40% total serum calcium	15% total serum calcium
Readily available for use	Bound to proteins	Complexed to anions such as chloride, citrate, bicarbonate, and phosphate
	Especially albumin	Ca^{++} is not available for use
	Ca^{++} is not available for use	

> **❯ HINT**
> Calcium is one of the electrolytes that does not want to live alone and will chelate or "marry" multiple substances. Once chelated or "married," it does not work. Only free (ionized) calcium is readily available to work (Box 7.18). Hypoalbuminemia also results in hypomagnesemia. Magnesium is also ionized or "free" and bound to proteins. Ionized levels are not frequently obtained.

Box 7.18 Calculation of Corrected Total Serum Calcium

Equation: Total Ca^{++} + 0.8 (4 - 2)
Example: Patient's total Ca^{++} is 7.0 and serum albumin is 2.0 7.0 + 0.8 (4 − 2) 7.0 + 0.8 (2) 7.0 + 1.6 = 8.6 as the corrected Ca^+

■ *What type of diuretic may cause hypercalcemia?*
■ **Thiazide diuretic**

Hypercalcemia is less common in ICU patients. Certain medications can cause hypercalcemia, including thiazide diuretics. Patients in the ICU require close monitoring of calcium levels and, if hypercalcemia occurs, determine the underlying cause; if it is the thiazide diuretic, the medication needs to be discontinued (Box 7.19).

Box 7.19 Causes of Hypercalcemia

Hyperparathyroidism	Drugs
Prolonged immobility	Thiazide diuretics
Neoplasm	Lithium
Orthopedic injuries	Sarcoidosis

■ *Does insulin infusion potentially cause hypokalemia or hyperkalemia?*
■ **Hypokalemia**

The majority of potassium is intracellular and certain situations and medications can shift potassium between intracellular and intravascular spaces. Insulin "drives" potassium into the cell, lowering the serum potassium levels (Box 7.20).

Box 7.20 Causes of Potassium Shifts

Intracellular Shifts (Hypokalemia)	Intravascular Shifts (Hyperkalemia)
Insulin	Lack of insulin
Beta agonists	Beta antagonists
Alkalosis	Acidosis
Sodium bicarbonate	Tissue injury
	Cardiac arrest

■ *Which electrolyte should be corrected to adequately replace potassium?*
■ **Magnesium**

Hypomagnesemia should be corrected before correcting hypokalemia due to increased renal losses of potassium. Magnesium is needed to regulate potassium, sodium, and calcium.

> **❯ HINT**
> Magnesium repletion is required to correct a potassium level of less than 3.0 mEq/L (Box 7.21).

Box 7.21 Causes of Hypokalemia

Low potassium intake	Diarrhea
Hyperalimentation	Diaphoresis
Diuresis	Pancreatitis and pancreatic abscesses
Hyperaldosteronism	Hypomagnesemia
Nasogastric (NG) tube to low wall suction	Delirium tremens
Vomiting	Hyperthyroidism

- ### *What is the cause of pseudohyperkalemia?*
- ### Clotted blood specimen

Hemolysis of blood in the tube can falsely elevate the potassium levels. Other causes of false elevation of potassium or pseudohyperkalemia are marked leukocytosis or thrombocytosis (Box 7.22).

Box 7.22 Causes of Hyperkalemia

Dilutional	Potassium-sparing diuretics
Muscle injury	Angiotensin converting enzyme inhibitors
Burns and trauma	and angiotensin receptor blockers
Renal failure	Rhabdomyolysis
Adrenal insufficiency	Tumor lysis

- ### *What is the mechanism of hypomagnesemia during periods of diuresis?*
- ### Decreased reabsorption

Magnesium reabsorption in kidneys has an inverse relationship to UO. High flow output results in a loss of magnesium in the urine.

> ❯ HINT
>
> In renal failure, magnesium is typically normal but can be elevated due to a low-flow state. So, AKI may cause hypermagnesemia and drugs high in magnesium should be avoided (Boxes 7.23 and 7.24).

Box 7.23 Causes of Hypomagnesemia

Malnutrition, starvation	Hyperglycemia, diabetes mellitus
NG suctioning	Acidosis
Parenteral nutrition	Hypercalcemia, hypophosphatemia
Decreased gastrointestinal absorption	Pancreatitis
Alcohol consumption	Sepsis
Diuretics	Alkalosis
Drugs binding magnesium	Insulin administration
Citrate	
Aminoglycosides	
Cyclosporine	
Digoxin	

Box 7.24 Causes of Hypermagnesemia

Renal failure
Excessive intake of magnesium-containing laxatives and antacids

■ *During initial refeeding, which electrolyte abnormality is most common?*
■ Hypophosphatemia

Following starvation, an abrupt increase in carbohydrates causes a spike in the release of insulin, which drives phosphate into the cell. This is similar to the shift of potassium and phosphate following administration of exogenous insulin (Box 7.25).

Box 7.25 Causes of Hypophosphatemia

Refeeding syndrome	Vitamin D deficiency
Insulin administration	NG suction
Diuretics	Chronic diarrhea
Respiratory alkalosis	Malabsorption syndrome
Hyperparathyroidism	Extreme catabolic states
Insufficient gastrointestinal absorption	

■ *What is the most common reason for hyperphosphatemia in an ICU patient?*
■ Acute kidney injury

Renal failure results in hyperphosphatemia due to inability of kidneys to excrete phosphates (Box 7.26).

Box 7.26 Causes of Hyperphosphatemia

Renal failure (acute and chronic)	Muscle injury
Excessive administration	Rhabdomyolysis
Hypoparathyroidism	Bisphosphonate therapy
Thyrotoxicosis	

■ *Which causes hyponatremia in the syndrome of inappropriate antidiuretic hormone (SIADH), hemodilution or a loss of sodium?*
■ Hemodilution

SIADH is the result of too much antidiuretic hormone. The kidneys reabsorb water, causing dilutional sodium. There is an excess of water in relation to sodium (Box 7.27).

Box 7.27 Causes of Hyponatremia

Hypoosmolar **euvolemic** hyponatremia	Syndrome of inappropriate antidiuretic hormone
	Glucocorticoid insufficiency
	Hypothyroidism
	Stress
	Medications: Haloperidol, vasopressin

(continued)

Box 7.27 Causes of Hyponatremia (*continued*)

Hypoosmolar **hypovolemic** hyponatremia	Cerebral salt wasting syndrome Vomiting Diarrhea Third spacing
Hypoosmolar **hypervolemic** hyponatremia	Nephrotic syndrome Hepatic cirrhosis Cardiac failure

> ❯ **HINT**
> Fluid status is the most important differentiation of the causes of hyponatremia.

■ *What are the two main alterations that can result in hypernatremia?*
■ **Free water deficit or excessive intake**

Hypernatremia can be caused by an abnormal water balance or excessive body sodium. A free water deficit is the loss of fluid, causing hemoconcentration and hypernatremia. Excessive body sodium may be due to greater intake of sodium, such as administration of too much hypertonic (3%) NaCl (Box 7.28).

Box 7.28 Causes of Hypernatremia

Hypovolemic hypernatremia	Diuretic excess Postobstructive uropathy Intrinsic renal disease
Euvolemic hypernatremia	Diabetes insipidus Hypodopsia Insensible fluid losses
Hypervolemic hypernatremia	3% NaCl Excessive intake of sodium Primary hyperaldosteronism Cushing's syndrome Hypertonic dialysis

SYMPTOMS/ASSESSMENT

■ *What effect does hypocalcemia have on blood pressure (BP)?*
■ **Lowers BP**

The cardiovascular effects of hypocalcemia include decrease in myocardial contractility (decreased cardiac output) and vasodilation (hypotension). The hypotension may be refractory to fluid administration and vasoconstrictive drugs. Bradycardia, which may progress to asystole or complete heart block, and prolonged QT interval are other cardiovascular effects of hypocalcemia.

> ❯ **HINT**
> When calcium channel blocker's cardiovascular effects are the same as of hypocalcemia it lowers the BP and decreases myocardial contractility.

■ *What is it called when the facial nerve is tapped lightly and produces involuntary twitching of facial muscles?*
■ **Chvostek sign**

Chvostek sign may be found in both hypocalcemia and hypomagnesemia patients. It is elicited by lightly tapping along the facial nerve. Trousseau's sign may also be present in both hypocalcemia and hypomagnesemia. This is a carpopedal spasm that occurs in response to hypoperfusion of the hand. It may be elicited with a BP cuff inflated to 20 mmHg for 3 minutes.

> **❯ HINT**
>
> Magnesium abnormalities are similar to calcium's (Box 7.29). Mild hypercalcemia and hypermagnesemia are relatively asymptomatic (Box 7.30).

Box 7.29 Signs of Hypocalcemia and Hypomagnesemia

Circumoral and distal paresthesia or tingling
Muscle cramps progressing to muscle spasm, tremors, twitching, tetany
Seizures
Positive Chvostek sign
Positive Trousseaus' sign
Hypotension
Bradycardia, ventricular tachycardia, and heart blocks

Box 7.30 Signs of Hypercalcemia and Hypermagnesemia

Lethargy, apathy, fatigue, depression	Nausea and vomiting
Excessive thirst	Abdominal pain
Muscle weakness, flaccidity	Hypertension
Decreased gastrointestinal motility	Shortened QT interval

■ *What is the most common symptom of both hypo- and hyperkalemia?*
■ **Ventricular arrhythmias**

Both hypo- and hyperkalemia may present with cardiovascular and neuromuscular symptoms. The neuromuscular symptoms include paresthesia and weakness of the extremities, which may progress to flaccid paralysis and respiratory arrest.

■ *What is the cardiovascular symptom of hypophosphatemia?*
■ **Ventricular dysfunction**

Hypophosphatemia can cause left ventricular dysfunction and may develop a dilated cardiomyopathy (Box 7.31).

Box 7.31 Symptoms of Hypophosphatemia

Weakened respiratory muscles	Acute hemolytic anemia
Confusion, lethargy	Acute left ventricular dysfunction
Gait disturbances and paresthesia	Reversible dilated cardiomyopathy

■ *Hyperphosphatemia mimics what other electrolyte abnormality?*

■ Hypocalcemia

Hyperphosphatemia causes hypocalcemia. There is an inverse relationship between the two. Symptoms of hypocalcemia are more prominent than signs of hyperphosphatemia.

■ *What system in the body is most affected by sodium abnormalities?*

■ Neurological system

Both hypo- and hypernatremia can cause altered mental status. Sodium abnormalities should be suspected in a patient who develops a change in mental status and altered fluid balance (Boxes 7.32 and 7.33).

Box 7.32 Signs of Hyponatremia

Nausea	Decreased mentation
Vomiting	Seizures
Lethargy	Cerebral edema
Confusion	Coma and death

Box 7.33 Signs of Hypernatremia

Confusion	Seizures
Weakness	Decreased mentation
Lethargy	Coma and death

DIAGNOSIS

■ *On the cardiac monitor, the nurse recognizes that the patient has developed U waves. What electrolyte abnormality commonly causes U waves?*

■ Hypokalemia

As potassium progressively decreases, the ECG demonstrates characteristic changes of hypokalemia. These changes include flattened T waves, ST depression, and U waves. Characteristic ECG changes of hyperkalemia include peaked T waves and widening of QRS complex. Arrhythmias include atrioventricular (AV) conduction blocks, ventricular fibrillation, and systole.

> ❯ HINT
> Hypokalemia develops "U" waves and hyperkalemia develops peaked "T" waves.

■ *What type of hyponatremia presents with a urine sodium level of more than 20 mmol/L?*

■ Hypoosmolar hypovolemia hyponatremia

Urine sodium levels of > 20 mmol/L indicate a renal loss of sodium as the cause for hyponatremia. This is not a dilutional hyponatremia and is not associated with hypervolemia. The increase in renal loss of sodium actually "pulls" water with the sodium and increases water excretion, resulting in hypovolemia. The patient would also exhibit signs of volume depletion.

MANAGEMENT

■ *When should calcium be replaced in a hypocalcemic patient?*
■ **Low-ionized or symptomatic patient**

Patients with low total serum calcium and normal ionized calcium levels typically do not require treatment. Patients who are symptomatic or have very low ionized calcium require treatment that includes replacing calcium.

■ *Should a patient with an ionized calcium level of 0.8 mmol/L who is hypotensive receive IV calcium gluconate or calcium chloride?*
■ **Calcium chloride**

This patient has a severely low ionized calcium level and is symptomatic of hypotension. Calcium chloride contains more calcium per 10% solution than calcium gluconate and physiologically is more readily available. Calcium gluconate requires hepatic deglucona-tion to make biologically usable calcium.

> ❯ HINT
> Calcium chloride is the replacement calcium of choice in a symptomatic patient. Treatment of a low electrolyte level is administration of the electrolyte.

■ *What are the treatments of a severe, acute hypercalcemia?*
■ **Hydration and diuresis**

Mild hypercalcemia may not require treatment. Calcium levels between 12 and 14 mg/dL may become symptomatic and levels higher than 14 mg/dL should be treated. Hydration will dilute the calcium and encourage diuresis with furosemide. Hemodialysis may be used in extreme cases. Chronic hypercalcemia may be managed with calcitonin or drugs that inhibit resorption of bone.

> ❯ HINT
> Three ways to treat an elevated electrolyte: dilute, diuresis, and bind it!

■ *What is used to bind potassium in a hyperkalemic patient?*
■ **Kayexalate**

Binding of potassium with kayexalate causes the excretion of potassium through the gas-trointestinal route. Hyperkalemia can be treated with hydration and administration of a potassium-wasting diuretic. Another way to manage hyperkalemia is to move the potassium from the serum into the intracellular space by administering a β-agonist (bronchodilator), insulin, or sodium bicarbonate. In severe cases of hyperkalemia or renal failure patients, removal of potassium is frequently with hemodialysis or continuous RRT.

> **HINT**
> Administer IV calcium chloride to patients experiencing lethal ventricular arrhythmias. This causes a direct antagonism of the hyperkalemic effect on cardiac cells.

■ *What infusion may benefit patients with hemodynamic instability due to hypermagnesemia?*

■ **IV calcium**

Hydration and renal excretion with administration of furosemide are the mainstays of treatment for hypermagnesemia. Administration of IV calcium may be used if the patient is hemodynamically unstable. Acute magnesium intoxication in renal failure can be managed with hemodialysis.

■ *What is the treatment of severe hyponatremia that is determined to be a true loss of sodium and not dilutional?*

■ **Hypertonic saline**

Dilutional hyponatremia is managed with fluid restrictions and diuresis. A euvolemic hyponatremia due to a renal loss of sodium should not have fluid restriction but replacement of sodium as the main treatment. Administration of a hypertonic solution too fast can cause a rapid shift in serum osmolality to a hyperosmolar state. This results in the irreversible demyelination of the neurons in the brain, particularly in the pons (Boxes 7.34 and 7.35).

Box 7.34 Treatment of Hyponatremia

Hypoosmolar **euvolemic** hyponatremia	Free water restrictions Loop diuretics Administer sodium
Hypoosmolar **hypovolemic** hyponatremia	Treat underlying cause Volume replacement
Hypoosmolar **hypervolemic** hyponatremia	Treat underlying cause Sodium restrictions Free water restrictions Loop diuretics

Box 7.35 Treatment of Hypernatremia

Hypovolemic hypernatremia	Correct volume deficits Correct free water deficits Treat underlying cause
Euvolemic hypernatremia	Correct free water deficits Treat underlying cause
Hypervolemic hypernatremia	Remove excess sodium Sodium restrictions Loop diuretics Hemodialysis (renal failure)

COMPLICATIONS

■ *Which neuromuscular blocking agent (NMBA) should be avoided in patients with crush injury or severe muscle trauma?*

■ **Succinylcholine**

Succinylcholine is a depolarizing NMBA. It has a rapid onset and short duration and so is frequently used for rapid sequence intubation. Depolarizing NMBA causes a rapid depolarization of all muscle, resulting in a paralysis. This can cause muscle cells to release intracellular substances such as potassium. A trauma patient with a crush injury or a patient who has sustained severe muscle trauma may already have increased release of potassium from injured muscle cells. Administering succinylcholine can cause a significant hyperkalemia and may progress rapidly to cardiac arrest.

> **HINT**
>
> An alternative NMBA that may be used in a patient at high risk for development of hyperkalemia is rocuronium, a short-acting, rapid-onset nondepolarizing NMBA.

■ *What is the most life-threatening complication of hypocalcemia?*

■ **Prolonged QT interval**

Hypocalcemia causes a prolonged QT interval that places the patient at a greater risk for an "R on T" phenomenon and Torsades de pointes. Measure the QTc on patients with electrolyte abnormalities that place them at a risk for development of a prolonged QT interval (Box 7.36).

> **HINT**
>
> Treat Torsades with magnesium.

Box 7.36 Electrolyte Abnormalities
That Prolong QT Interval

Hypomagnesemia
Hypocalcemia
Hyperkalemia
Hyperphosphatemia

■ *What is the most significant complication of hypophosphatemia in ICU patients?*

■ **Diaphragm weakness**

Hypophosphatemia contributes to acute and chronic respiratory failure and has been associated with failure of ventilatory weaning.

■ *Following the onset of AKI, which electrolyte abnormality may cause seizures?*

■ **Hyponatremia**

Hyponatremia is a result of a combination of dilutional hyponatremia and a true loss of sodium in the renal tubules. Low sodium is one of the electrolyte abnormalities that can cause seizures (Box 7.37).

Box 7.37 Electrolyte Abnormalities That Cause Seizures

Hypocalcemia
Hypomagnesemia
Hyponatremia
Hypernatremia
Hypoglycemia

Questions

1. Which of the following, if lasting longer than 6 consecutive hours, is an indication of acute kidney injury?

   A. Urine output < 2 mL/kg/hr
   B. Urine output < 1.5 mL/kg/hr
   C. Urine output < 1 mL/kg/hr
   D. Urine output < 0.5 mL/kg/hr

2. Which of the following definitions is considered end-stage renal disease (ESRD)?

   A. A threefold increase in SCr
   B. A decrease in GFR by 75%
   C. Complete loss of function for > 4 weeks
   D. Complete loss of function for > 3 months

3. Which of the following drugs cause prerenal failure by blocking the vasoconstriction of the efferent arterioles?

   A. NSAIDs
   B. Aminoglycosides
   C. Contrast medium
   D. ACE inhibitor

4. Which of the following is characteristic of rhabdomyolysis?

   A. Tea-colored urine
   B. Bloody urine
   C. White cell casts in urine
   D. Tubular epithelial casts

5. Which of the following laboratory findings could be expected in ATN?

   A. Hypophosphatemia
   B. Decreased urine osmolality
   C. Decreased urine sodium
   D. Elevated BUN:creatinine ratio

6. Which of the following descriptions best describes ultrafiltration?

   A. Movement of water by pressure gradient and transport of small and larger molecular-weight solutes
   B. Movement of solutes from area of higher to an area of lower concentration
   C. Water is transported by gradient pressure across a semipermeable membrane
   D. Countercurrent is used to pull solutes across a semipermeable membrane

7. An ICU patient with sepsis develops elevated creatinine and BUN levels. The urine output is 10 mL/hr and has potassium of 5.6 mEq/L. Continuous venovenous hemodialysis (CVVHD) as well as mechanical ventilation are initiated as a result of onset of

acute respiratory distress syndrome (ARDS). Over the next 24 hours, the patient develops significant hypophosphatemia. Which of the following is the most likely cause of the hypophosphatemia?

A. CRRT
B. Azotemia
C. Mechanical ventilation
D. Hyperkalemia

8. A patient in the ICU develops increased muscle tremors and spasms. He is found to have a positive Chvostek sign. Which of the following electrolyte abnormalities is the most likely cause of the increased muscle tone?

A. Hyperkalemia
B. Hypercalcemia
C. Hypomagnesemia
D. Hypophosphatemia

9. A hyponatremia develops following a traumatic brain injury in the ICU. Which of the following laboratory values would indicate hemodilution as the cause of the hyponatremia?

A. Normal serum chloride level
B. Hyperosmolality
C. Low serum chloride level
D. Elevated hematocrit

10. A patient in the ICU has failed weaning trials the past 2 days. Which of the following electrolytes need to be assessed and optimized to facilitate weaning and respiratory muscles?

A. Magnesium
B. Potassium
C. Sodium
D. Phosphate

Multisystem Review

In this chapter, you will review:

- Sepsis and septic shock
- Distributive shock: Anaphylaxis
- Toxic ingestions/drug overdose/toxin exposure
- Asphyxia/anoxic brain injury
- Therapeutic hypothermia
- Moderate sedation

SEPSIS AND SEPTIC SHOCK

- *What is the presence of bacteria in the bloodstream called?*
- **Bacteremia**

A bacteremia is the viable presence of bacteria in the bloodstream. Blood cultures are positive for bacteria. A fungemia is the presence of fungus in the bloodstream. A positive culture is one of the signs of an infection. An infection initiates the inflammatory response and onset of sepsis (Box 8.1).

Box 8.1 Signs of an Infection

Presence of white cells in normal sterile body fluid
Positive culture (urine, blood, sputum)
Perforated viscous
Radiographic evidence of pneumonia in association with purulent sputum

- *What is the white blood cell (WBC) criteria used to define sepsis?*
- **WBC greater than 12, 000 or less than 4,000 or greater than 10% bands**

Sepsis is the inflammatory response to a known infection. Sepsis occurs if two or more of the defined criteria are present. Systemic inflammatory response syndrome (SIRS) is the systemic inflammatory response to a variety of severe clinical insults. SIRS is defined by the same criteria used to define sepsis but without signs of infection and a negative blood culture (Box 8.2).

> **〉 HINT**
> Sepsis is a disease process managed in all areas of the hospital and is not exclusive to critical care. SIRS has negative blood cultures.

Box 8.2 Criteria for Sepsis

Temperature > 38.3°C (101°F) or < 36°C

Heart rate > 90 beats/min

Respiratory rate > 20 breaths/min or $PaCO_2$ < 32 mmHg

WBC > 12,000 cells/mm³ or < 4,000 mm³ > 10% immature granulocytes (bands)

■ *What is severe sepsis?*

■ **Sepsis with hypotension and/or hypoperfusion**

Severe sepsis is sepsis accompanied by hypotension and/or hypoperfusion. Severe sepsis is also called sepsis-induced tissue hypoperfusion or organ dysfunction. Hypotension is systolic blood pressure (BP) less than 90 mmHg, mean arterial pressure (MAP) less than 70 mmHg, or a decrease in BP by greater than 40 mmHg from baseline or MAP less than 70 mmHg. Hypoperfusion may include but is not limited to oliguria, increased lactate levels higher than 4 mmol/L, or acute alteration in mental status. The sepsis bundles use a lactate level greater than 4 mmol/L to recognize hypoperfusion (Box 8.3).

Box 8.3 Signs of Hypoperfusion

Acute altered mental status	Coagulation abnormalities (international normalized ratio [INR] > 1.5 or activated partial thromboplastin time (aPTT) > 60 sec)
Blood glucose > 140 mg/dL in patients without diabetes	
Arterial hypoxemia (PaO_2/FiO_2 ratio < 300)	Ileus
Acute oliguria (< 0.5 mL/kg/hr for at least 2 hours)	Thrombocytopenia (platelet count < 100,000)
	Hyperbilirubinemia (total bilirubin > 2 mg/dL)
Creatinine increase > 0.5 mg/dL above baseline	

> **HINT**
> Septic shock is defined by hypotension and hypoperfusion despite adequate resuscitation.

■ *What causes multiple organ dysfunction in sepsis?*

■ **Hypoperfusion**

Multiple organ dysfunction syndrome (MODS) is the presence of altered organ function, involving two or more organs, in an acutely ill patient such that homeostasis cannot be maintained without intervention. It is progressive but potentially reversible and is a result of hypoperfusion and injury to the organs.

> **HINT**
> The incidence of mortality is related to the number of organs involved in MODS and the severity of organ dysfunction (Box 8.4).

Box 8.4 Signs of Organ Dysfunction

System	Major Sign
Pulmonary	PaO_2/FiO_2 ratio < 300
Renal	Increased serum creatinine > 2.0 or creatinine increase > 0.5 mg/dL or 44.2 µmmol/L
Hepatic	Increased bilirubin levels > 4 mg/dL
Hematology	Decreased platelet counts < 100,000/µL INR > 1.5 aPTT > 60 sec
Central nervous system	Altered Glasgow Coma Scale (GCS)

PATHOPHYSIOLOGY

■ *What is the most common microorganism that causes sepsis?*
■ **Gram-positive bacteria**

Gram-positive bacteremia has surpassed the gram-negative bacteria. A common gram-positive bacteria found in hospitals is methicillin-resistant *Staphylococcus aureus* (MRSA; Box 8.5).

Box 8.5 Gram-Negative Bacteria

Escherichia coli	Enterobacter
Klebsiella pneumoniae	Serratia
Pseudomonas aeruginosa	Proteus

> **HINT**
> Gram-negative bacteria colonize the gastrointestinal (GI) tract and oral secretions (Box 8.6). Central-line sepsis is a result of gram-positive bacteremia.

Box 8.6 Gram-Positive Bacteria

Staphylococcus
Streptococcus

■ *Which microorganism is the most common cause of a secondary infection?*
■ **Fungus (Candida)**

Fungal infections frequently present as a second episode of an infection. This is due to the use of antibiotics to treat the first infection, which alter the normal flora and allow opportunistic infections to develop. Another high-risk patient is an immunosuppressed patient. Fungal sepsis (fungemia) has a higher mortality than bacteremia and is harder to diagnose. The presence of a fungemia may not result in a positive blood culture. Management is frequently based on presumptive therapy, which is to "presume" there is a fungemia and treat with antifungal medication. New tests may be used to assist with the diagnosis of Candida (1,3 β-d-glucan assay [Grade 2B], mannan, and antimannan antibody assays).

SIRS is frequently caused by fungal infections due to an inflammatory response without a known infection or positive blood culture.

SYMPTOMS/ASSESSMENT

■ *An increase in bands greater than what percentage indicates severe sepsis?*
■ **Greater than 10%**

Bands are immature WBCs. If more than 10% of the circulating WBCs are bands this indicates an overwhelming infection and sepsis. Other WBC changes potentially indicating sepsis include WBC count greater than 12,000 or less than 4,000.

> ❯ HINT
>
> For example, if the complete blood count (CBC) differential finds 45% bands it indicates that 45% of the circulating WBCs are immature and not functional.

■ *In severe sepsis/septic shock, does the left ventricular (LV) ejection fraction (EF) increase or decrease?*
■ **Decrease**

Proinflammatory cytokine, tumor necrosis factor (TNF), is released following the presence of a microorganism and initiates the inflammatory response. TNF has a negative contractility effect of the myocardium and results in a decrease in EF. The cardiac output (CO) is usually high in sepsis because of systemic vasodilation lowering the resistance (Box 8.7).

> ❯ HINT
>
> Use of a right ejection fraction–oximetry (REF-ox) pulmonary artery catheter in sepsis patients has shown a decrease in EF even during periods of high COs. Right ventricular EF commonly ranges from 30% to 40% during early sepsis.

Box 8.7 Symptoms of Sepsis/Sepsis Shock

Tachycardia	Metabolic acidosis
Tachypnea	Respiratory alkalosis
Leukocytosis or leukopenia or increased bands	Pulmonary artery hypertension
Fever	Altered mental status
Decreased systemic vascular resistance (SVR)	Edema or positive fluid balance
Hypotension (vasodilation)	Hyperglycemia (> 140 mg/dL or 7.7 mmol/L) in a nondiabetic patient
Increased CO	
Decreased EF	Signs of organ dysfunction
LV dilation	

DIAGNOSIS

■ *What diagnostic determines the microorganism(s) involved in causing an infection and the best antibiotics needed to treat the infection?*

■ **Culture and sensitivity**

Diagnosis of sepsis is the presence of two or more of the defining criteria for sepsis. Once sepsis is recognized, cultures determine the causative microorganisms and their susceptibility to certain antibiotics. Recommendation is at least two sets of blood cultures (both anaerobic and aerobic bottles) with at least one drawn percutaneously and one drawn from a vascular access device that is more than 48 hours old. Both sets of blood cultures can be obtained at the same time as long as they are from two different sites. Cultures from other potential sites of infection (urine, sputum, cerebrospinal fluid [CSF], wounds) are obtained and are sent with the blood cultures for testing.

> ❯ HINT
> If the same organism is recovered from both the samples, there is a better likelihood that the organism is responsible for the sepsis.

■ *What other lab tests beside the CBC can be used to determine the presence of an infection?*

■ **Plasma C-reactive protein and prolactin**

Plasma C-reactive protein and prolactin are biomarkers for diagnosis of infection. They may be used as additional information but are not, at this time, shown to distinguish from infection and other causes of inflammation.

> ❯ HINT
> Procalcitonin levels may be beneficial in determining when to discontinue the antibiotics.

MEDICAL MANAGEMENT

■ *What is the overall best management goal for sepsis?*

■ **Prevention**

Prevention of an infection or sepsis is still the best management. Hand washing is the main area of prevention found to lower the incidence of infections across the continuum of patient types and ages (Box 8.8).

Box 8.8 Sources of Hospital-Associated Infections

Catheter-associated urinary tract infection	Hospital-acquired pneumonia
Central line–associated bloodstream infections	Intra-abdominal source
Ventilator-associated pneumonia	

■ *What is the current recommendation to prevent a catheter-associated urinary tract infection (CAUTI)?*

■ **Minimize the use and duration of the urinary catheter**

Urinary tract infections are the most common type of health care-associated infections. Current practice is to mostly avoid a Foley catheter insertion, if possible. If a bladder catheter is required in surgery, the goal is to discontinue it within 24 hours. Removing the indwelling catheter as soon as possible will lower the incidence of urinary tract infections. The most common causative microorganisms are *Escherichia coli* and *Candida* (Box 8.9).

> ❭ **HINT**
> Remember all lines and tubes in the patient are a source of infection and should be removed as soon as possible. It is not recommended to change bags or indwelling catheters on a routine basis. The catheter can be changed if clinical indications are present, including infection or contamination of the system (Box 8.10).

Box 8.9 Appropriate Reasons for Urinary Catheter Use

Accurate input and output in critically ill patients Need to monitor urine output	Large volume of fluid infusions or diuretics
	Urological surgical patients
Unable to use bedpan or urinal	Urinary retention or obstruction
Coma	
Sedation and paralytics	

Box 8.10 Prevention of Urinary Tract Infections

Aseptic insertion technique and use of sterile equipment	Maintain a closed drainage system
	Empty collecting bag regularly
Keep bag off the floor	May use antiseptic/antimicrobial-impregnated catheters
Keep bag lower than the bladder	
Properly secure to prevent movement of bladder	

■ *What nursing intervention has been found to lower the incidence of ventilator-associated pneumonia (VAP)?*

■ **Oral care with chlorhexidine**

Oropharyngeal decontamination with chlorhexidine gluconate is recommended to lower the incidence of VAP. Selective digestive decontamination has also been proposed to lower the risk of VAP (Box 8.11).

Box 8.11 Methods of Prevention of VAP

Proper hand washing	Subglottic suctioning
Oral decontamination	Prevent unplanned extubations/reintubations
Digestive decontamination	Avoid saline lavages
Head of the bed (HOB) elevated	

■ *How quickly should antibiotics be started following a diagnosis of sepsis?*

■ **Within 1 hour**

Antibiotics are the main treatment of sepsis and may halt its progression and improve outcomes if administered early in the course of sepsis. Cultures should be obtained prior to the administration of antibiotics unless doing so would cause significant delay in the administration of antibiotics. Antibiotics can result in sterilization of the cultures within a few hours, making identification of the causative organisms more difficult. They should be obtained sooner than 45 minutes after the diagnosis of sepsis. Broad-spectrum antibiotics should be used to be effective against all likely organisms. Once culture results are obtained, antibiotics should be changed to a more specific antibiotic for the organism's susceptibility with the goal being within 3 to 5 days.

> ❯ **HINT**
>
> Recommendation is to maintain a 5- to 7-day course of antibiotic therapy. May increase the number of days in case of slow clinical response or continued presence of the infected source.

■ *In early goal-directed therapy of severe sepsis, what is the central venous pressure (CVP) goal of the initial fluid resuscitation in a spontaneous breathing patient?*

■ **CVP 8 to 12 mmHg**

Severe sepsis is persistent hypotension or hypoperfusion after the initial bolus of fluid. Early goal-directed strategy includes monitoring CVP and $ScvO_2$ to determine the adequacy of resuscitation. A CVP of 8 to 12 mmHg is recommended for spontaneous breathing patients and slightly higher on ventilated patients (12–15 mmHg) because of positive pressure effects in the chest. $ScvO_2$ can be monitored intermittently or continuously. The goals should be obtained within 6 hours on recognition of sepsis. Goals can be obtained with fluid administration, blood products, dobutamine infusion, and/or lower oxygen demands with sedation or paralysis. Another parameter used to monitor hemodynamics is stroke volume variance (SVV), which will determine fluid responsiveness.

> ❯ **HINT**
>
> Lactate levels may also be monitored with a goal to normalize serum lactate (Box 8.12). A decrease in heart rate is also a good indication of successful resuscitation.

Box 8.12 Goals of Resuscitation in Severe Sepsis

CVP 8–12 mmHg in spontaneous breathing
CVP 12–15 mmHg ventilated
MAP $\geq$ 65 mmHg
Urine output $\geq$ 0.5 mL/kg/hr
$ScvO_2$ 70% or SvO_2 65%

■ *What fluids are recommended for initial resuscitation in sepsis?*

■ **Crystalloids**

Current recommendation for fluid resuscitation in severe sepsis or sepsis-induced hypoperfusion is crystalloids. This is recommended because of lack of benefit for albumin used initially, which is more expensive than a crystalloid. If the patient requires substantial amounts of fluid to meet the goals of volume resuscitation, then albumin administration is recommended with crystalloids. Initially, the fluid challenge should be a minimum of 30 mL/kg bolus with more fluids, if needed, to meet the predetermined goals of volume resuscitation.

> **HINT**
Hydroxy ethyl starches (Hetastarch) are not recommended in resuscitation of sepsis patients because of their worsening effect on kidneys.

■ *What vasopressor is considered to be the first choice in maintaining MAP greater than 65 mmHg?*
■ **Norepinephrine (Levophed)**

Vasopressor therapy is recommended to maintain MAP greater than or equal to 65 mmHg. Below this perfusion pressure, autoregulation in the critical vascular beds is lost. The vasopressor recommended as a first-line treatment is norepinephrine. If an additional vasopressor is required, epinephrine or vasopressin may be added to maintain pressure or to lower the dose of norepinephrine. Vasopressin is not recommended as a single first-line vasopressor in sepsis. Dopamine may be an alternative vasopressor to norepinephrine but only in certain patients who are at very low risk for tachyarrhythmias. Low-dose dopamine should not be used for renal protection. A patient with absolute or refractory bradycardia may receive dopamine as the first-line vasopressor. Phenylephrine is not recommended in the treatment of septic shock unless associated with serious arrhythmias or CO is known to be high or when other vasopressor agents have failed to achieve the target MAP.

> **HINT**
An arterial line is recommended for continuous and more accurate BP readings. Central venous access is required for the administration of vasopressors.

■ *When should corticosteroid therapy be considered in a patient with sepsis?*
■ **Refractory to vasopressors**

A patient who responds to fluids and/or vasopressor therapy by improving hemodynamic parameters (BP) and lactate levels does not require corticosteroid treatment. If hemodynamic stability cannot be achieved, even after resuscitation and vasopressors, 200 mg/day of hydrocortisone as a continuous infusion is recommended. Continuous infusions may control blood glucose more effectively than intermittent boluses with less significant hyperglycemia. Once vasopressors are not required, hydrocortisone may be tapered down and discontinued. The adrenocorticotropin hormone (ACTH) test is not recommended to determine indication for corticosteroid therapy.

> **HINT**
Side effects of hydrocortisone are hypernatremia and hyperglycemia.

■ *According to the Sepsis Campaign guidelines, when should the insulin protocol be initiated in a sepsis patient?*

■ **Glucose greater than 180 mg/dL**

Current recommendations for glucose control are to treat with sliding-scale insulin if blood glucose levels are greater than 180 mg/dL at two consecutive times. Maintain glucose less than 180 mg/dL while avoiding hypoglycemia. Blood glucose levels may be checked every 4 hours when stable and every 1 to 2 hours while elevated. Maintaining strict glucose levels of less than 110 mg/dL is not recommended because of the incidence of hypoglycemia.

> ❯ **HINT**
> Point-of-care glucose tests may not be as accurate as plasma glucose levels from the laboratory and should be interpreted cautiously especially in patients with low hematocritis.

■ *At what serum pH would sodium bicarbonate therapy be administered in septic shock patients with lactic acidosis?*

■ **Less than 7.15**

There is no benefit to treating pH with sodium bicarbonate until pH decreases less than 7.15. The side effects of sodium bicarbonate cause the risks of administration to be greater than the benefit (Box 8.13).

Box 8.13 Complications of Sodium Bicarbonate

Fluid overload	Hypercarbia
Hypernatremia	Decrease serum ionized calcium
Increased lactate levels	Greater affinity of hgb to red blood cells (RBCs)

SURGICAL MANAGEMENT

■ *In the case of a known source of infection, what is the best management?*

■ **Remove the source of infection**

Radiographics are frequently used to find the location of the infection. If the infectious source is amendable, then drainage, percutaneous drainage, or surgical excision may be required. Source control as rapidly as possible can lower the incidence of mortality (Box 8.14).

> ❯ **HINT**
> If the source is determined to be an intravenous (IV) access source, the catheter must be removed promptly after obtaining other access.

Box 8.14 Foci Infections That Are Surgically Amendable

Abscesses (including intra-abdominal)	Intestinal ischemia
Gastrointestinal perforation	Necrotizing soft tissue
Cholangitis	Empyema
Pyelonephritis	Septic arthritis

COMPLICATIONS

■ *What is the primary physiology for a hypoperfused state in sepsis?*
■ **Inability of the cells to use oxygen**

Initial hypoperfusion is a result of distributive shock (vasodilation) and hypovolemia (increased vascular permeability). Even after fluid resuscitation and BP are restored, hypoperfusion may persist. It is largely attributed to an inability of the cells to use the oxygen delivered to the tissues. Another major contributing factor is maldistribution of blood flow, which occurs at the regional level (splanchnic, renal, and mesenteric) as well as at the microvascular level.

> **❯ HINT**
> Remember the aphorism, "You can lead a horse to water but you cannot make it drink." In sepsis, you can optimize the delivery of oxygen to the tissues/cells, but you cannot make them take in the oxygen (Box 8.15).

Box 8.15 Causes of Inadequate Tissue Oxygenation

Decreased oxygen delivery (DO_2)	Inability to offload O_2 from hgb
Inability to extract oxygen	Arteriovenous shunt
Blockage of normal cellular metabolism	Endothelial injury
Greater distance between capillary and tissue (edema)	Loss of vascular tone

■ *What is the GI complication due to use of multiple antibiotics in treating sepsis?*
■ *Clostridium difficile*

C. difficile is a superinfection that may occur as a result of using multiple antibiotics, broad-spectrum antibiotics, and lengthy duration of treatment. Narrowing the spectrum and shortening the time of antibiotics therapy may lower the risk of opportunistic infections such as Candida or superinfections such as *C. difficile* and resistant bacteria (vancomycin-resistant enterococcus faecium).

> **❯ HINT**
> Antibiotics can change the normal GI flora. Probiotics may be used to limit some of this altered flora.

■ *What is the most common cause of death in septic shock?*
■ **Multiple organ dysfunction syndrome**

MODS is a complication of tissue and organ hypoperfusion that occurs in severe sepsis and septic shock. MODS is defined as the presence of altered organ functions in acutely ill patients such that homeostasis cannot be obtained without intervention. The number of organs affected predicts mortality. Any organ can be affected by sepsis-induced hypoperfusion (Box 8.16).

> **HINT**

This is also commonly called multisystem organ failure (MSOF).

Box 8.16 Common Organs Involved in MODS

Acute respiratory distress syndrome	Septic encephalopathy
Acute kidney injury	Systolic and diastolic dysfunction of myocardium
Hepatic failure	Disseminated intravascular coagulation
Gastrointestinal tract	Metabolic dysfunction with hyperglycemia

■ *What plays a central role in microvascular dysfunction that occurs in MODS?*
■ **Endothelium**

The endothelium regulates vasomotor tone, coagulation, vascular permeability, and balance between pro- and anti-inflammatory cytokines. Biomarkers that measure endothelial activity (plasminogen activator inhibitor-1) demonstrate increased levels following activation of the inflammatory system and correlate the severity of MODS.

■ *What tool can be used to determine the rate and extent of organ failure?*
■ **Sequential organ failure assessment (SOFA)**

The SOFA scoring system is used to determine the extent of organ function or rate of failure.

> **HINT**

When scoring, if none match the patient, the score is set at 0 for that section. If more than one match, then the highest score is used (Box 8.17).

Box 8.17 SOFA

Respiratory System	
PaO$_2$/FiO$_2$	SOFA Score
< 400	1
< 300	2
< 200 **and** mechanically ventilated	3
< 100 **and** mechanically ventilated	4
Nervous System	
Glasgow Coma Scale	SOFA Score
13–14	1
10–12	2
6–9	3
<6	4

(continued)

Box 8.17 SOFA (*continued*)

Cardiovascular System	
MAP or Vasopressor Requirement	SOFA Score
MAP < 70 mmHg	1
Dopamine < 5 *or* dobutamine (any dose)	2
Dopamine > 5 *or* epinephrine ≤ 0.1 *or* norepinephrine ≤ 0.1	3
Dopamine > 15 *or* epinephrine > 0.1 *or* norepinephrine > 0.1	4
Liver	
Bilirubin	SOFA Score
1.2–1.9	1
2.0–5.9	2
6.0–11.9	3
> 12	4
Coagulation	
Platelets × 10³	SOFA Score
< 150	1
< 100	2
< 50	3
< 20	4
Renal System	
Creatinine or Urine Output	SOFA Score
1.2–1.9	1
2.0–3.4	2
3.5–4.9	3
> 5	4

DISTRIBUTIVE SHOCK: ANAPHYLAXIS

- *How is anaphylaxis different from an anaphylactoid reaction?*
- Immunoglobulin E (IgE) mediated

Anaphylaxis and anaphylactoid reactions are both acute, life-threatening hypersensitivity reactions, but anaphylaxis is immune-related, whereas an anaphylactoid reaction is not. Anaphylaxis involves IgE binding to an antigen that the person was previously exposed to. Anaphylactoid does not have the immune component but is similar in assessment, diagnosis, and treatment.

> **HINT**
> Both are called life-threatening hypersensitivity reactions.

- *How quickly can the symptoms of hypersensitivity reactions occur following exposure to the provoking agent?*
- Within minutes

The onset of symptoms can occur within minutes to hours. Typically, symptoms will peak in severity within 5 to 30 minutes. The episode frequently lasts fewer than 24 hours but can be protracted or reoccur after initial resolution.

PATHOPHYSIOLOGY

■ *In both hypersensitivity reactions, what is triggered causing the release of chemical mediators?*
■ **Mast cells**

Mast cells are activated in both anaphylaxis and anaphylactoid reactions, releasing several chemical mediators. Overall, the mediators increase capillary permeability and cause peripheral vasodilation. Increased capillary permeability can cause airway swelling and angioedema. Peripheral vasodilation results in hypotension, which is labeled as distributive shock (Box 8.18).

> ❯ **HINT**
> The most life-threatening component of a hypersensitivity reaction is angioedema.

Box 8.18 Chemical Mediators Released in Anaphylaxis

Bradykinin
Platelet-activating factor
Prostaglandins
Leukotrienes

■ *What are the two most common causes of anaphylaxis?*
■ **Food and insect stings**

Food sensitivities, insect stings, and antibiotics are the most common causes of an IgE-mediated anaphylaxis reaction. These occur after previous exposure to a provoking agent. Stinging insects such as bees, wasps, and fire ants contain a substance in their venom that initiates the IgE antibody response. Penicillin is the most common antibiotic to cause an anaphylaxis reaction. Other common antibiotics include cephalosporin and sulfonamides (Box 8.19).

Box 8.19 Common Food Allergies That Cause Anaphylaxis

Peanuts	Milk
Shellfish	Eggs
Fish	Seeds
Tree nuts	

> **❯ HINT**
> Some food allergens are so severe that just touching or inhaling the odor of those foods can cause a hypersensitivity reaction (Boxes 8.20 and 8.21).

Box 8.20 Causes of IgE-Mediated Hypersensitivity Reactions

Food allergies	Muscle relaxants
Insect stings	Latex
Pollen	Snake bites
Antibiotics	

Box 8.21 Causes of Nonimmunological Hypersensitivity

Contrast media
Opioids
Aspirin and nonsteroidal anti-inflammatory drugs (NSAIDs)

SYMPTOMS/ASSESSMENT

■ *What is the most life-threatening symptom of anaphylaxis reactions?*

■ **Angioedema**

Angioedema can cause the loss of the airway from edema and is the most life-threatening symptom of anaphylaxis. Symptoms include wheezing and dyspnea. Urticaria is a common associated symptom. Sudden loss of consciousness can also be an initial sign and patients may report a feeling of "impending doom" (Box 8.22).

Box 8.22 Symptoms of Anaphylaxis

Airway swelling	Abdominal pain
Hoarseness	Hypotension
Urticaria and pruritus	Dizziness and syncope
Dyspnea	Chest tightness and pain
Wheezing	Headache
Nausea and vomiting	Seizure
Diarrhea	Flushing

MEDICAL MANAGEMENT

■ *What is the initial drug used to treat an anaphylaxis reaction?*

■ **Epinephrine**

Epinephrine 1:1,000 dilution 0.2 to 0.5 mg dose can be administered subcutaneously or intramuscularly. If there is severe hypotension, epinephrine can be administered as a continuous infusion. It is an α- and β-agonist, but it will also decrease release of mast cells. Hypotension is treated with fluid resuscitation and vasopressors, and supplemental oxygen is administered. Steroids and antihistamines (Benadryl) sometimes provide even greater relief of symptoms.

> **HINT**
Antihistamines block the H_1 receptor, so adding an H_2 receptor blocker (Ranitidine) can enhance effectiveness.

■ *What drug can limit the effectiveness of epinephrine?*
■ **β-blockers**

Patients taking β-blockers may be resistant to epinephrine demonstrating continued hypotension and bradycardia. The bradycardia may require atropine to manage. Other drugs that may interfere include angiotensin-converting enzyme (ACE) inhibitors and monoamine oxidase (MAO) inhibitors.

■ *A patient states he has an allergy to contrast dye but requires a diagnostic procedure. What can be given prior to administration of contrast to decrease the allergic reaction?*
■ **Steroids and antihistamines**

Pretreatment can be performed with steroids and antihistamines prior to giving contrast dye in a sensitive patient who requires a diagnostic procedure.

COMPLICATIONS

■ *What is a potential cardiovascular complication caused by hypotension and hypoxia?*
■ **Myocardial infarction**

Airway obstruction is the most common complication of anaphylaxis. Other complications are not common. Severe hypotension and hypoxia from airway edema can cause acute myocardial infarction (AMI).

TOXIC INGESTIONS/DRUG OVERDOSE/TOXIN EXPOSURE

■ *What mixed-drug combination is the most common overdose?*
■ **Opioids, alcohol, and sedatives**

Opioids, sedatives, and alcohol include a mixed combination of drugs and are the most common overdose in the emergency department (ED). The hallmark symptom is a depressed level of consciousness (LOC). Acetaminophen is the most common single-drug overdose. Overdoses may be intentional and unintentional.

> **HINT**
Most overdoses involve more than one class of drugs and may have a mixed presentation.

PATHOPHYSIOLOGY

- *What is the physiology for the development of metabolic acidosis with cyanide poisoning?*
- Inhibits cytochrome oxidate

Inhibition of cytochrome oxidate results in interference in oxidative phosphorylation and cellular energy production. The anaerobic metabolic pathway produces lactic acid with the development of lactic acidosis. Cyanide also interferes with oxygen consumption with the development of tissue hypoperfusion.

> ❯ HINT
> Nipride infusions can induce methemoglobinemia and elevated thiocyanate levels.

SYMPTOMS/ASSESSMENT

- *What are the two most important assessments in the initial evaluation of drug or toxin overdoses?*
- Vital signs and neurological assessment

Vital signs are important in assisting with the determination of the causative substance, severity of the overdose, and in guiding initial management. Tachypnea is a nonspecific finding but a respiratory depression guides the need for immediate intubation. Neurological assessment, including LOC, pupils, ocular movement, and motor skills, is useful in determining the substance and acuity of the patient. Frequent neurological assessments are recommended to follow changes over time (Box 8.23).

> ❯ HINT
> Bowel sounds may also be used.
> Hypoactive = opioids or anticholinergics
> Hyperactive = organophosphates

Box 8.23 Symptoms of Common Toxins

Drug	Blood Pressure (BP)	Heart Rate (HR)	Respiratory Rate (RR)	Temp.	Pupils	Nystagmus	Seizures
Anticholinergics	I	I	I	I	I	U	I
Sympathomimetics cocaine, amphetamines	I	I	I	I	I	U	I
Cyclic antidepressants	D	I		I			I
Salicylates		I	I				I
Opioids	D		I	D	D (except meperidine)		
Carbon monoxide		I	I	D		I	

(continued)

Box 8.23 Symptoms of Common Toxins (*continued*)

Drug	Blood Pressure (BP)	Heart Rate (HR)	Respiratory Rate (RR)	Temp.	Pupils	Nystagmus	Seizures
Organophosphates	D	D	I		D		I
Alcohol			D		I	I	I
Sedatives, hypnotics	D	D	D	D		I	

I, increase; D, decrease; U, unchanged.

■ *Which two alcohol ingestions have the greatest morbidity and mortality?*
■ Ethylene glycol and methanol

Ethylene glycol and methanol ingestion can result in significant metabolic abnormalities, seizures, and coma. Visual disturbances are "red flags" for methanol ingestion and the presence of calcium oxalate crystals in urine are "red flags" for ethylene glycol (Box 8.24).

> ❯ HINT
> Ethylene glycol = antifreeze
> Methanol = solvent, antifreeze, fuel
> Acetone = paint thinners, nail polish remover
> Isopropyl alcohol = disinfectant
> Ethanol = drinking alcohol, fuel

Box 8.24 Symptoms of Ethylene Glycol and Methanol Ingestion

Pulmonary edema	Nausea and vomiting
Hypotension	Visual disturbances (methanol)
Ataxia	Photophobia, blindness, blurred vision
Seizures	Calcium oxalate crystals in urine (ethylene glycol)
Coma	Anion gap metabolic acidosis
Abdominal pain	Osmolal gap

> ❯ HINT
> Anion gap metabolic acidosis may not be present initially.

■ *Which of the overdoses presents with "wet" symptoms?*
■ Cholinergic overdose

A cholinergic overdose presents with "wet" symptoms of increased lacrimation, salivation, urination, emesis, and diarrhea (Box 8.25).

Box 8.25 Symptoms of Cholinergic Overdose

"Wet" symptoms	Fasciculations
GI upset	Confusion
Bronchorrhea	Miosis
Bradycardia	

> HINT
>
> SLUDGE: salivation, lacrimation, urination, defecation, GI upset, emesis.

■ *A sympathomimetic overdose causes what BP changes?*

■ **Hypertension**

Sympathomimetic drugs (such as cocaine, amphetamines, methamphetamines) cause a sympathetic response. Extreme hypertension and tachycardia are common cardiovascular symptoms of overdose. Presentation of new-onset seizure should warrant a toxicology screen for a sympathomimetic drug.

> HINT
>
> In a sympathomimetic drug overdose, everything "speeds up," including mentation (Box 8.26).

Box 8.26 Symptoms of Sympathomimetic Overdose

Hypertension	Hallucinations (visual and tactile)
Tachycardia	Acute psychosis
Arrhythmias	Mydriasis
Seizures	Diaphoresis
Central nervous system (CNS) excitation	Hyperthermia

■ *A patient presents with decreased LOC and depressed respirations. What is the most likely overdose?*

■ **Sedatives or hypnotics**

Sedatives and hypnotics are the most widely prescribed drugs. An overdose presents with decreased LOC and respiratory depression. Hypotension may also be present. These patients frequently require emergency intubation to protect an airway.

> HINT
>
> Opioid overdose presents very similarly to sedative overdose. Opioids also frequently present with miosis (constricted pupils).

■ *A patient overdoses with Benadryl. Would the pupils be constricted or dilated?*

■ **Dilated (mydriasis)**

Benadryl is an anticholinergic drug. Anticholinergic overdose presents with mydriasis, hyperthermia, and tachycardia. Anticholinergic drugs block the neurotransmitter acetylcholine and inhibit the parasympathetic nervous system. This results in greater sympathetic stimulation, causing papillary dilation (Box 8.27).

> HINT
>
> Miosis = small pupils
> Mydriasis = dilated pupils

Box 8.27 Symptoms of Anticholinergic Overdose

Dry skin	Tachycardia
Hyperthermia	Delirium
Mydriasis	Thirst
Diaphoresis	Urinary retention

■ *A patient presents to the ED with nausea and vomiting, headache, and decreased LOC. A pulse oximetry shows 100% saturation, but the arterial blood gas (ABG) comes back only 88% saturated. What is the most likely cause of this presentation?*

■ **Carbon monoxide poisoning**

Carbon monoxide is a colorless and odorless gas that can cause headache, dizziness, nausea, seizures, and coma. Carbon monoxide binds with hemoglobin to form carboxyhemoglobin. It has a 240 times greater affinity for hemoglobin than oxygen so it reduces the amount of hemoglobin available to carry oxygen. Pulse oximetry cannot distinguish between oxygen and carboxyhemoglobin, so it will typically demonstrate 100% saturation. Laboratory blood gases can determine what is bound to hemoglobin and provide an accurate oxygen saturation level. The discrepancy is indicative of carbon monoxide poisoning. Confirmation of the diagnosis is increased arterial or venous carboxyhemoglobin levels.

> **HINT**
> History of possible exposure to carbon monoxide is also important for determining the diagnosis.

DIAGNOSIS

■ *What is the initial diagnosis typically based on?*

■ **Clinical presentation**

The clinical presentation is typically used to make an initial diagnosis of drug overdose or toxin exposure. The exact substance may not be known initially and determining the substance is not a priority over resuscitation and treatment. Blood and urine will be sent for drug and toxin screens to assist with a more specific diagnosis. Qualitative toxicology screens are performed on urine samples and indicate only the presence or absence of the substance. A quantitative study provides the substance as well as the serum levels and can direct treatment in some cases. Blood alcohol levels are also obtained.

> **HINT**
> Treatment is not delayed awaiting toxicology screens to come back. Qualitative toxicology screens do not change the initial management (Box 8.28). Cyclic antidepressants can be measured but do not correlate with the severity of toxicity.

Box 8.28 Quantitative Studies Assist in the Management of the Following Overdoses

Acetaminophen	Phenytoin
Carbamazepine	Lithium
Carboxyhemoglobin	Digoxin
Ethanol	Valproic acid
Methanol	Antidepressants
Ethylene glycol	

- *If information about an overdose can be obtained, what is the most important information for determining the significance of toxin levels?*
- **Time of ingestion**

History should include the substance ingested or exposed to, amount ingested, and the time of ingestion. The time of ingestion is important to determine how significant the presenting clinical symptoms are and to interpret the drug or toxin levels. Note any unusual odors on the patient's breath, clothing, emesis, and nasogastric aspiration.

> ❭ **HINT**
> Also determine whether the drug is regular or of sustained-release form. Sustained-release drugs will need to be monitored and treated longer until the drug is out of the system.

- *What two lab results are important to determine the presence of anion gap metabolic acidosis?*
- **ABG and electrolytes**

ABG provides information of oxygenation and ventilatory ability. Hypoxemia, hypercarbia, and metabolic acidosis are common findings that may need correcting. If there is metabolic acidosis, calculate the anion gap.

> ❭ **HINT**
> Obtain a 12-lead electrocardiogram (ECG) if cardiotoxic drug ingestion is suspected.

- *What is an osmolal gap?*
- **Comparison of serum osmolality to calculated serum osmolality**

Calculate an osmolality and compare it to the serum osmolality obtained from the laboratory. A positive osmolal gap is greater than 10 mOsm/kg (Boxes 8.29 and 8.30).

Box 8.29 Osmolal Gap Calculation

$(2 \times Na^+ + Glucose/18) + (blood\ urea\ nitrogen\ [BUN]/2.8)$

Box 8.30 Example of Positive Osmolal Gap Toxins

Methanol
Ethanol
Ethylene glycol
Acetone
Isopropyl alcohol

MEDICAL MANAGEMENT

■ *What is the priority of care in drug overdoses?*
■ **Airway**

Initial priorities in managing drug overdoses follow the ABCs: airway, breathing, and circulation. Emergency management may include intubation and mechanical ventilation to protect the airway. The most common reason for hypotension in toxic ingestions is venous pooling, so treatment is fluid resuscitation.

> ❯ HINT
> Exceptions include skin contamination with organophosphates, which can incapacitate health care providers, and cyanide poisoning, which requires a cyanide antidote kit.

■ *What three interventions are commonly recommended in a patient with decreased LOC?*
■ **Glucose, thiamine, and naloxone**

Following ABCs, a patient presenting with a decreased LOC may receive glucose, thiamine, and naloxone as initial treatment. To treat potential hypoglycemia, 50% glucose (25–50 g IV) is administered because hypoglycemia can cause unresponsiveness. Thiamine (100 mg IV) and naloxone (0.4–2 mg IV) are given to reverse potential opioid overdose. Flumazenil can reverse benzodiazepines but is not typically given routinely for an overdose or decreased LOC. Rapid reversal of benzodiazepine overdose can cause seizures from withdrawal.

> ❯ HINT
> Naloxone is indicated in the classic presentation of opioid overdose: miosis, respiratory depression, and decreased LOC.

■ *What is the recommended primary GI decontamination method following oral ingestion of a drug overdose or toxin?*
■ **Activated charcoal (AC)**

AC absorbs the substances and allows greater elimination through the GI tract. The best results occur when administered within 1 hour of ingestion of the substance. The dose is 1 g/kg and it is most commonly administered through gastric tubes. Cathartics, such as sorbitol, may be given in conjunction with AC to shorten transit time in the GI tract and to lower the amount of drug absorbed. Induced vomiting with ipecac is not recommended in most patients due to risk of aspiration or protracted vomiting. Caustic agents should never be managed with induced vomiting. Gastric lavage is not recommended for all patients and should only be done within 1 hour of ingestion. Whole-bowel irrigation can be performed with large volumes of polyethylene glycol electrolyte solutions.

> HINT

A contraindication for AC is a perforated bowel. Contraindications for lavage are acid or alkali ingestions.

■ *What is the procedure for accelerating renal excretion of drugs?*
■ **Diuresis and alteration of urine pH**

Diuresis with IV fluids and diuretics can accelerate elimination through the kidneys. Certain drugs will increase excretion if the urine is alkaline. Sodium bicarbonate infusions are used to alkalinize the urine. Hemodialysis may be considered in life-threatening ingestions involving substances excreted by kidneys.

■ *What is the antidote for acetaminophen?*
■ **N-acetylcysteine (NAC)**

Glutathione normally metabolizes toxic metabolites of acetaminophen. NAC is a substitute for glutathione causing a greater metabolism of toxic byproducts. NAC can be administered by oral or IV route within 24 hours of ingestion (most effective within 8 hours). The oral route has a strong sulfur smell and is not well tolerated without episodes of vomiting. IV route is a bolus followed by an infusion for 21 hours. It has a higher incidence of an anaphylactoid reaction. Acetaminophen levels can be obtained and are used to determine the need for administration of NAC. Levels greater than 10 µmmol/L are considered high, and in combination with elevated liver enzymes, they indicate the need for NAC.

> HINT

Rumack–Matthew nomogram is used to plot the levels to determine the need for NAC.

■ *What are the drugs that inhibit metabolism of ethylene glycol or methanol to toxic metabolites?*
■ **Ethanol or fomepizole**

Alcohol dehydrogenase metabolizes ethanol alcohol over other alcohols. Administration of ethanol will prevent metabolism of ethylene glycol or methanol to toxic metabolites. Ethanol infusion will worsen decreased LOC. Fomepizole is a competitive inhibitor of alcohol dehydrogenase and allows elimination through renal excretion or hemodialysis without a decrease in LOC. Methanol ingestion may also receive folic acid to eliminate formic acid.

> **HINT**
AC does not bind alcohols but may be administered if suspected drug overdose is combined with alcohol consumption. Hemodialysis is more effective in managing metabolic acidosis than sodium bicarbonate (Box 8.31).

Box 8.31 Indications for Hemodialysis

Visual impairment
Renal failure
Pulmonary edema
Severe or refractory metabolic acidosis
Alcohol level > 25 mg/dL

■ *What drug may be given to reverse the cardiovascular effects of a β-blocker overdose?*

■ **Glucagon**

Beta-adrenergic blockers produce bradycardia and hypotension in an overdose. Glucagon is considered the first-line treatment because of its positive chronotropic and inotropic effects. It can be administered by IV bolus or as a continuous infusion until the symptoms are corrected. Calcium gluconate may be used to reverse the hypotension. The management of a calcium channel blocker overdose is similar and requires frequent monitoring of ionized calcium levels.

> **HINT**
Consider placing a transcutaneous pacemaker during initial treatment.

■ *What is the primary treatment for carbon monoxide poisoning?*

■ **Administration of 100% oxygen**

Administration of 100% oxygen should be initiated as soon as a possible diagnosis of carbon monoxide poisoning is made. The patient may need to be intubated if he shows a decreased LOC. The use of hyperbaric oxygen may be used in certain situations if the patient is unresponsive to the initial treatment of 100% oxygen.

> **HINT**
Hyperbaric oxygen may decrease the incidence of cognitive deficits associated with carbon monoxide exposures.

■ *What class of drugs may be avoided in managing hypertension of acute cocaine intoxication?*

■ **β-1 selective β-blocker**

Hypertension of cocaine intoxication is caused by pure α stimulation. Administering a β-1 selective β-blocker results in unopposed α-adrenergic activity and complications of coronary artery vasoconstriction and possibly worsening of hypertension. Labetalol may be the drug of choice due to its combination of an α-blocker and a β-blocker. The first-line treatment for anginal chest pain is nitroglycerin followed by either phentolamine or calcium channel blockers.

> **HINT**
Treat complications of cocaine toxicity with, for example, IV hydration to prevent rhabdomyolysis.

■ **What is the treatment for wide QRS complexes in cyclic antidepressant overdoses?**
■ **Sodium bicarbonate**

Cyclic antidepressant overdose can cause wide QRS complexes (> 0.10 seconds) and can result in ventricular tachycardia (Torsades de pointes). The intraventricular delays are caused by the cyclic antidepressant slowing the influx sodium into myocardial cells. Sodium bicarbonate uncouples the cyclic antidepressant from myocardial cells. Sodium bicarbonate also treats myocardial depression. Recent studies have found success with hypertonic saline in treating the wide QRS complex and hypotension. An overdose of selective serotonin reuptake inhibitors (SSRIs) is usually not as severe as the cyclic antidepressants and are managed similarly.

> **HINT**
Magnesium is used to manage Torsades de pointes.

COMPLICATIONS

■ **What is the major complication of an acetaminophen overdose, both intentional and unintentional?**
■ **Liver failure**

Liver failure is caused by an accumulation of the toxic metabolite N-acetyl-p-benzoquinone imine (NAPQI) in excess of the substance glutathione that is required to conjugate NAPQI for easier removal. Conjugation of the metabolite into a water-soluble state allows for renal excretion. The excess unconjugated substance binds to the hepatocytes causing inflammation, necrosis, and cell death. This can occur with an acute overdose of acetaminophen or with chronic abuse with accumulation over time.

> **HINT**
Nonintentional overdose usually occurs because of lack of education regarding the dose limit of acetaminophen in a 24-hour period coupled with all the medications that contain acetaminophen.

■ **What is an acute cardiovascular complication of a sympathomimetic overdose?**
■ **AMI**

Sympathomimetic drug overdose causes stimulation of the sympathetic nervous system with extreme hypertension and tachycardia. This significantly increases the workload of the heart and myocardial resistance. Tachycardia decreases diastolic time and coronary artery perfusion. The increase in demand and decrease in supply results in myocardial ischemia. Other life-threatening complications are intracerebral hemorrhage, stroke, rhabdomyolysis, necrotizing vasculitis, and death. Dilated cardiomyopathy is a long-term cardiovascular complication.

> **HINT**
> AMI can occur even in young people without coronary artery disease who have had a sympathomimetic overdose.

■ *What syndrome can occur with an overdose of SSRI?*
■ **Serotonin syndrome**

Serotonin syndrome can be life threatening and may be caused by other drugs as well as SSRIs (MAO inhibitors, lithium, meperidine). The syndrome can present with hyperthermia, hypertension, tachycardia, tremors, and seizures (Box 8.32). It is best prevented by administering AC soon after an initial overdose. If it does occur, manage the life-threatening symptoms, which includes intensive cooling, antihypertensives, anticonvulsants, sedation, and intubation with mechanical ventilation. Cyproheptadine is a serotonin antagonist that may be given to treat serotonin syndrome but efficacy has not been proven at this time.

> **HINT**
> Serotonin syndrome does not require administration of dantrolene or bromocriptine.

Box 8.32 Symptoms of Serotonin Syndrome

Agitation	Diarrhea
Decreased LOC	Tremor
Hypertension	Muscle rigidity
Tachycardia	Myoclonus
Diaphoresis	Seizures
Hyperthermia	

ASPHYXIA/ANOXIC BRAIN INJURY

■ *What is different about hypoxic–ischemic brain injury (HI–BI) when compared to an ischemic stroke?*
■ **Global ischemia**

An ischemic stroke results in a more regional ischemia based on the vascular territory. HI–BIs affect blood flow to the entire brain so HI–BI has a more global effect on the ischemia.

> **HINT**
> HI–BI has also been called anoxic injury or anoxic encephalopathy.

■ *What is the most predominant outcome following survival of HI–BI?*
■ **Coma or vegetative state**

Generalized brain hypoxia or anoxia results in greater injury to the cortical structures such as the lobes of the cerebral cortex and the memory center of the hippocampal area, then to the brainstem structures. Patients may have a decreased LOC but still have reflexes and spontaneous respirations due to the intact brainstem.

> **HINT**
> These patients are not brain dead because of the continued brainstem function.

PATHOPHYSIOLOGY

■ *What is the excitatory neurotransmitter that increases following an anoxic brain injury?*
■ **Glutamate**

Following an anoxic injury, the inhibition of adenosine triphosphate (ATP) occurs, resulting in anaerobic metabolism leading to efflux of glutamate. Glutamate is a neuroexcitatory substance that causes further damage of the neurons, influx of calcium, apoptosis, and cellular death.

> **HINT**
> Calcium channel blockers have been used during periods of hypoxia as a neuroprotectant by blocking the influx of calcium (Figure 8.1).

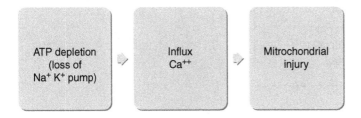

Figure 8.1 Physiology of ischemia.

■ *What is released following reperfusion resulting in further cellular death?*
■ **Free radicals**

A reperfusion injury occurs once blood flow is reestablished to an organ or tissue. Affected mitochondria produce oxygen free radicals during periods of ischemia. Following reperfusion, free radicals and inflammatory mediators are released and exacerbate tissue necrosis by lipid peroxidation (Box 8.33).

Box 8.33 Causes of Anoxic Brain Injuries

Postcardiopulmonary resuscitation (CPR)
   Respiratory arrest
   Cardiac arrest
Near drowning
Strangulation
	Attempted suicide by hanging
	Loss of airway in significant amount of time
	Airway obstruction
	Carbon monoxide poisoning
	Profound hypotension

■ *What type of cerebral edema occurs with a HI–BI?*

■ **Cytotoxic cerebral edema**

Cytotoxic cerebral edema indicates the extra water is intracellular. This is typically caused by a hypoxic–ischemic injury. The lack of ATP (energy source at the cellular level) interferes with the $Na^+ K^+$ pump, allowing a greater amount of sodium to influx into the cell. Water follows sodium and results in intracellular swelling and edema.

SYMPTOMS/ASSESSMENT

■ *What are tested to evaluate brainstem function?*

■ **Cranial nerves**

Neurological evaluation of the cerebral cortex includes assessment of the level of arousal and mentation. Brainstem assessment includes cranial nerves and reflexes.

> **❯ HINT**
> It is important to exclude factors that may affect the neurological examination (Box 8.34).

Box 8.34 Factors That Obscure Neurological Examination

Hypothermia	Ongoing nonconvulsant seizure
Illicit drugs prior to hospitalization	Postictal
Ongoing cerebral hypoperfusion	Electrolyte abnormalities
Sedatives and analgesics	Metabolic derangements
Neuromuscular blocking agents	

DIAGNOSIS

■ *What diagnostic test has been most widely used to assess LOC and guide prognosis after a HI–BI?*

■ **Electroencephalogram (EEG)**

An EEG has been used most frequently in conjunction with clinical neurological examinations to determine LOC and to assist with determining the prognosis after an HI–BI. The reactivity of EEG waves to external stimulation is more important than the baseline reading in HI–BI evaluations. Sedation, metabolic derangements, and sepsis can alter the EEG findings, making them less prognostic.

> ### 〉 HINT
> The presence of reactivity on EEG with an external stimulus indicates a better prognosis.

■ *What diagnostic test may be used to assess the integrity of afferent pathways?*

■ **Somatosensory evoked potentials (SSEPs)**

SSEPs assess the integrity of afferent pathways from the brain stem and thalamocortical pathways to the primary somatosensory cortex. Injury in the subcortical area of the brain may cause a slowing of the pathway, whereas injury in the cortical portion causes an absence of impulses within the pathway. This is not influenced by sedation or metabolic derangements like EEG.

■ *How long after an insult will a computed tomography (CT) scan demonstrate diffuse cerebral edema?*

■ **Within 48 hours**

CT scans may find diffuse cerebral edema due to cytotoxicity. Generally, cerebral edema is found within 48 hours following the insult. MRI, with diffusion weighted imagery (DWI) and FLAIR capabilities, may be used to determine the extent of injury within 24 hours.

MEDICAL MANAGEMENT

■ *What is the primary medical management of an anoxic brain injury?*

■ **Therapeutic hypothermia (TH)**

TH has been found in postcardiac arrest resuscitation to improve outcomes if initiated early and maintained for 12 to 24 hours. This technique is also frequently used on HI–BI patients as adjunctive treatment in addition to maintaining an airway, treating cerebral edema, administering anticonvulsants, and preventing complications. Hyperbaric oxygen may be tried as an adjunctive therapy following stabilization of the patient.

COMPLICATIONS

■ *What is a common complication of a HI–BI that typically occurs soon after an insult?*

■ **Seizure**

There is a relatively high incidence of seizures within 24 hours following a global ischemic injury to the brain. They may also occur within several weeks of the insult. This is because of an increase in excitatory neurotransmitters (glutamate) following an injury, which has been found to lower the seizure threshold (Box 8.35).

> ### 〉 HINT
> The seizure is typically a complex partial seizure or a myoclonic seizure.

Box 8.35 Complications of HI–BI

Seizure
Movement disorders
Parkinsonism
Dystonia
Tremor
Athetosis
Motor weakness, paresis, or paralysis
Cognitive impairment
Impaired attention
Memory impairment
Language difficulties
Posthypoxic leukoencephalopathy (demyelination)
Neuropsychiatric problems (delirium, psychosis, akinetic mutism)

TESTABLE NURSING ACTIONS

THERAPEUTIC HYPOTHERMIA

■ *What is the primary indication for TH?*
■ **Out-of-hospital cardiac arrest**

Therapeutic temperature modulation (TTM) encompasses mild hypothermia and maintenance of normothermia. Out-of-hospital cardiac arrest with ventricular fibrillation is the primary indication for TH (mild). The American Heart Association also includes in-house postcardiac arrest with any arrhythmia for comatose patients with return spontaneous circulation and out-of-hospital cardiac arrest with pulseless electrical activity and asystole.

> **HINT**
> TH can cause a coagulopathy and may not be as great a benefit
> following traumatic brain injuries or intracerebral hemorrhages.

■ *What is the primary mechanism of TH in preventing brain injury during reperfusion?*
■ **Decreases metabolism**

The reduction in metabolism in the brain results in a decrease in oxygen demand. Immediately following resuscitation, during the reperfusion stage, this decrease in oxygen demand improves brain oxygenation. Other benefits of TH may include stabilization of cell membranes and the blood–brain barrier, inhibition of oxygen free radicals during reperfusion, and reducing brain inflammation.

> **HINT**
> Hypothermia reduces cerebral oxygen consumption by a rate of 6% per
> 1°C change in temperature.

■ *What is the temperature goal for TH following a cardiac arrest?*
■ **32°C to 34°C**

Cooling a patient's core temperature from 32°C to 24°C has shown an increase in survival rates and improved neurological outcomes. Early initiation following successful resuscitation improves success of therapy. TH is maintained for 12 to 24 hours. It is recommended that at least two sites be used for monitoring body temperature. Core temperatures are recommended, and axillary and tympanic sites should be avoided.

> **HINT**
> Cooling below 32°C is difficult due to shivering and may increase risk of arrhythmias.

■ *What are the three phases of TH?*
■ **Induction, maintenance, and rewarming**

Induction is the rapid reduction of body temperature with internal and/or external cooling methods. The maintenance-phase goal is to maintain hypothermic temperature for 12 to 24 hours. The rewarming phase is controlled and is purposeful rewarming of the patient. Avoid too rapid of rewarming due to potential neural axonal injury.

> **HINT**
> Rewarming is recommended to occur at a rate of 0.2° to 0.3°C/hr (Box 8.36).

Box 8.36 Three Phases of TH

Induction	Maintenance	Rewarming
Obtain baseline Hemodynamic profile Electrolytes	Maintain body temperature within goal range	Controlled and purposeful Goal is to rewarm within 12–24 hours Prevent overshooting of temperature
Rapid reduction in body temperature Surface cooling Internal cooling	Manage electrolyte abnormalities Avoid overshooting electrolyte correction	Monitor Hemodynamics Electrolytes
Prevent shivering	Frequent vital signs	Administer fluids if hypotensive
	Monitor electrolytes and coagulation studies	Monitor temperature for rebound hypothermia
	Provide sedation and analgesia	
	Prevent or manage shivering	

■ *Which cooling method, surface or intravascular, has been shown to cool faster during the induction phase?*
■ **Intravascular cooling**

Intravascular cooling can use the technique of either metal or circulating cold water-filled balloon conductors or infusion of cold saline. The advantage of intravascular cooling is more rapid cooling, which is more effective in the induction phase than surface cooling. The disadvantages are it is invasive and more expensive. Surface cooling may use air, volatile liquids, or cold water and/or ice. It is less invasive but may cause greater fluctuations in body temperature. Selective brain-cooling devices are now available, such as intranasal cooling and devises that specifically cool the head.

> **HINT**
Some studies have shown that a more rapid induction has a greater success with improving neurological outcomes.

■ *What is the most common complication of TH?*
■ **Shivering**

Shivering is a natural response to hypothermia but can impede induction and maintenance of goal body temperature. Shivering generates heat and increases consumption two to five times greater than normal. Lowering body temperature produces vasoconstriction, which is a compensatory mechanism to prevent heat loss. It keeps core organs 2°C to 4°C higher than the peripheral ones. Once vasoconstriction is no longer working to maintain heat, then shivering begins as a compensatory mechanism to increase body temperature (Box 8.37).

> **HINT**
A higher rate of shivering is found in males and patients with low magnesium levels.

Box 8.37 Adverse Effects of Shivering

Increase body temperature	Tachycardia
Patient discomfort	Hypertension
Increase metabolism	Tachypnea
Increase oxygen demand and consumption	Increased intracranial pressure (ICP)
Increased production of CO_2	

■ *What is the purpose of counter surface warming?*
■ **To prevent shivering**

Counter surface warming can be used to prevent shivering. Skin temperature influences at least 20% of the shivering threshold so blowing warm air on skin (across the face or body) at 40°C to 43°C will increase the shivering threshold (Box 8.38).

Box 8.38 Prevention of Shivering

Counter surface warming
Rapid cooling past the threshold of 35°C
Keep hands and feet covered with gloves and socks
Adequate sedation

■ *What assessment tool may be used to determine the presence and degree of shivering?*

■ **Bedside Shivering Assessment Tool (BSAT)**

BSAT is a validated four-point scale that has been found to accurately predict energy expenditure. It quantifies the assessment of shivering and can be used to determine the efficacy of current management. It is easy to use (palpate neck and chest region) and can be performed hourly and more often during the induction and rewarming phases.

> **HINT**
> Shivering begins in the trunk and spreads to the extremities (Box 8.39).

Box 8.39 BSAT

Score		
0	None	No shivering noted on masseter, neck, or chest wall
1	Mild	Localized to neck and/or thorax only
2	Moderate	In addition, involves gross motor movements of upper extremities
3	Severe	Gross motor movements of trunk, upper, and lower extremities
P	Paralyzed	Pharmacologically paralyzed

■ *Which analgesic is used most frequently to manage shivering?*

■ **Meperidine (Demerol)**

Meperidine has been found to decrease shivering and vasoconstriction thresholds. It has the adverse effects of neurotoxicity and lowering of the seizure threshold. Meperidine may be used in combination with other drugs, including buspirone (Buspar) and/or propofol (Diprivan) to work synergistically to lower the threshold. Buspar is a 5-HT 1a agonist and has been found to be effective in reducing shivering. Other drugs that may be used include tramadol (Ultram), ondansetron (Zofran), and magnesium infusions. Neuromuscular blocking agents may be used to stop shivering but are typically used only if other methods are ineffective.

> **HINT**
> The goal is to decrease the shivering threshold, that is, lower the point at which shivering begins.

■ *What happens to potassium levels during the induction of hypothermia?*

■ **They decrease**

Potassium shifts intracellularly during the induction of hypothermia. This lowers serum potassium levels. Other electrolyte abnormalities include hypophosphatemia and hypomagnesemia (Box 8.40).

> **HINT**
> Avoid overreplacing electrolytes because during rewarming the electrolytes will shift back into the serum, causing hyperkalemia, hypermagnesemia, and hyperphosphatemia.

Box 8.40 Complications of Hypothermia

Shivering	Cardiac arrhythmias
Electrolyte disturbances	Lowers drug metabolism rates in liver
Coagulopathy	Pneumonia
Bradycardia	Hyperglycemia
Decreased myocardial contractility	Sepsis

■ *What are two ECG changes that may occur with hypothermia?*

■ **Elevated J point and Osborne wave**

There is elevation of the J point (backside of the QRS complex) 1 to 2 mm from baseline. An Osborne wave is a positive deflection occurring immediately behind the QRS complex. Either of these ECG changes may be found with hypothermia.

> **HINT**
> An elevated J point should not be mistaken as an elevated ST segment.

MODERATE SEDATION

■ *What is the level of arousal when a patient is given a moderate sedation?*

■ **Respond purposefully to verbal commands**

Moderate sedation is used for diagnostic and therapeutic procedures. There are different levels of sedation, ranging from minimal sedation to anesthesia. A patient's response to stimulation determines the level of sedation. The ability to maintain an airway and ventilate is also included in the definitions of the levels of sedation (Box 8.41).

Box 8.41 Levels of Sedation

Level of Sedation	Arousal	Airway/Ventilation
Minimal	Responds normally to verbal commands Impaired cognitive function and coordination	Unaffected
Moderate	Responds purposefully to verbal commands or light tactile stimulation Amnesia may be present	No intervention required Protected reflexes are present (cough, gag)
Deep	Cannot be easily aroused or responds purposefully to stimulation Amnesia may be present	May require assistance to maintain airway Spontaneous ventilation may be inadequate
Anesthesia	Drug-induced loss of consciousness Unarousable even with painful stimulation	Often requires intubation and ventilation

> **HINT**
Anesthesia is not considered moderate sedation.

■ *What are the two major goals of moderate sedation?*
■ **Provide relief of anxiety and pain control**

The major goals of moderate sedation, at all levels, include providing relief from anxiety (sedation) and pain control. Deep sedation may be used also to minimize or prevent patient movement during the procedure.

■ *What is the greatest concern when providing moderate sedation?*
■ **Respiratory depression**

Maintaining the ability to have effective spontaneous ventilation is an important aspect of moderate sedation. Medications administered to obtain moderate sedation have side effects of respiratory depression, and multiple drug administration may have a synergistic effect. The ability to maintain an airway and effective ventilation are goals during moderate sedation and both should be monitored closely (Box 8.42).

Box 8.42 Risk Factors for Moderate Sedation

Morbidly obese
Elderly
History of severe cardiovascular or pulmonary disease
Obstructive sleep apnea
Substance abuse
Smoking history

■ *Prior to initiation of moderate sedation, what must be obtained from the patient or family?*

■ **A signed consent form**

An informed consent from must be obtained that explain the benefits and risks of administration of moderate or deep sedation (Box 8.43).

Box 8.43 Preprocedure Assessment

Relevant history
Assessment of systems (emphasis on pulmonary and cardiovascular systems)
Airway assessment
Ensuring nothing by mouth (NPO) status
Pain assessment
Determine level of anxiety

> **❯ HINT**
> An airway assessment is recommended prior to a procedure in case complications of moderate sedation occur and the patient requires emergency intubation.

■ *During the procedure, how frequently should vital signs be assessed and documented when using moderate sedation?*

■ **Every 5 minutes**

The assessment and documentation of vital signs, oxygen saturation, $EtCO_2$ (if in use), and level of sedation should be done every 5 minutes during the procedure or more frequently if significant changes or events occur.

> **❯ HINT**
> Alarms should be on at all times and documented.

■ *What are the two most commonly used classes of medications used to obtain moderate sedation?*

■ **Opioids and benzodiazepines**

Opioids not only provide analgesia but also sedation. They may be used alone or in combination with a benzodiazepine. Benzodiazepine is an anxiolytic used to control anxiety and provide amnesia and hypnotic effects for the procedure. Commonly used opioids are morphine and fentanyl. Diazepam and lorazepam are frequently used benzodiazepines. Other sedatives that may be used include ketamine, methohexital, and propofol. Naloxone is used to reverse complications of opioids, and flumazenil is used for the reversal of benzodiazepines.

> **❯ HINT**
> Administer reversal agents slowly in small increments to reverse the side effect (respiratory depression) without reversing the sedation or analgesic effect of the medication.

■ *In addition to respiratory depression, what other complication can commonly occur with the administration of moderate sedation?*

■ **Hypotension**

Airway and ventilation complications are the most common, but hypotension can also occur. This is commonly a result of histamine release causing vasodilation and hypotension (Box 8.44).

Box 8.44 Complications of Moderate Sedation

Respiratory depression
Loss of airway
Hypotension
Drug overdose
Anaphylaxis
Nausea and vomiting
Aspiration

BIBLIOGRAPHY

Dellinger, R., et al. (2012) Surviving sepsis campaign: International guidelines for management of severe sepsis and septic shock. *Critical Care Medicine, 41*(2).

Presciutti, M., Bader, M., & Hepburn, M. (2012). Shivering management during therapeutic temperature modulation: Nurse's perspective. *Critical Care Nurse*, 32(1) 33–42.

Questions

1. A patient with complete spinal cord injury at the C4 level has bladder atony and requires catheterization. Which of the following bladder catheterizations is the recommended goal in the acute care of a spinal cord–injured patient?

   A. Indwelling catheter
   B. Intermittent catheterization
   C. External catheters
   D. Stents placed in the urethra

2. Ms. J has been in the ICU for 3 days following a motor vehicle collision. She is now febrile (temperature 38.5°C) with an elevated WBC count (20,000). The following are her vital signs:

   BP 124/64
   HR 112
   RR 24
   Lactate 2 mmol/L

   Which of the following best describes the complication Ms. J is experiencing?

   A. Sepsis/SIRS
   B. Severe sepsis
   C. Septic shock
   D. Multisystem organ dysfunction

3. Mr. M is in the ICU for management of exacerbation of his congestive heart failure. He develops fever and his WBC count has elevated to 14,000. What is the recommended time frame to initiate antibiotics?

   A. Within 1 hour
   B. 2 to 3 hours
   C. Within 6 hours
   D. Antibiotics are not indicated at this time

4. A physician orders an initial bolus of fluids to be administered in a sepsis-induced hypoperfused patient. Which of the following fluids would be recommended for an initial bolus?

   A. Albumin
   B. Normal saline
   C. Hetastarch
   D. Packed red blood cells

5. Which of the following is recommended before initiating a hydrocortisone infusion in septic shock patients?

   A. Low cortisol levels
   B. ACTH test
   C. Hypotension despite vasopressors
   D. Presence of three organs in failure

6. Which of the following electrolytes need to be monitored closely during infusion of hydrocortisone?

   A. Sodium and chloride
   B. Sodium and magnesium
   C. Phosphate and glucose
   D. Glucose and sodium

7. A patient with severe sepsis is receiving fluid boluses. The physician has ordered that vasopressor therapy be initiated according to the sepsis bundles. Which of the following vasopressors is considered the first-line vasopressor for treating hypotension in severe sepsis?

   A. Phenylephrine
   B. Dopamine
   C. Norepinephrine
   D. Vasopressin

8. A patient presents with airway edema, wheezing, nausea, and vomiting after eating dinner at a seafood restaurant. Which of the following is the most likely cause for this presentation?

   A. Anaphylactoid reaction
   B. Anaphylaxis
   C. Drug-induced angioedema
   D. Food poisoning

9. A patient presents to the emergency room with vomiting, incontinence, and increased salivation. The family states that the patient took an overdose of pills but they are not sure what the pills were. Based on the presentation, what type of overdose is most likely in this patient?

   A. Cholinergic
   B. Anticholinergic
   C. Sedative
   D. β-blocker

10. A patient in the ICU has been on a lorazepam infusion for 4 days and is noted to have a new anion-gap metabolic acidosis. Which of the following accumulations is most likely the cause of the metabolic acidosis?

    A. Ketones
    B. Propylene glycol
    C. Thiocyanate
    D. Lactic acid

11. Which of the following methods of inducing TH is associated with a faster decrease to goal temperature?

    A. Surface cooling devices
    B. Ice packs
    C. Intravascular cooling
    D. Cooling blankets

12. Which of the following is recommended to prevent shivering during the induction and maintenance phase of TH?

    A. Administer anticonvulsant medications
    B. Cover patient with warm blankets
    C. Administer thorazine before induction
    D. Blow warm air across the face

13. Following a near-drowning, a patient is intubated and on mechanical ventilation. Her neurological examination demonstrates no response to painful stimulation. She has a gag-and-swallow reflex. She also has positive cold calorics and doll's eye sign. Her CT scan reveals diffuse edema. Which of the following is the most accurate statement regarding her injury?

    A. The organ donation agency should be notified because she has met criteria for brain death.
    B. This is a global injury due to anoxia and may be treated with TH.
    C. Near-drowning typically produces vasogenic cerebral edema and should be monitored with an ICP catheter.
    D. The most important issue with her is the potential for pulmonary complications.

14. What is the temperature goal for the maintenance phase of TH?

    A. 34°C to 36°C
    B. 32°C to 34°C
    C. 30°C to 32°C
    D. Less than 30°C

15. A patient being managed with TH is noted to have a score of 2 on the BSAT. Which of the following would be the best description of severity of shivering based on the score?

    A. Shivering involves gross movement of upper and lower extremities
    B. Shivering is localized to the neck and chest regions only
    C. Shivering involves gross movement of upper extremities
    D. There is no shivering noted at this time

Behavioral/Psychological Review

In this chapter, you will review:

- Substance dependence
- Pain, agitation, and delirium
- Dementia
- Suicidal behavior
- Mood disorders: Depression
- Aggressive behaviors/violence
- Failure to thrive
- Elder abuse
- Restraint use in the ICU

SUBSTANCE DEPENDENCE

- **What is the major difference between an addiction and a dependence on a drug?**
- **Compulsive cravings**

An addiction is an acquired chronic disorder characterized by compulsive use of drugs with a craving resulting in physical, psychological, and social harm. This craving and abuse continue despite the evidence of harm. It is a loss of control and denial of potential for harm and is characterized by the persistent use of dysfunctional drugs. The definition for addiction includes a compulsion or an overpowering drive to take the drug in order to experience the psychological effects.

> **HINT**
> Chronic use of an opioid does not mean the patient is addicted.

- **What is the adaption to drugs at the cellular level such that when the drug is removed abruptly, withdrawal symptoms occur?**
- **Dependence**

Dependence on a substance is the result of chronic drug administration and has a characteristic set of signs and symptoms called withdrawal syndrome. Dependence can occur with and without addiction. The incidence of physical dependence on substances (including alcohol) is greater than most health care workers realize and needs to be monitored closely to prevent complications of withdrawal.

> HINT
Abuse can coexist independently from both dependence and addiction.

■ **What is the illicit use of a substance outside the legitimate medical practice called?**
■ **Abuse**

Abuse is when a substance is used, either prescribed or illicit, outside of normal practice or without medical justification.

■ **When a person has multiple prescriptions for pain and anxiety prescribed by several different physicians, what is this typically called?**
■ **Drug seeking**

There are three main reasons for people seeking drugs. One is because they have a drug addiction and are seeking substances for their cravings and a "high." Other drug seekers may be obtaining drugs to sell but are not actually taking the substances themselves. There are also a large number of drug seekers who are people truly in pain but are not being managed appropriately for their pain. They are commonly seen as addicts but actually have a pseudoaddiction on the drug because of unrelieved pain or fear of reemergence of the pain.

> HINT
People in pain may do extraordinary things to obtain pain medications to adequately control their pain.

■ **What are the most commonly prescribed addictive drugs in the world?**
■ **Hypnotics and sedatives**

Hypnotics and sedatives are the most commonly prescribed drugs in the world with addicting properties. Alcohol is the most widely used substance.

> HINT
Alcohol is a sedative/hypnotic so there is cross-tolerance and cross-dependence between alcohol and other sedatives.

■ **What is the major characteristic of alcohol abuse (not just use)?**
■ **Dangerous behaviors**

Alcohol abuse is defined as a pattern of recurrent alcohol use associated with dangerous behaviors (e.g., driving while intoxicated, fighting, or being sexually promiscuous) or a failure to meet one's obligations at home or work.

> HINT
Abuse is not determined by a set amount or frequency of alcohol consumption.

PATHOPHYSIOLOGY

■ *What part of the brain is responsible for "addictions" to substances?*
■ **Subcortical region**

Addiction affects the subcortical areas of the hypothalamus. The subcortical areas of the brain are not involved in higher cognitive processing; but these are areas of the brain that motivate and mediate instinctual drive-based and emotionally charged behaviors. Despite the different types of drugs that are addicting, the common characteristic of all of the potentially addictive drugs is a specific neuronal pathway called the mesolimbic dopamine pathway. It is located in the "reward center" of the brain. Drugs that affect this pathway cause a release of dopamine, which then stimulates the release of endogenous opioids, the result of which is profound euphoria and elevated moods associated with drug intoxication and drug-seeking behavior.

■ *When does physical dependence on a substance become apparent?*
■ **Sudden cessation**

Physical dependence occurs over time as the body adapts to the repeated dosing of the drug. Physical dependence becomes apparent with withdrawal or sudden reversing and rapid fall in drug levels. Suddenly, unopposed by the drug's effects, the adaptive changes become nonadaptive and physical symptoms appear.

> ❯ HINT
> Some drugs have minimal to no physical dependence or withdrawal symptoms even in addicted people.

■ *What is the excitatory neurotransmitter receptor that alcohol inhibits?*
■ **N-methyl-D-asparate (NMDA)**

Acute alcohol ingestion inhibits NMDA receptors, reducing excitatory glutamate transmission, and has an agonist (enhancing) effect on gamma aminobutyric acid (GABA), the inhibitory neurotransmitter. Initially, alcohol produces euphoria, exaggerated feelings of well-being, and reduced self-control, and then produces sedation. Long-term use of alcohol causes chronic suppression of excitatory receptors (NMDA), so the brain increases the synthesis of excitatory neurotransmitters. Abrupt cessation of alcohol use causes a rebound stimulatory effect and accounts for the symptoms of withdrawal (Box 9.1).

> ❯ HINT
> Alcohol withdrawal syndrome (AWS) is a result of unopposed hyperexcitable neurons. This contributes to delirium tremens (DT) and withdrawal seizures.

Box 9.1 Neurotransmitters in the Brain

Gamma-aminobutyric acid (GABA)	Inhibitory neurotransmitter
Glutamate	Excitatory neurotransmitter
N-methyl-D-aspartate (NMDA)	Excitatory receptors
Serotonin	Excitatory transmission
Dopamine	Excitatory transmission
Norepinephrine	Excitatory transmission

SYMPTOMS/ASSESSMENT

■ *What is an important component of the initial assessment of all patients admitted into the intensive care unit (ICU)?*

■ **Obtain accurate history**

Prevention of AWS is the first step to decreasing mortality. An accurate drinking history to determine potential dependence on alcohol assists with prevention and early recognition of the symptoms of AWS. Ask the patient about his alcohol use, including the frequency and number of drinks daily (Box 9.2).

> ❯ **HINT**
> Consider obtaining further information regarding the amount of alcohol intake from a family member.

Box 9.2 Questions to Ask Regarding Alcohol Consumption

What alcoholic beverages are consumed?	How many years have you been drinking?
How many per occasion are consumed?	Any history of alcohol withdrawal?
How often do you drink?	History of other substance abuse?
When was the time of your last drink?	History of major psychological conditions?

■ *What is a commonly used assessment/screening tool for alcohol use/abuse?*

■ **CAGE questionnaire**

The CAGE questionnaire is short and easy-to-use screening tool to be incorporated into a routine admission history of alcohol use. One "yes" answer to these questions suggests that the patient needs to be observed more closely and two "yes" answers is highly correlated with alcohol abuse or dependence, and three "yes" answers indicates alcohol abuse with an increase in sensitivity to 100%.

> ❯ **HINT**
> One of the problems with the CAGE assessment is that it does not distinguish between past and present alcohol use (Box 9.3).

Box 9.3 CAGE Questionnaire

C	Have you felt you can **cut** down on your drinking?
A	Have people **annoyed** you by criticizing your drinking?
G	Have you ever felt bad or **guilty** about your drinking?
E	Have you ever had a drink first thing in the morning to steady your nerves or to get rid of a hangover? (**eye opener**)

■ *What do most people do when asked about how many drinks they have had per day or when asked about taking illicit substances?*

■ **Deny or minimize**

Most people want to either deny or minimize the amount they drink when discussing their alcohol intake or use of illicit substances. Ask questions in a nonjudgmental and matter-of-fact way with other general questions. For example, ask about the alcohol intake following questions on caffeine consumption (Box 9.4).

> **⟩ HINT**
> Ensure the patient knows that everyone is being asked these questions.

Box 9.4 Definition of "One" Drink

12 ounces of beer	2½ ounces cordial or liqueur
8½ ounces of malt liquor or fortified beer, ale (40-ounce bottle)	2½ ounces cordial or liqueur
5 ounces of wine	1½ ounces of spirits, 80-proof vodka, gin, whiskey, or brandy
3½ ounces fortified wine (sherry or port)	

DIAGNOSIS

■ *What laboratory test will elevate within 4 to 8 weeks with alcohol ingestion?*

■ **Mean corpuscular volume (MCV)**

Elevated MCV may indicate alcohol abuse. Index of red blood cell (RBC) size (macrocytosis) increases with alcohol intake within 4 to 8 weeks. This occurs in 90% of all alcoholics. The mechanism is unknown but it may be caused by poor nutrition.

■ *What pattern of elevated liver enzymes indicates alcohol-induced liver failure?*

■ **Aspartate aminotransferase (AST) is two times higher than alanine aminotransferase (ALT)**

Alcohol-induced liver dysfunction will elevate both AST and ALT. The pattern specific for liver failure is an AST two times greater than ALT. This pattern is generally not seen in other causes of liver failure. Homocysteine levels are elevated in nonabstinent alcoholics and the levels may be associated with withdrawal seizures.

> **⟩ HINT**
> Homocysteine levels may be a useful biomarker of risk of alcohol withdrawal seizures.

■ *When do symptoms of AWS peak following the last drink?*

■ **24 to 48 hours**

Autonomic hyperactivity appears within hours of the last drink and usually peaks within 24 to 48 hours. Withdrawal signs typically start between 5 and 10 hours after the last drink. Symptoms of AWS can range from mild, self-limiting to severe and life threatening (Box 9.5.) Chronic alcoholics typically experience progressively shorter intervals between their last drink and progressive worsening symptoms of AWS during each subsequent episode. This phenomenon is called a "kindling effect" (Figure 9.1)

Box 9.5 Symptoms of AWS

Mild	Major
Autonomic hyperactivity	Hallucinations
Tachycardia	Tactile
Mild anxiety	Visual
Hypertension	Auditory
Gastrointestinal (GI) disturbances	Seizures
Diaphoresis	Tonic–clonic
Insomnia	Delirium tremens (DTs)
Vivid dreams	Confusion
Headaches	Disorientation
Anorexia, nausea, and vomiting	Impaired attention
Hyper-reflexia	Severe autonomic activity
Hyperventilation	Hallucinations
Low-grade fever	Respiratory or cardiovascular collapse

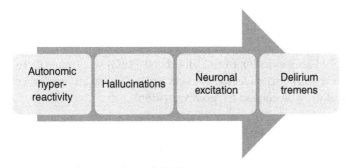

Figure 9.1 Progression of AWS.

- *What tool is used clinically to determine the severity of AWS?*
- **Clinical Institute Withdrawal Assessment for Alcohol Scale, Revised (CIWA-Ar)**

CIWA-Ar is a tool used to determine the severity of AWS and to guide therapeutic intervention. A score of less than 9 indicates that the patient must be observed. If the score is greater than 9, a benzodiazepine should be administered. Determination of the score is then repeated each hour until less than 10 and dosing of benzodiazepine is continued until less than 9. At this point, scoring can be every 8 hours, then discontinued when score is less than 6 on four consecutive assessments.

> HINT

Use of a symptom-triggered dosing protocol with the use of CIWA-Ar may reduce treatment time and amount of drug used versus administering a fixed dose (Box 9.6).

Box 9.6 CIWA-Ar

Patient: _____ Date: _____ Time: _____ (24-hour clock, midnight = 00:00)
Pulse or heart rate, taken for 1 minute: _____ Blood pressure:

NAUSEA AND VOMITING: Ask: "Do you feel sick to your stomach? Have you vomited?" Observation.
0 no nausea and no vomiting
1 mild nausea with no vomiting
4 intermittent nausea with dry heaves
7 constant nausea, frequent dry heaves and vomiting

TACTILE DISTURBANCES: Ask: "Have you any itching, pins-and-needles sensations, any burning, any numbness, or do you feel bugs crawling on or under your skin?" Observation.
0 none
1 very mild itching, pins and needles, burning or numbness
2 mild itching, pins and needles, burning or numbness
3 moderate itching, pins and needles, burning or numbness
4 moderately severe hallucinations
5 severe hallucinations
6 extremely severe hallucinations
7 continuous hallucinations

AUDITORY DISTURBANCES: Ask: "Are you more aware of sounds around you? Are they harsh? Do they frighten you? Are you hearing anything that is disturbing to you? Are you hearing things you know are not there?" Observation.
0 not present
1 very mild harshness or ability to frighten
2 mild harshness or ability to frighten
3 moderate harshness or ability to frighten
4 moderately severe hallucinations
5 severe hallucinations
6 extremely severe hallucinations
7 continuous hallucinations

VISUAL DISTURBANCES: Ask: "Does the light appear to be too bright? Is its color different? Does it hurt your eyes? Are you seeing anything that is disturbing to you? Are you seeing things you know are not there?" Observation.
0 not present
1 very mild sensitivity
2 mild sensitivity
3 moderate sensitivity
4 moderately severe hallucinations
5 severe hallucinations
6 extremely severe hallucinations
7 continuous hallucinations

HEADACHE, FULLNESS IN HEAD: Ask: "Does your head feel different? Does it feel like there is a band around your head?" Do not rate for dizziness or lightheadedness. Otherwise, rate severity.
0 not present
1 very mild
2 mild

(continued)

Box 9.6 CIWA-Ar (*contiuned*)

---

3 moderate
4 moderately severe
5 severe
6 very severe
7 extremely severe

TREMOR: Arms extended and fingers spread apart. Observation.
0 no tremor
1 not visible, but can be felt fingertip to fingertip
4 moderate, with patient's arms extended
7 severe, even with arms not extended

PAROXYSMAL SWEATS: Observation.
0 no sweat visible
1 barely perceptible sweating, palms moist
4 beads of sweat obvious on forehead
7 drenching sweats

ANXIETY: Ask: "Do you feel nervous?" Observation.
0 no anxiety, at ease
1 mildly anxious
4 moderately anxious, or guarded, so anxiety is inferred
7 equivalent to acute panic states as seen in severe delirium or acute schizophrenic reactions

AGITATION: Observation.
0 normal activity
1 somewhat more than normal activity
4 moderately fidgety and restless
7 paces back and forth during most of the interview or constantly thrashes about

ORIENTATION AND CLOUDING OF SENSORIUM: Ask: "What day is this? Where are you? Who am I?"
0 oriented and can do serial additions
1 cannot do serial additions or is uncertain about date
2 disoriented for date by no more than 2 calendar days
3 disoriented for date by more than 2 calendar days
4 disoriented for place/or person

Total **CIWA-Ar** Score _____ Rater's initials _____ Maximum possible score 67
The **CIWA-Ar** is *not* copyrighted and may be reproduced freely. This assessment for monitoring withdrawal symptoms requires approximately 5 minutes to administer. The maximum score is 67 (see instrument). Patients scoring less than 10 do not usually need additional medication for withdrawal.

MEDICAL MANAGEMENT

▪ *What is the drug of choice for preventing and/or treating AWS?*
▪ Benzodiazepines

The mechanism of action for benzodiazepines is to enhance depression of neurotransmitter GABA, which replaces the effect of alcohol. Lorazepam or diazepam may be used to reduce the risk of AWS. Neuroleptics have also been used to manage AWS but may not be as effective as benzodiazepines. They do not treat the autonomic effects of AWS. Pregabalin or tiapride are nonbenzodiazepine drugs that may be used in AWS. They prevent the hypersecretion of excitatory neurotransmitters found in AWS.

> **HINT**

Lorazepam has a shorter half-life than diazepam, which may help prevent oversedation.

- **■** *The administration of thiamine to patients with a history of alcohol use is done to prevent which syndrome?*
- **■** **Wernicke–Korsakoff's syndrome**

Wernicke's encephalopathy (WE) and Korsakoff's syndrome are a result of thiamine deficiency. Administration of intravenous (IV) thiamine is used routinely to prevent Wernicke–Korsakoff's syndrome. Multivitamins are frequently added in the management of patients with a history of alcohol use (Box 9.7).

Box 9.7 Causes of Thiamine Deficiency in Alcohol Use

Dietary deficiency	Increased excretion
Reduced absorption	Interrupts metabolism of thiamine

- **■** *A patient with AWS develops tetany and positive Chvostek's sign. What common electrolyte abnormality seen with alcohol use may present with these symptoms?*
- **■** **Hypomagnesium**

Hypomagnesium is a common electrolyte abnormality of patients with alcohol use and AWS. Symptoms of low magnesium include tetany and positive Chvostek's sign. Other electrolyte abnormalities that need to monitored and corrected include hyponatremia, hypokalemia, and hypophosphatemia.

- **■** *What are the two problems that occur with managing pain in a substance abuse patient?*
- **■** **Give too little or too much**

There are *two major errors* that occur in the hospital when managing pain in patients with a history of drug and/or alcohol addiction. The errors can be at both extremes of the spectrum. The patient's reported pain is not believed by the health care providers and the request for pain medication is denied. Or the patient is treated as a nonaddictive patient and opioid intake is allowed to escalate beyond reasonable estimates to control the pain (Box 9.8).

Box 9.8 Hints for Managing Pain in Substance Abusers

Avoid excessive negotiation but allow some decisions to be made by the patient
Be prepared to administer higher doses (development tolerance)
Give nonopioids in combination with opioids
Accept patient's reported pain and treat following appropriate assessments
Do not try to treat the addiction while the patient is in pain
Substance abusers may have a low tolerance for pain
Do not administer an agonist antagonist opioid (sudden reversal of opioids)
Monitor for symptoms of withdrawal
Avoid detoxification during treatment of acute pain

> ❯ HINT
> When opioids are no longer required, taper slowly to minimize the emergence of withdrawal symptoms.

COMPLICATIONS

■ *What is the primary symptom of the complication of Korsakoff's syndrome?*
■ **Amnesia**

Without treatment of thiamine, 75% of WE patients develop permanent severe amnestic syndrome (Korsakoff's syndrome; Boxes 9.9 and 9.10).

Box 9.9 Symptoms of Korsakoff's Syndrome

Retrograde amnesia
Anterograde amnesia (inability to assimilate new information)
Decreased spontaneity
Decreased initiative
Confabulation (filling in memory gaps with distorted facts)

Box 9.10 Symptoms of Wernicke's Encephalopathy

Delirium	Ophthalmoplegia (paralysis of eye muscles)
Nystagmus	Memory abnormalities
Ataxia	

Source: With permission from Gelinas, et al. (2006). Validity of the Critical Care Pain Observation Tool in adults: *American Journal of Critical Care, 15*: 420–429.

■ *What is a common high-risk complication of AWS?*
■ **Seizures**

Patients who are at high risk for AWS-induced seizures include those with a prior history of withdrawal seizures, high alcohol consumption, and multiple previous detoxifications. Many alcohol-dependent patients have causes other than alcohol withdrawal that contribute to or cause seizures. An electroencephalogram (EEG) can differentiate between AWS seizures and epilepsy. The EEG of AWS patients demonstrates normal low-amplitude waves, whereas EEGs of patients with epilepsy shows generalized spike and wave points.

■ *What is the complication of AWS that has exacerbation of autonomic symptoms?*
■ **DTs**

DTs is one of the most serious manifestations of AWS. It is characterized by fluctuating disturbances of consciousness and change in cognition occurring over a short period of time. Symptoms are due to exacerbation of autonomic system and can result in death (Box 9.11).

Box 9.11 Symptoms of DTs

Sweating	Hypertension
Nausea	Tachycardia
Palpitations	Hyperthermia
Tremor	Tachypnea

PAIN, AGITATION, AND DELIRIUM

■ *What type of pain is typically undertreated in critically ill patients?*

■ **Procedural pain**

Procedures are frequently performed in the ICU and result in periods of intense pain. Frequently analgesia is present for maintenance in ICU following a trauma, surgery, or burns, but treatment of intermittent pain due to procedures is not consistent and is ineffective. Removal of chest tubes is an example of a painful procedure commonly not adequately managed.

> **HINT**
> Preemptive analgesia should be administered before the procedure to alleviate pain.

■ *What is the primary goal in managing agitation and delirium?*

■ **Control at the lightest level of sedation**

Maintaining light levels of sedation is associated with improvements in clinical outcomes of ICU patients. These improvements include shorter ICU stays, shorter overall hospital days, lower ventilator days, and fewer complications from mechanical ventilation. Sedation is titrated with the goal of light sedation instead of deep, unless clinically contraindicated.

> **HINT**
> Lighter levels of sedation (as well as unrelieved pain) may increase signs of stress response (i.e., tachycardia and hypertension) and should be monitored closely.

■ *What is an acute change in neurological function with alterations of mental status with disorganized thinking?*

■ **Delirium**

Delirium is a syndrome characterized by an acute onset of cerebral dysfunction with a change of fluctuation in baseline mental status, inattention, and either disorganized thinking or an altered level of consciousness (LOC). The cardinal signs of delirium are a disturbed LOC and a change in cognition. Presence of delirium is an independent predictor of poor outcome (Box 9.12).

Box 9.12 Cardinal Signs of Delirium

Disturbed level of consciousness (LOC)	Decreased awareness of environment Reduced ability to sustain focus or attention
Change in cognition	Memory deficit Disorientation Language disturbances Hallucinations or delusions

> **HINT**
> A misconception of delirium is that it requires hallucinations or delusions. Delirium can be present without these symptoms. Hyperactive delirium is more often associated with hallucinations and delusions.

■ *Which medications are commonly associated with delirium?*
■ **Sedatives**

Administration of sedatives and opioids to ICU patients contributes to the development of delirium. Disease states such as sepsis may induce delirium (Box 9.13).

Box 9.13 Factors Contributing to Delirium

Sedatives	Immobilization
Opioids	Sensory overload
Physical restraints	Certain medications
Sleep deprivation	Drug or alcohol withdrawal
Disease states (i.e., sepsis, multiple organ dysfunction syndrome)	Mechanical ventilation

■ *What medical history may increase the risk of developing delirium in the ICU?*
■ **Dementia**

There are four known risk factors and many other suspected risks for the development of delirium in the ICU (Box 9.14). Pre-existing dementia is the medical history known to be a significant risk factor for the development of delirium.

> **HINT**
> Delirium that occurs in a dementia patient is frequently called "sundowner's syndrome." Age (older patients) is a known risk factor in non-ICU patients and probably is a contributing risk in ICU delirium.

Box 9.14 Known Risk Factors for Delirium

Dementia	History of alcoholism
History of hypertension	High severity of illness on admission to the ICU

SYMPTOMS/ASSESSMENT

■ *When should pain assessment be performed on an ICU patient?*
■ **Routinely, on all ICU patients**

Pain assessment should be routinely performed on a regular basis. It is considered to be the fifth vital sign and should be performed as frequently as obtaining vital signs (as frequently as hourly in an ICU patient). Good management of pain is dependent on the assessment for pain on a frequent basis. Patients in the ICU can experience pain even at rest. Pain levels increase with movement, coughing, and procedures. Pain is frequently remembered after discharge from the ICU and contributes to posttraumatic stress disorder (PTSD).

> **❯ HINT**
> Women have greater pain following a cardiac surgery as compared to men.

■ *A patient who is restless and agitated in the ICU may have what complication?*
■ **Delirium**

Delirium is defined as a temporary state of mental confusion, whereas psychosis is a severe mental disorder characterized by loss of contact with reality. Delirium is characterized by restlessness and agitation (Box 9.15).

Box 9.15 Symptoms of Delirium

Short attention span	Sleep disturbances
Restlessness and agitation	Abnormal psychomotor activity
Persecutory delusions	Emotional disturbances (fear, anxiety, anger, depression, apathy)
Vivid hallucinations	

> **❯ HINT**
> Patients with delirium may be agitated, calm, or lethargic (Box 9.16).

Box 9.16 Signs of Agitation

Exhibits continual movement	Pulling out lines and tubes
Fidgeting	Disorientation
Moving from side to side	Does not follow simple commands

DIAGNOSIS

■ *What are two pain assessment tools used in the ICU to determine pain in nonverbal patients?*
■ **Behavioral Pain Scale (BPS) and Critical Care Pain Observation Tool (CPOT)**

BPS and CPOT are two tools commonly used in the ICU to assess for the presence of pain in nonverbal patients who are unable to self-report pain but who are capable of motor activity. BPS and CPOT have been found to be the most valid behavioral assessment scales (Boxes 9.17 and 9.18). Reliable assessment of pain is the basis of pain management. Although self-report is preferred over observation, patients on mechanical ventilation, those with decreased LOC, and/or sedation may not have the ability to self-report pain. The least reliable assessment of pain is change in vital signs and should not be used to determine pain levels. Vital sign changes can be a red flag to perform a pain assessment.

> HINT

Behavioral assessment tools may not be as reliable in brain-injured patients.

Box 9.17 BPS

Facial expression	Relaxed	1
	Partially tightened	2
	Fully tightened	3
	Grimacing	4
Upper limbs	No movement	1
	Partially bent	2
	Fully bent with finger flexion	3
	Permanently retracted	4
Compliance with ventilation	Tolerating movement	1
	Coughing but tolerating ventilation most of the time	2
	Fighting ventilator	3
	Unable to control ventilation	4

Source: With permission from Gelinas, et al. (2006). Validity of the Critical Care Pain Observation Tool in adults: *American Journal of Critical Care, 15*: 420–429.

Box 9.18 CPOT

Indicator	Description	Score	
Facial expression	No muscular tension observed	Relaxed, neutral	0
	Presence of frowning, brow lowering, orbit tightening, and levator contraction	Tense	1
		Grimacing	2
	All of the above facial movements plus eyelids tightly closed		
Body movements	Does not move at all (does not necessarily mean absence of pain)	Absence of movement	0
		Protection	1
	Slow, cautious movement, touching or rubbing the pain site, seeking attention though movements	Restlessness	2
	Pulling tubes, attempting to sit up, moving limbs/thrashing, not following commands, striking at staff, trying to climb out of bed		
Muscle tension (evaluation by passive flexion and extension of upper extremities)	No resistance to passive movement	Relaxed	0
	Resistance to passive movements	Tense, rigid	1
	Strong resistance to passive movement, inability to complete them	Very tense or rigid	2
Compliance with ventilator (intubated patients) *or* vocalization (extubated patients)	Alarms not activated, easy ventilation	Tolerating ventilator or movement	0
	Alarms stop spontaneously		1
	Asynchrony, blocking ventilation, alarms frequently activated	Coughing but tolerating ventilator	2
			1
	Talking in normal tone or no sound	Fighting with ventilator	2
	Sighing, moaning	Talking in normal tone or no sound	0
	Crying out, sobbing		
		Sighing, moaning	1
		Crying out, sobbing	2
Total range		0–8	

■ *What is the Ramsey Scale used for in the ICU?*
■ **Determine sedation levels**

There are several tools used in the ICU to determine sedation levels. Sedation scales can be used to titrate the level of sedation, maintaining a lighter sedation except in certain situations that require deeper sedation. The Ramsey Scale is one of the sedation assessment tools used in the ICU (Box 9.19).

> **❯ HINT**
> These sedation scales are not accurate in comatose patients or patients receiving neuromuscular blocking agents. The Richmond Agitation Sedation Scale (RASS) and Sedation Agitation Scale (SAS) are two of the more valid and reliable assessment tools with high inter-rater reliability (Boxes 9.20 and 9.21).

Box 9.19 Sedation Scales

Ramsey Scale	New Sheffield Sedation Score
Motor Activity Assessment Scale (MASS)	Adaption to the Intensive Care Environment (ATICE)
SAS	Minnesota Sedation Assessment Tool
RASS	Vancouver Interaction and Calmness Scale (VICS)
Sedation Intensive Care Score (SEDICS)	

Box 9.20 RASS

Score	Term	Description
+4	Combative	Overtly combative, violent, immediate danger to staff
+3	Agitated	Pulls or removes tube(s) or catheter(s); aggressive
+2	Very agitated	Frequent nonpurposeful movement, fights ventilator
+1	Restless	Anxious, but movements not aggressive or vigorous
0	Alert and calm	
−1	Drowsy	Not fully alert but has sustained awakening (eye-opening/eye contact) to voice (>10 sec)
−2	Light sedation	Briefly awakens with eye contact to voice (< 10 sec)
−3	Moderate sedation	Movement or eye opening to voice (but no eye contact)
−4	Deep sedation	No response to voice, but movement or eye opening to physical stimulation
−5	Unarousable	No response to voice or physical stimulation

Box 9.21 SAS

Score	Term	Descriptor
7	Dangerous agitation	Pulling at endotracheal tube (ETT), trying to remove catheters, climbing over bedrail, striking at staff, thrashing side to side
6	Very agitated	Requiring restraint and frequent verbal reminding of limits, biting ETT
5	Agitated	Anxious or physically agitated, calms to verbal instructions
4	Calm and cooperative	Calm, easily arousable, follows commands
3	Sedated	Difficult to arouse but awakens to verbal stimuli or gentle shaking, follows simple commands but drifts off again
2	Very sedated	Arouses to physical stimuli but does not communicate or follow commands, may move spontaneously
1	Unarousable	Minimal or no response to noxious stimuli, does not communicate or follow commands

■ *What objective measurement of brain function is used to measure depth of sedation in patients receiving neuromuscular blocking agents?*

■ **Bispectral Index (BIS) monitor**

The BIS monitor is available for monitoring brain function and can be used as an objective measurement of sedation levels. It is more commonly used on mechanically ventilated patients on neuromuscular blocking agents. Once paralyzed for therapeutic purposes, the nurse is unable to use assessment scales for sedation. Other objective measures of brain function include auditory evoked potentials or Narcotrend Index.

> ❯ HINT
>
> The subjective sedation scores are recommended in patients not receiving a neuromuscular blocking agent.

■ *What tool is available for monitoring delirium in the ICU?*

■ **Confusion Assessment Method for ICU (CAM-ICU)**

CAM-ICU is a valid and reliable tool used in the ICU to monitor for delirium. It is recommended that all patients in the ICU be monitored routinely for delirium.

MANAGEMENT

■ *Which opioid analgesic has a complication of neurotoxicity?*

■ **Meperidine**

Meperidine administration can result in the accumulation of the neurotoxic metabolite normeperidine. Neurotoxic findings include tremors, shakiness, myoclonus, and seizures. Meperidine is not frequently used for pain management in the ICU because of neurotoxicity. IV opioids are recommended as first-line drugs to manage pain in the ICU. Nonopioids can be used to supplement and lower the dose of the opioid (Box 9.22).

> ❯ HINT
>
> Combining a nonopioid with an opioid can decrease the side effects of the opioid. When treating neuropathic pain, administer either an anticonvulsant (gabapentin) or an antidepressant (carbamazepine).

Box 9.22 Common Analgesics Used in the ICU

Morphine	Remifentanil
Fentanyl	Ketorolac
Hydromorphone	Intravenous (IV) acetaminophen
Methadone	Local and regional anesthetics

■ *What is the recommended mode of delivery for analgesics following abdominal aortic aneurysm repair?*
■ **Thoracic epidural**

Abdominal aortic surgeries have shown excellent pain management with a thoracic epidural catheter being placed prior to surgery. This route is superior to IV opioids with fewer complications in certain patient populations. Thoracic epidural pain management may also benefit patients with multiple rib fracture. This allows the patient to breathe deeply and cough without pain, which lowers the incidence of developing pneumonia.

■ *What is the purpose of daily "wake up" on patients receiving sedation?*
■ **Maintain lighter level of sedation**

Daily "wake up" ensures the patient is at a lighter level of sedation. Protocols are used in most hospitals to interrupt sedation daily until the patient awakens, and then resedate. The interruption has not been found to cause significant physiological stress and may decrease length of stay (LOS) in the ICU and mechanical ventilator days. Deep sedation is one reason for delayed emergence from sedation. Other causes include prolonged infusion, older age, hepatic dysfunction, or renal failure.

> **❯ HINT**
> This technique is frequently called "sedation vacation."

■ *Which of the sedatives frequently used in the ICU is recommended in patients requiring intermittent awakenings?*
■ **Propofol**

Propofol is a nonbenzodiazepine frequently used to provide sedation in mechanically ventilated patients. It has a very quick onset and short half-life so patients will wake up faster once the propofol infusion has been stopped. Benzodiazepines may also be used for sedation in the ICU but may have a longer half-life (Box 9.23).

> **❯ HINT**
> Propofol is commonly used in neurological patients requiring frequent neurological assessments due to its shorter emergence. However, propofol's duration of clinical effect is much shorter because propofol is rapidly distributed into the peripheral tissues.

Box 9.23 Agents Used for Sedation in the ICU

Agent	Onset (IV Route; min)	Half-Life (hr)
Lorazepam	15–20	8–15
Diazepam	2–5	20–120
Midazolam	2–5	3–11
Propofol	1–2	2–24
Dexmedetomidine	5–10	2–3

■ *Which sedative does not have respiratory depression and can be used on a nonintubated patient?*

■ **Dexmedetomidine**

Dexmedetomidine is a selective α-receptor agonist. It is different from other sedatives because it has been found to have analgesic effects and may lower the dose of the opioid. It does not affect the respiratory system and so may be given to nonventilated patients. It is the only sedative approved by the Food and Drug Administration (FDA) in nonintubated ICU patients. Propofol is not recommended for nonventilated patients. Benzodiazepines and propofol have sedating, hypnotic, amnesic, and anxiolytic effects without analgesic effects. Their primary side effects include hypotension and respiratory depression. Dexmedetomidine's side effects include hypotension and bradycardia.

> **HINT**
> Patients sedated with dexmedetomidine wake up with minimal stimulation and are more interactive.

■ *What nonpharmacological intervention may lower the number of ICU days and decrease the incidence of delirium?*

■ **Early mobilization**

Early and aggressive mobilization of ICU patients reduces the depth of sedation, decreases length of hospital stay and ICU days. Mobilization and ambulation of patients on mechanical ventilation have been found to lower the number of mechanical ventilation days. Pharmacological management has included haloperidol but there is no study confirming that haloperidol reduces delirium in ICU patients. Use of dexmedetomidine for sedation in mechanically ventilated patients may lower the incidence of delirium when compared to benzodiazepines (Box 9.24).

> **HINT**
> A complication of haloperidol is prolonged QT interval with increased incidence of Torsades de pointes.

Box 9.24 Interventions to Promote Sleep in the ICU

Control lighting at night
Cluster patient activities (allow periods of undisturbed sleep)
Decrease stimuli at night

COMPLICATIONS

■ *What physiological occurrence leads to the majority of the complications of unrelieved pain?*

■ **Stress response**

Unrelieved pain results in the activation of the stress response and the sympathetic nervous system. This produces tachycardia, vasoconstriction, and reduced arterial and tissue oxygenation (Box 9.25).

Box 9.25 Complications of Unrelieved Pain in the ICU

Stress response	Immunosuppression
Hypermetabolic catabolism	Chronic neuropathy pain
Impaired wound healing	Posttraumatic stress disorder
Increased risk of wound infections	Myocardial ischemia

■ *Which patient population is more likely to be sensitive to benzodiazepines?*
■ **Elderly**

Elderly patients are more sensitive to the sedating effects of benzodiazepines and can have adverse reactions, including agitation and delirium. The patient may have a different reaction to a different benzodiazepine.

■ *What food allergies would indicate that a patient is at risk for an allergic reaction to propofol?*
■ **Egg or soybean**

Propofol is dissolved in a 10% lipid emulsion that contains egg lecithin and soybean oil. This can precipitate allergic reactions if a person has an allergy to either eggs or soybeans. Other potential complications of propofol that are due to the lipid emulsion are hypertriglyceridemia and acute pancreatitis.

> ❯ **HINT**
> Propofol infusion syndrome (PRIS) is a rare but life-threatening condition (Box 9.26). Complications of PRIS include acute kidney injury, rhabdomyolysis, and liver dysfunction.

Box 9.26 Symptoms of PRIS

Worsening metabolic acidosis	Arrhythmias
Hypotension despite vasopressors	Hyperkalemia
Hypertriglyceridemia	

■ *What is a potential complication of agitation in an intubated patient?*
■ **Self-extubation**

Agitation can cause harmful effects on the patient and, potentially, health care providers (Box 9.27).

Box 9.27 Complications of Agitation

Self-extubation	Injury to self
Increased oxygen consumption	Injury to health care providers
Hemodynamic instability	Unable to participate in care

DEMENTIA

■ *What is the most common type of dementia?*
■ **Alzheimer's disease (AD)**

AD is the most common type of dementia. AD is subdivided into dementia with early onset (< 65 years of age) and with late onset (> 65 years of age). Vascular dementia is the second most common form of dementia and is the result of a stroke. There are multiple other types and causes of dementia (Box 9.28).

Box 9.28 Types and Causes of Dementia

Alzheimer's disease	Huntington's disease
Vascular dementia	Normal pressure hydrocephalus
Frontotemporal dementia	Wernicke–Korsakoff syndrome
Parkinson's disease	HIV/AIDS dementia
Creutzfeldt–Jacob disease	Alcohol-induced dementia

■ *What are the two known risk factors for AD?*
■ **Age and genetics**

There is not a single risk factor but it is likely that there are multiple factors that result in AD. The two known risk factors for AD are age and genetic predisposition. The risk of AD doubles every 10 years after the age of 65.

PATHOPHYSIOLOGY

■ *Is AD a cortical or a subcortical dementia?*
■ **Cortical**

Cortical dementia is characterized by loss of neurons and synapses in the cerebral cortex and certain subcortical regions resulting in gross atrophy. It typically involves degeneration of temporal and parietal lobes. AD involves cortical dysfunction involving memory (Box 9.29).

Box 9.29 Contrasting Characteristics of Cortical and Subcortical Dementia Syndromes

	Subcortical Dementia	Cortical Dementia
Language	No aphasia	Aphasia early
Memory	Recall impaired; recognition normal or better preserved	Recall and recognition impaired
Visiospatial skills	Impaired	Impaired
Calculation	Preserved until late	Involved early
Speed of cognitive processing	Slowed early	Normal until late in disease course
Personality	Apathetic	Unconcerned

(continued)

Box 9.29 Contrasting Characteristics of Cortical and Subcortical Dementia Syndromes (*continued*)

	Subcortical Dementia	Cortical Dementia
Mood	Depressed	Euthymic
Speech	Dysarthric	Normal articulation until late in disease course
Posture	Bowed	Upright
Coordination	Impaired	Normal until late in disease course
Adventitious movements	Present: chorea, tremor, tics, dystonia	Absent
Motor speed	Slowed	Normal

■ *What two areas of the brain play a critical role in memory?*

■ **Hippocampus and amygdala**

The hippocampus is located in the deep portion of the brain above the brainstem. It is responsible for acquiring and temporarily storing memory. Declarative memory is stored in the hippocampus. The amygdala is located under the temporal lobe and receives input from the sensory system. These structures are a part of the limbic system.

> **〉 HINT**
> Information must be stored temporarily (short term) for it to become a long-term memory.

■ *What type of memory is used when performing a familiar task without actually having to think about it?*

■ **Declarative memory**

There are several different types of memory. Declarative memory is being able to perform a task or activity without having to think about it or think about the steps. An example is driving to and from work every day (Box 9.30).

Box 9.30 Types of Long-Term Memory

Semantic memory	Involves the conscious involvement of the learner	Example, skill in using a telephone book
Implicit memory	Information learned without the conscious involvement of the person Memories established through early and frequent repetitions	Example, singing the *Happy Birthday* song
Motor memory	Memory of tasks involving motor skills	Example, riding a bike
Affective memory	Memory that is triggered by feelings or emotions	Example, memories brought back through the sense of smell

> **〉 HINT**
> Memory and learning are not two different processes, and memory is required for learning to occur.

■ *What are the two pathophysiologic changes in the brain that are characteristic of AD?*

■ **Amyloid plaque and neurofibrillary tangles**

The pathological changes that occur in AD are caused by the production of amyloid plaque and neurofibrillary tangles in the brain. Plaques are dense, insoluble deposits of β-amyloid peptide. Neurofibrillary tangles are aggregates of twisted protein thread found inside the nerve cells. These protein threads consist of a main component called "tau."

SYMPTOMS/ASSESSMENT

■ *What are the two primary symptoms of AD?*

■ **Memory loss and cognitive decline**

The symptoms seen in AD are the result of the death of many neurons in the hippocampus and cerebral cortex. This results in memory loss, impaired cognition, and behavioral changes. Memory is required for cognitive capabilities. Memory deficits are the early signs of the onset of AD and progress with the disease process. AD affects semantic memory first. Motor memory is eventually affected, with the person feeling frustration over not being able to do even simple tasks. He or she may lose both fine and gross motor skills.

> ❯ HINT
> Affective memory may remain intact as long as the person can communicate.

■ *At what stage of AD does the patient begin to pace and wander?*

■ **Stage II**

There are four stages of AD. Each stage demonstrates a progressive loss, including mental, physical, or emotional changes. The onset may be insidious and can frequently be frustrating for the person in the early stages. Stage I may not be recognized as an onset of dementia. After the diagnosis, the family may look back and identify these symptoms retrospectively. Memory loss (recent memories) is the first symptom (Box 9.31).

Box 9.31 Stages of AD

Stage I	Short-term memory losses (long-term memory remains intact) Loss of spontaneity (less joy or enthusiasm) Sporadic loss of words (loss of words or substitution of inappropriate words) Easy to anger (may be physical as well as verbal) Less discrimination with choices (messy or unkempt, not as meticulous with clothing)
Stage II	Disorientation to time and place (may be the first alarm for family members) Impaired communication (unable to express thought) Difficulty in making decisions or plans (takes longer to make minor decisions) Loss of impulse control (may act on all thoughts regardless of consequences) Mistakes in judgment (social situations or money management) Decreased concentration (difficulty to finish a task or activity) Increased self-absorption Avoidance of new situations

(continued)

Box 9.31 Stages of AD *(continued)*

	Delusions (may be based on a reality in past history)
	Rummaging and pillaging (may hoard or stock items excessively or may pick items up that do not belong to him or her and put them somewhere)
	Wandering and pacing (wanders aimlessly for hours without fatigue; pacing is accompanied by signs of anxiety, tension, and strain)
Stage III	Sundowning (sleep disrupted with wandering in the middle of the night)
	Catastrophic reactions (to various events and can result in verbalization, pacing, and physical reaction)
	Failure to recognize family and friends
	Hyperorality (unexplained movements of mouth and tongue)
	Preservation (continual activity after the stimulus is removed; i.e., continue to chew even though the food is ready to swallow)
	Latency (inability to begin an activity)
	Agnosia (inability to recognize commonly used tools; i.e., toothbrush)
	Apraxia (inability to perform a task with an item; i.e., unable to brush teeth with a toothbrush)
Stage IV	Unable to communicate in a meaningful way
	No recognition of self or others
	Total dependence

DIAGNOSIS

■ *What is the primary test used to diagnose memory losses and dementia?*
■ **Mini-Mental State Examination (MMSE)**

MMSE is a neurophysiologic test used to determine the onset or presence of dementia. It involves copying drawings, remembering words, reading, and subtracting serial numbers.

■ *What is the definitive diagnosis of AD?*
■ **Autopsy**

Definitive diagnosis is on autopsy only. Autopsy reveals plaque formation and neurofibrillary tangles to confirm the diagnosis. A probable diagnosis is made based on history and physical examination, diagnostic tests, cognitive testing, and mental status evaluation.

MANAGEMENT

■ *What is the primary pharmacological management for AD?*
■ **Cholinesterase inhibitors**

Cholinesterase is an enzyme that breaks down acetylcholine (ACh) after it crosses the synapse. The drug suppresses this enzyme so that acetylcholine is not broken down as rapidly thereby increasing the concentration of ACh. This may temporarily slow the rate of decline in memory and thinking ability in early stages (mild to moderate). Examples include donepezil hydrochloride (Aricept), galantamine (Razadyne), rivastigmine (Exelon), and Exelon patch. The other drugs approved to treat AD are NMDA receptor antagonists. NMDA receptors are for glutamate, which is an excitatory neurotransmitter. Excessive amounts of glutamate can lead to cell death (excitotoxicity). An example includes memantine (Akatinol).

> **HINT**
> A common side effect of cholinesterase inhibitors is nausea and vomiting (cholinergic excess).

COMPLICATIONS

■ *What is a common complication of a dementia patient that occurs in the evening and can increase the likelihood of falls in hospital?*

■ **Sundowning**

Sundowning is a type of agitation that occurs with older patients and patients with dementia. In the evenings or during the night they become more disoriented and agitated. This agitation can frequently contribute to patient falls in the hospital.

> **HINT**
> Turning on lights well before sunset and closing the curtains at dusk will minimize shadows and may help diminish confusion that occurs with sundowning.

SUICIDAL BEHAVIOR

■ *Which patient population should receive a screening for depression or suicidal thoughts?*

■ **All patients**

The Joint Commission (TJC) has urged hospital and health care providers to watch for attempted suicides in patients with no history of psychiatric problems or history of previous attempts. The alert stresses that it is not just psychiatric patients who kill themselves, citing as an example someone recently diagnosed with cancer going into the emergency room (ER) because the cancer-related pain has become unbearable and commits suicide in the ER. Almost 25% of suicides within the hospital occur in nonpsychiatric settings, such as ERs, oncology units, ICU, and long-term care hospitals. Screen all patients for depression and suicidal thoughts when they are admitted to a hospital or into the ICU.

> **HINT**
> The methods most often used were hanging, suffocation, intentional drug overdose, and strangulation.

PATHOPHYSIOLOGY

■ *What is the most common underlying belief of a person who attempts or commits suicide?*

■ **Hopelessness**

Suicide occurs in response to feelings of hopelessness. Feelings of hopelessness result from the belief that suffering will never stop and, as a result, nothing positive will ever come of the future. Death is viewed as an option to end the suffering and prevent a future without hope.

■ **What increases the likelihood of suicidal thoughts in patients with medical illnesses?**

■ **Pain**

Patients diagnosed with cancer or those who are in intense, intractable pain may feel worn out and hopeless. There is a need for routine evaluation and monitoring of suicidal behavior in both severe acute and chronic pain. Medical illness raises the risk for suicide because the presence of an illness or injury, especially associated with persistent pain, strains coping abilities. It increases the likelihood the patient will attribute the failures to cope with as personal inadequacy. There is an uncertainty about the future and worry that the medical condition will cause further loss and deterioration of the self.

> ⟩ **HINT**
> The presence of an illness, injury, or pain often leads to feelings of depression, especially in individuals sensitive to loss of control (Box 9.32). Thirty to forty percent of people who commit suicide have made a previous attempt.

Box 9.32 Increased Risks for Suicidal Behavior

Family history of suicide	Substance abuser
Previous suicide attempt	History of psychiatric problems
Prescription of potentially lethal medications	Suicidal ideation
Diagnosis of cancer or chronic illness	Suicidal behavior
Physical health problems	PTSD
Traumatic brain injury	Delirium or dementia
Severe pain (chronic or acute)	Social stressors: financial strain, unemployment
Poor prognosis or prospect of certain death	Disability

SYMPTOMS/ASSESSMENT

■ **A patient in the ICU is recovering from surgery. The patient states his family would "be better off without him." What is this statement?**

■ **Verbal suicide threat**

Verbal suicide threats need to be recognized. When performing suicide risk assessment, start with questions that assess the person's feelings about life. Then ask specific questions about death, self-harm, and suicide. Examples of verbal suicide threats include: "Life is not worth living," "I wish I would go to sleep and not wake up."

> ⟩ **HINT**
> The nurse should take seriously all statements made by a patient that indicate, either directly or indirectly, the desire to die.

■ *A patient in an acute care hospital may have different warning signs than a patient in a psychiatric hospital. What is an important assessment that should be ongoing with all ICU patients?*

■ **Watch for warning signs**

Frequently, patients who commit suicide or self-harm in an acute care environment, like an ICU, may not have significant risk factors but typically will have demonstrated warning signs. In critically ill or injured patients, coping skills that normally have been functional may not be effective. The threat is perceived as being overwhelming and feelings of hopelessness and depression become more common. Most in-hospital suicides are impulsive, without apparent planning. At least once a shift, ask about suicidal intent in patients with warning signs (Box 9.33).

> **❯ HINT**
> Suicide assessment by the ICU nurses should become a part of the daily assessment (Boxes 9.34–9.35).

Box 9.33 Warning Signs

Irritability	Anxiety
Verbal suicide threat	Impulsiveness
Agitation	Global insomnia
Complaints of unrelenting pain	Lack of interest in future plans or current treatment
Refusing visitors or medications	
Refusing to eat	Excessive fear and worries
Acute signs of depression	Delusions or hallucinations
Expressing feelings of hopelessness and helplessness	Requesting early discharge

Box 9.34 Questions Regarding Suicidal Thoughts

In the past 2 weeks, have you had thoughts you would be better off dead?
In the past 2 weeks, have you had thoughts of hurting yourself in any way?
Have you made a suicide attempt in the past?
Do you have a current plan?
When you have thought of hurting yourself, what would you do?
How often have those thoughts occurred?

Box 9.35 Use of Mnemonic "In Sad Cases" in Depression Signs

IN	Interest (life not worth living)	C	Concentration
S	Sleep	A	Agitation/slowed
A	Appetite	S	Stricken with guilt
D	Depressed	E	Energy
		S	Suicide (thinks, plans, has means)

MANAGEMENT

■ *If a patient mentions feeling hopeless, what would be the best response?*

■ **Talk openly**

Talk openly about depression, death, and suicide with patients. Communications needs to include listening to the patient. Ask direct questions without being judgmental. Determine whether the patient has a plan to carry out the suicide. Do not counsel the patient yourself but get professional help (Box 9.36).

> ❯ HINT
> The more detailed the plan, the greater the risk. Do not leave a person who is talking about suicide alone.

Box 9.36 Interventions to Prevent Suicide

Remove items that could be used for suicide
  Sharp objects
  Cleaning solvents
Place patient on 1:1 observation
Initiate elopement precautions
	Referral to mental health professional for
	  further assessment
	Follow up appropriately at the time of
	  discharge

■ **What is a common method for attempting suicide in an acute care hospital environment?**

■ **Hanging**

Hanging has been a common method for suicide or self-harm in the acute hospital setting. The availability of means to perform self-harm by hanging is present in ICU and other areas of the hospital. This includes cords, call button cords, sheets, bandages, and IV tubing. Staff training should include knowledge of potential means of suicide in the ICU and how to prevent access to these means (Box 9.37).

> ❯ HINT
> Perform close observation, at least every 15 minutes, in high-risk patients and document the observations. Remove potentially hazardous items from the patient's room and secure patient's belongings.

Box 9.37 Methods of Suicide in the Hospital

Hanging	Drug overdose
Jumping out of windows	Strangulation
Cutting with a sharp object	

MOOD DISORDERS: DEPRESSION

■ **What are periods of profound depression and/or mania that interfere with living called?**

■ **Mood disorders**

Mood disorders include bipolar disease and depression. These are considered pervasive alterations in temperament characterized by profound periods of depression or exaggerated mania or both. These extreme variations of mood interfere with the daily lives of those afflicted with these mood disorders, potentially causing problems with interpersonal relationships and livelihood of those involved.

> HINT
Mood disorders are the most commonly diagnosed psychiatric disorder in which those affected attempt or commit suicide.

■ **How is a major depressive disorder different from feeling "down" for several days?**
■ **More severe**

Major depressive disorders are more severe than feeling "down" for several days, which commonly occurs in most people. It is a severe state of despair and gloom that is a debilitating condition. In major depressive disorder, there is a significant change from the person's normal behavior and functioning for several weeks or more. They typically experience feelings of hopelessness and joylessness with thoughts that life is not worth living. Without treatment, symptoms may recede over time but can reoccur in time.

> HINT
Major depressive disorder is different from chronic, long-term depression, which is called dysthymia.

■ **What are two coexisting disorders that are associated with a high increased risk of depression?**
■ **Medical disorders and psychiatric disorders**

Medical disorders may include any medical diagnosis or severe life-threatening disorders. People with medical disorders are more likely to develop depression than they would if they were in a healthy state. There is a high rate of depression in patients with chronic illnesses, pain, diagnosis with poor prognosis, and end of life. Some degree of depression is actually normal in bereavement but severe feelings of "darkness" and ideation of suicide are considered a major depressive disorder. Psychiatric disorders are also commonly associated with major depression. Depression can lead to an increase in mortality from other diseases such as coronary artery disease and cancer.

> HINT
Elderly living in nursing homes have a high rate of major depression due to loneliness, loss, illness, pain, and facing death as a reality.

PATHOPHYSIOLOGY

■ **What is the theory called in which a person is depressed because this person believes her problems are her own fault and there is nothing she can do to change them?**
■ **Learned helplessness**

Learned helplessness is a theory that considers the reason that people experience depression. The theory proposes that anxiety about situations or problems leads to depression. The patients believe they are at fault for their problems (guilt). According to the theory, they also believe that there is nothing they can do to change their own situation or problems. Other theories that consider major depressive disorders include cognitive and psychoanalytic theories.

> ❯ HINT
> Genetic factors may play a role in the development of depressive disorders but are not completely responsible without other factors involved.

▪ **Are serotonin levels found to be low or high in major depressive disorders?**
▪ **Low**

Serotonin is a neurotransmitter that has many roles in behavior, mood, cognition, and aggressiveness. Major depressive disorders are found to have a deficiency of serotonin and it's precursor, tryptophan. Serotonin, norepinephrine, and dopamine are destroyed by an enzyme called monoamine oxidase (MAO) (Box 9.38). MAO inhibitors are antidepressants that increase serotonin levels by inhibiting the enzyme MAO. Neuroendocrine function has been found to play a role in depressive disorders. Adrenal cortisol secretion is increased during periods of depression.

> ❯ HINT
> Selective serotonin reuptake inhibitors (SSRIs) are antidepressants that increase serotonin levels by inhibiting presynaptic reuptake.

Box 9.38 Neurochemical Involvement in Depression

Neurochemical	Role	Level of Depression
Serotonin	Affects mood, behavior, and cognition	Low
Norepinephrine	Energizes body in stress	Low
Dopamine	Motivation and pleasure center of brain	Low
Acetylcholine	Alters mood, sleep, and neuroendocrine function	High

SYMPTOMS/ASSESSMENT

▪ **What are three key elements that should be included in a brief assessment for depression?**
▪ **Mood, energy, and pleasure**

Mood is an individual's overall current outlook on life. A low mood is gloomy, down-hearted, and sad. Findings of low energy levels include listlessness, and patients frequently state they are tired for no reason. The element of pleasure is assessed by determining the patient's feelings of self-worth and hope. Low pleasure (anhedonia) is found if the patient is feeling hopeless, joyless, helpless, and worthless. Low findings in all three of these key elements indicate a current state of depression, and a more comprehensive assessment is recommended (Box 9.39).

> **HINT**

When obtaining an assessment history, listen to what and how the patient provides the information as well as his body language. Many patients with low self-esteem and depression have poor hygiene on admission to hospital and show signs of self-neglect.

Box 9.39 Components of Comprehensive Assessment of Depression

Personal history of depression, suicide attempts, psychiatric disorders
Family history of depression, suicide, and psychiatric disorders
Obtain more details of current episode of depression
General appearance
Motor activity during interview
Determine affect
Ability to process information
Decision making and problem solving
Self-concept

■ *The psychotic features of a major depressive condition may include false perceptions and false ideas. What are these two conditions called?*

■ **Hallucinations and delusions**

Psychotic features may sometimes occur with major depression. These include experiencing hallucinations, which are false perceptions of reality, and delusions, which are false ideas. Other symptoms that may occur during profound depression include catatonic and melancholic features (Box 9.40).

Box 9.40 Symptoms of Major Depressive Disorder

Catatonic features	Peculiar movements
	Stupor
	Meaningless repetition of words
	Repetition of movements
Melancholic features	Lack of pleasure in anything
	Excessive or inappropriate guilt
	Marked slowness
Common symptoms	Extreme negativism
	Appetite changes
	Weight loss
	Insomnia
	Lack of energy
	Slow mental processing
	Withdrawn and inactive
	Fixed facial expression
	Limited movement
	Minimal eye contact
	Flat affect
	Apathy
	No verbal responses at times
	Poor judgment
	Diminished ability to concentrate

(continued)

Box 9.40 Symptoms of Major Depressive Disorder (*continued*)

Atypical symptoms	Agitation
	Anxiety
	Easily provoked to anger
	Restlessness
	Hyperinsomnia
	Leaden feelings in legs

> **HINT**
> Depression may be greatest in the morning or on awakening (diurinal).

DIAGNOSIS

- **What is a common rating scale used to assess depression?**
- **Beck's Depression Inventory II**

Beck's depression scale is frequently used in the acute care setting to rate the degree of depression. It is a 21-item assessment tool that takes approximately 5 minutes to administer. The Geriatric Depression Scale and the Patient Health Questionnaire are also depression screening tools used in acute care settings.

> **HINT**
> In 2008 the American Heart Association (AHA) recommended screening for depression in all patients with acute coronary syndrome.

MANAGEMENT

- **A patient on a tricyclic antidepressant (TCA) presents with dry mouth, sweating, and blurred vision. What is the most likely cause of these symptoms?**
- **Anticholinergic syndrome**

TCAs produce anticholinergic syndrome as a side effect. TCAs cause a higher incidence than SSRIs. Anticholinergic syndrome includes dry mouth, sweating, blurred vision, weight gain, and sexual dysfunction. TCAs inhibit reuptake norepinephrine and serotonin, allowing for more time at postsynaptic receptor.

> **HINT**
> TCA takes up to 2 to 6 weeks to begin being effective (Box 9.41).

Box 9.41 Common Side Effects of TCAs

Orthostatic hypotension	Weight gain
Sedation	Dry mouth
Tachycardia	Constipation
Headache	Urinary hesitancy
Blurred vision	Sweating
Tremor	

■ *What class of drug is considered to be a first-line agent to treat major depression and has less cardiovascular effects than TCAs?*

■ **SSRIs**

SSRI is recommended to treat major depressive disorders. They have lower cardiotoxicity than TCA and are safer for older patients. SSRIs have a lower rate of anticholinergic symptoms (Box 9.42).

Box 9.42 Common Side Effects of SSRIs

Anxiety	Tremor	Sexual dysfunction
Sedation	Nausea and vomiting	Constipation or diarrhea
Headaches		

■ *Which antidepressant has a potential significant side effect of hypertension?*

■ **MAO inhibitors (MAOIs)**

MAOIs are responsible for inhibiting the enzyme MAO, allowing an increase in serotonin levels. Drugs and foods high in tyramine can interact with the MAOI, causing hypertension and strokes. Foods high in tyramine include smoked or fermented products such as bacon, ham, and most cheeses. Therapeutic drug levels may take up to 4 weeks after initiation of MAOI therapy.

■ *What is the major goal of the nurse when speaking to a depressed patient?*

■ **Affirm patient's worth**

When speaking with a patient experiencing depression, establish a trusting relationship (Box 9.43).

Box 9.43 Interpersonal Skills With a Depressed Patient

Establish a trusting relationship
Convey message of "being" there for the patient
Affirm the patient is valuable
Allow patient time to talk about his or her feelings
Display unconditional positive regard for patient
Empathy

COMPLICATIONS

■ *What is the major complication of severe major depressive disorder?*

■ **Suicide**

Recurrence rates of depression and suicides are high in people with severe major depressive disorder. Suicide precautions should be initiated and the patient must be monitored closely (Box 9.44).

Box 9.44 Other Complications of Major Depression

Compulsive behaviors (eating disorders, gambling, substance abuse)	Malnutrition
	Social isolation
Substance abuse	

AGGRESSIVE BEHAVIORS/VIOLENCE

■ *What acts constitute violence in the workplace?*

■ **Verbal to physical assault**

Violence in the hospital can range from verbal to physical assault. Workplace violence is an act in which a person is abused, intimidated, threatened, or assaulted while working at his or her place of employment. The health care setting leads all other industries in the percentage of nonfatal assaults against workers (Box 9.45).

Box 9.45 Examples of Aggressive Behaviors/Violence in the Workplace

Verbal threats	Sarcastic comments
Shouting or yelling	Belittling gestures
Pushing, hitting, kicking, or physical harm	Aggressive body postures
Cursing and offensive language	Spitting or biting
Slamming doors, throwing objects, or punching walls	

■ *What is an example of a patient who would be considered "inherently" violent?*

■ **Prison inmate**

A prison inmate being cared for in the ICU may have what is called an inherent risk for violence. Other cases may include known psychotic patients. Continual observation for aggression or violence may be indicated in these cases. Other cases of patient or family violence are situational. Something in the situation causes the nonviolent person to become aggressive and even violent. This occurs more frequently in hospital settings (Box 9.46).

> ❯ **HINT**
> Provoking situations include issues that cause frustration such as delays in patient care.

Box 9.46 Types of Violence in the Workplace

Violence by stranger	Violence by coworker
Violence by patient or family member (client)	Violence by someone in a personal relationship

■ *What is a common reason in the ICU that can result in anger and aggressive behaviors?*

■ **Stress**

The ER and ICU are high-dependency areas prone to being very stressful and causing stress to patients and family members. Stress can lead to anxiety, anger, and aggression.

Anxiety can result in frustration and feelings of helplessness. In the ICU, family members often are anxious and exhibit frustration regarding visitation rules, wanting to talk to the doctors, and fear for their loved ones. They often feel powerless about the situation and about loss of their own autonomy. Anger often follows these feelings and may even bring some perceived "power" back to the person.

> ❯ HINT
> Health care providers may experience aggression from clients influenced by drugs, alcohol, stress, or physical trauma.

ASSESSMENT/SYMPTOMS

- ◼ *A family member begins to raise his voice and pound on the table. What are these signs?*
- ◼ **Signs of anger**

There are five warning signs of escalating behaviors leading to violence. These include confusion, frustration, blame, anger, and hostility. Anger is characterized by visible changes in body posture and very risky behaviors that lead to violence (Boxes 9.47 and 9.48).

Box 9.47 Signs of Anger

Argumentative	Cursing
Difficult to please	High-pitched voice
Sarcasm	Acting-out behavior
Pacing and motor agitation	

Box 9.48 Warning Signs of Escalating Behaviors

Confusion	Bewilderment Distracted
Frustration	Impatience Feelings of sense of defeat
Blame	Placing responsibilities on other people Find fault in others' actions Place blame directly on health care providers
Anger	Visible changes in body posture Threatening behaviors
Hostility	Threats of physical action Actual acts of physical harm

MANAGEMENT

- ◼ *What is the best management for aggressive behaviors?*
- ◼ **Prevention**

One of the most important aspects of managing aggressive behaviors is to recognize signs that signal distress and intervene before these aggressive behaviors occur. Most situations of aggressive behavior and violence have warning signs of escalating emotions (such as anger) and may be diffused with appropriate interventions.

> **❯ HINT**
> Learn how to recognize, avoid, or diffuse potentially violent situations
> (Box 9.49). When dealing with angry or hostile patients/family members,
> always be prepared to evacuate or isolate. Do not get cornered in the
> room; remain near the door for faster exit.

Box 9.49 Interventions for Warning Signs

Confusion	Listen to concerns Provide honest answers and accurate information
Frustration	Clarify questions Reassure them
Blame	Obtain consultations of experts Use other health care providers Arrange family conferences Refocus on facts
Anger	Allow venting or expressing feelings Do not argue Do not offer solutions
Hostility	Evacuate to safety Call security

■ *What is a commonly taught technique used as an early intervention in potentially aggressive incidents?*

■ **De-escalating**

Certain behaviors and responses can help de-escalate situations that can escalate to violence. These responses should be routinely practiced in dealing with patients and family members. If at any time the situation appears to escalate beyond the comfort zone, disengage and walk away. Hospital security should be called for assistance in those situations (Box 9.50).

Box 9.50 De-escalating Techniques

Remain calm, speak slowly and clearly
Be confident
Focus on what the person is saying
Listen with empathy
Encourage the person to talk
Acknowledge the person's feelings
Establish ground rules and calmly describe consequences of violent behavior
Break down the problem into smaller, more manageable issues
Ask for his or her recommendations to correct the situation
Do not allow the person to block your exit
Acknowledge concerns and accept criticism
Avoid physical contact and long periods of fixed gazes
Avoid sudden movements that might be interpreted as being threatening
Acknowledge the seriousness of the situation
Maintain space between yourself and the person
Do not bargain with the person
Maintain an open posture
Be vigilant throughout the encounter

■ *If a patient becomes angry at the nurse for having to attempt to start an IV a second time, what is the best reaction of the nurse?*

■ **Validate the patient's anger**

Anger is a human emotion and a rational expression of anger can be appropriate in some situations. Discouraging angry feelings may cause the person discomfort and escalate his or her feelings. Acknowledge the person's angry feelings. Responding with anger back at the patient will only escalate the situation. Understanding anxiety and addressing the underlying cause of anger will decrease the chance of escalating anger (Boxes 9.51 and 9.52).

> ❯ **HINT**
> Nurses need to avoid personalizing the anger, even if directed at them.

Box 9.51 Interventions for Angry Behaviors

Listen to the patient or family member	Attempt mutual problem solving
Do not dismiss the person's concerns	Assist with identifying the source of anger
Recognize anxiety and intervene early	Call in a second staff member when there are
Avoid being defensive	signs of patient getting agitated
Allow the person to express anger	May use the call button to call for assistance
Encourage patients to have more control	

Box 9.52 Actions to Minimize Security Risks

Be aware of your surroundings
Trust your instincts
Remove yourself from uncomfortable situations
Remain close to the door during incidents

COMPLICATIONS

■ *What potential negative effects on the workplace environment occur over time with repeated incidences of dealing with violence?*

■ **Low morale**

Frequent experience with anger and violence in the hospital can lead to low morale among nursing staff, increased stress, and burnout in nurses. Working in a hostile environment leads to staff turnover (Box 9.53).

Box 9.53 Effects of Violence in Hospitals

Minor or major physical injuries	Low morale of nurses
Physical disability	Increased job stress
Psychological trauma	Increased nursing turnover

FAILURE TO THRIVE

■ *What is the greatest concern for a patient with a failure to thrive (FTT) syndrome?*

■ **Nutrition**

FTT syndrome has been described as weight loss by greater than 5%, decrease in appetite, poor nutrition, and dehydration. This is accompanied by inactivity, social withdrawal, loneliness, and depression.

> **〉 HINT**
> The weight loss and lack of intake are unintended.

■ *What is a common cause for older adults to develop an FTT?*

■ **Chronic illness**

FTT in an older adult patient may be a result of chronic illness with a decline in functional activities. This commonly results in physical and emotional deprivation. The occurrence of FTT increases with age and may be found in both community and nursing home residents. It may also be due to depression, which is frequently caused by a recent loss or a change in the person's living situation.

> **〉 HINT**
> FTT is not considered a part of the normal aging process and should not be labeled as a "geriatric" problem.

PATHOPHYSIOLOGY

■ *How does FTT affect a patient's ability to think and make decisions?*

■ **Decreased cognitive ability**

FTT can cause a decrease in a patient's cognitive and decision-making ability. This can lead to a devastating cycle of being unable to recognize that lack of food and water intake is causing the current dysfunction. The patient is unable to reason and make decisions to prepare and cook meals or consume food and water regularly (Box 9.54).

Box 9.54 Four Main Areas of Concern With FTT

Malnutrition	Impaired cognition
Impaired physical function	Depression

■ *A patient with a history of stroke is admitted with FTT syndrome. What is a potential physical reason for the lack of food and water intake?*

■ **Dysphagia**

Stroke patients commonly experience dysphagia. This can restrict the patient's diet, increase difficulty in preparing appropriate foods, make foods less appealing, and limit fluid intake.

Physical problems, such as dysphagia, can also contribute to the FTT syndrome. Other physical problems that can interfere with eating and functional activity include hearing and visual losses, and poorly fitting dentures.

> ❯ **HINT**
> Overly restrictive diets (renal, diabetes, cardiac diets) can contribute to the lack of appetite and limited caloric intake in these patients.

SYMPTOMS/ASSESSMENT

- **Besides the physical assessment and medical evaluation, what is an important aspect of assessment with FTT patients?**
- **Living conditions**

The assessment and history taking includes a thorough evaluation of the living situation (home or in a nursing home), financial situation (can they afford to buy food), and whether the patient is living in an abusive environment (physical or emotional). Alcohol and substance abuse may also lead to malnutrition and isolation of the patient and should be asked about during the interview. Evaluation of functional ability to perform activities of daily living and nutritional status with a referral to a registered dietician are recommended.

> ❯ **HINT**
> Obtain the patient's current list of medications and look for possible drug interactions or side effects that could be contributing to the FTT syndrome (Box 9.55). Combinations of any of these drugs increase the likelihood of FTT syndrome.

Box 9.55 Common Drugs Associated With FTT

Steroids	Anticholinergics
Tricyclic antidepressants	Neuroleptics
Selective serotonin reuptake inhibitors	High-dose diuretics
Antiepileptics	Antihypertensives
Benzodiazepines	Beta-blockers
Opioids	

DIAGNOSIS

- **What is the primary focus of the evaluation in a patient with FTT syndrome?**
- **Find underlying medical disease**

FTT is not a disease but is typically a result of an underlying medical illness. There is not an actual diagnosis of FTT but findings of unintentional malnutrition should trigger a thorough evaluation for a medical disease. A diagnosis of the medical illness allows for the determination of whether it is treatable or has a reversible cause. Treatment of FTT is to frequently treat or manage the underlying disease (Box 9.56).

> ❯ **HINT**
> FFT is not an intentional desire for death and should not be considered a sign of end of life. Following a fall with a hip or pelvic fracture,

an elderly person frequently experiences a loss of function and independence compared to his prior level.

Box 9.56 Potential Underlying Medical Causes of FTT

Cancer	Chronic steroid use
Cardiac diseases (coronary artery disease [CAD], congestive heart failure [CHF])	Onset of dementia or depression
	Continence issues
Chronic pulmonary disorders	Inflammatory bowel disease
End-stage renal disease	Cerebrovascular disease
Diabetes mellitus	Brain tumor
Systemic lupus erythematosus	History of pelvic or hip fracture
Liver dysfunction (cirrhosis, hepatitis)	
Systemic infection	

MANAGEMENT

■ **What is the primary goal in managing FTT syndrome in the acute care setting?**

■ **Ensure adequate caloric intake**

Patients admitted with FTT are typically malnourished and require nutritional consults. A primary goal is to ensure adequate caloric and protein intake. This may require an individualized menu, using a less restrictive diet, providing more appetizing food, and encouraging supplementation with high-protein drinks. In critically ill patients, the calories and protein may be provided with enteral or parenteral feeding. They frequently require administration of vitamins and mineral supplements.

> ❯ **HINT**
> A goal is to prevent further loss of muscle mass with increased protein in the diet. Sarcopenia is the name for loss of muscle mass that occurs with aging.

■ **What physical complications of lack of intake could be contributing to cognitive decline?**

■ **Dehydration and electrolyte abnormalities**

With FTT syndrome, the patient may not be drinking adequate fluids and this could lead to dehydration and electrolyte abnormalities. These can contribute to the decline in cognitive function. Adequate fluid replacement is required to correct the complications of dehydration. IV fluids may be indicated if the patient is unable to consume a sufficient amount of water by mouth. Monitoring and treating electrolyte abnormalities may also prevent some complications of FTT.

■ **What has a synergistic effect with nutrition to provide a sense of well-being?**

■ **Exercise**

Exercise can work with nutrition to improve the overall feeling of well-being. Older people benefit from low-impact exercise and flexibility exercises. Exercise can stimulate appetite and decrease the rate of muscle loss. Encourage physical activity on discharge.

> **HINT**
> While in the hospital, ensure physical therapy and occupational therapy
> are involved in the care of patients with FTT.

COMPLICATIONS

- *A malnourished state can increase a person's likelihood of what complication with wound management?*
- **Delayed wound healing and infections**

Malnourishment can impair the immune system, decreasing wound healing and increasing risk for wound infections (Box 9.57).

Box 9.57 Complications of FTT

Falls	Anemia
Impaired immune response	Fatigue
Poor wound healing	Dehydration
Decreased immunity	Electrolyte abnormalities
Increased infection rates	Muscle wasting
Pressure ulcers	Increased surgical mortality
Decreased independence	

ELDER ABUSE

- *Who is frequently the first person to report elder abuse in home situations?*
- **Health care providers**

Older people are less likely to self-report abuse. It is typically the health care providers who recognize the signs of elder abuse and report the situation to adult protective services. They may be the only people outside of the family to interact with the person (Box 9.58). Suspected as well as confirmed cases should be referred. Identifying, reporting, and treating elder abuse is a responsibility of all health care providers. If it is severe enough, call the police and assure that the perpetrator does not have access to the patient.

> **HINT**
> Mandatory reporting laws for confirmed elder abuse exist in all
> 50 states and 44 states have mandatory laws to report suspected cases.

Box 9.58 Reasons for Lack of Self-Report of Abuse

Fear of retaliation	Protecting their family
Fear of being placed in a nursing home	Being ashamed or feelings of guilt
Feelings of being powerless	Lack of knowledge on how to report

- *What constitutes elder mistreatment or abuse?*
- **Physical, emotional, or sexual abuse**

Persons 60 years of age or older may experience physical, emotional, and/or sexual mistreatment or abuse. According to the World Health Organization (WHO), elder abuse is "a single, or repeated act, or lack of appropriate action, occurring within any relationship where there is an expectation of trust which causes harm or distress to an older person." Neglect and financial exploitation are both considered elder abuse. Neglect is not meeting the patient's needs and failure to protect the person from harm. Emotional abuse may include threats, humiliation, and verbal abuse.

> ❯ HINT
>
> Remember these patients frequently rely on the perpetrator to provide them with shelter, food, money, and clothing.

■ **What is the most common reason for lack of reporting elder abuse in the critical care areas?**

■ **High acuity or unconsciousness**

Critical care nurses usually have only brief periods of time with the patient and due to the criticality of the patient's status, they may not have explored the potential for elder abuse. Patients may be unconscious and unable to report to the nurse. Screening for elder abuse routinely will assist with identifying abuse cases. Abuse can occur in domestic or institutionalized settings.

> ❯ HINT
>
> Families may know of the situation or are the ones actually abusing the patient so may deny the abuse.

PATHOPHYSIOLOGY

■ **What underlying illness of the patient has been found to increase risk of abuse?**

■ **Dementia**

Patients with dementia are at a greater risk of being physically and emotionally abused. Short-term memory losses, agitation, and aggression associated with dementia place high stress on the primary caregivers and increase the risk of abuse.

> ❯ HINT
>
> Keep the risk factors in mind as a "red flag" for potential elder-abuse situations (Box 9.59). A greater workload and responsibility of the primary caregiver increases the risk of abuse.

Box 9.59 Risk Factors for Elder Abuse

Presence of dementia	History of mental illness of primary care provider
Shared living conditions	Alcohol misuse/abuse of primary care provider
Social isolation	Physical impairment
Financial difficulties	Lack of support for the primary caregiver
Greater dependence on primary care provider	Older

SYMPTOMS/ASSESSMENT

- ■ *When would be the ideal time to talk with an alert and oriented elderly patient about potential abuse?*
- ■ **When alone**

Establishing a good rapport and a trusting relationship with elderly patients will allow them to feel safer about disclosing mistreatment and abuse. Most of the time, they will not talk about the abuse while the family is present. Once the family leaves, opening the conversation about abuse may help the patients discuss their situation.

> ❭ **HINT**
> Encourage patients to talk and empower them to prevent further abuse. Document everything pertinent from the interview. It may be used later in a court of law for criminal or guardianship proceedings. In elderly patients, use similar rules that are used when assessing pediatric abuse. Always think, do the injuries match the story?

MANAGEMENT

- ■ *What should the critical care nurse do if she suspects an elderly patient was in an abusive situation at home?*
- ■ **Report the suspected abuse**

The report of the suspected abuse can be directly to the adult protective services or to the ICU manager or social worker. Nurses should know hospital policy and whether there is a protocol in place for reporting suspected or confirmed cases of elder abuse. Legally and ethically, nurses have a responsibility to protect the patients from further harm or injury.

> ❭ **HINT**
> Nurses need to continually be aware of their suspicions and intuitions regarding potential abuse.

COMPLICATIONS

- ■ *What psychological disorder can be caused by an abusive situation?*
- ■ **Depression**

Elder abuse diminishes self-respect, pride, and dignity. This leads to depression, social isolation, and higher rates of dementia. It may contribute to FTT syndrome and higher mortality from illnesses or injuries.

> ❭ **HINT**
> Elder abuse places the person at a higher risk of suicide.

TESTABLE NURSING ACTIONS

RESTRAINT USE IN THE ICU

- *What restraining therapy should be used in ICU?*
- **Least restrictive but effective**

Restraints can cause issues with patient comfort and dignity as well as complications of falls, limb injuries, and skin breakdown. The recommended restraint is the one that is least restrictive but still effective. Alternatives to restraints should be considered when appropriate and underlying problems treated that may decrease the need for restraints. Bed alarms may be used to alert the nurse of the patient getting out of bed and may lower the need for restraints (Box 9.60).

> **❯ HINT**
> Restraints should not be routinely used on all ICU patients. The need should be determined on a case-by-case basis.

Box 9.60 Interventions to Lower the Need for Restraints

Adequate pain management	Involvement in activities
Treat delirium or agitation	Adequate lighting in room
Assess for fever or hypoxia	Frequent toileting offered
Ambulate (if possible)	Allow family to sit with patient
Alternative therapy (pet therapy, aromatherapy, massage)	

- *How often should restraint renewal be reordered?*
- **Every 24 hours**

Restraining orders are limited to 24 hours and require daily orders for renewal. The rationale for the need for restraints should also be documented daily. An order should be obtained within 1 hour of initiating restraints.

- *What type of restraint is an analgesic when administered for sedation purposes?*
- **Chemical restraint**

Analgesics, sedative, hypnotics, and neuroleptic drugs may assist with decreasing the need for restraints but these are still considered chemical restraints. These drugs are not purely chemical restraints but are a part of therapeutic treatment that may lower the need for physical restraints.

- *What is the primary purpose of restraints in the ICU?*
- **Patient safety**

Restraint use in the ICU is primarily for patient safety to prevent inadvertent discontinuation of endotracheal tubes or other invasive lines or tubes. Restraints may also be used to prevent falls and injuries in patients with delirium or dementia. Restrained patients require frequent observation to prevent complications. Families and patients need to receive information about the purpose of the restraints.

> ❯ HINT
> The nurse must balance responsibility to protect the patient's rights and the obligation to prevent injury to the patient.

BIBLIOGRAPHY

Barr, J., et al. (2013). Clinical practice guidelines for the management of pain, agitation and delirium in adult patients in the intensive care unit. *Critical Care Medicine, 41*(1), 263–295.

Gelinas, et al. (2006). Validity of the Critical Care Pain Observation Tool in Adults: *American Journal of Critical Care, 15*: 420–429.

Hartsell, Z., Drost, J., Wilkens, J., & Budavari, I. (2007). Managing alcohol withdrawal in hospital patients. *Journal of the American Academy of Physician Assistants, 20*(9), 20–25.

Rittenmeyer, L. (2012). Aggression in high dependency care environment. *Critical Care Nursing Clinics of North America, 24*, 41–51.

World Health Organization. (n.d.). *Ageing and life course: Elder abuse*. Retrieved from http://www.who.int/ageing/projects/elder_abuse/en/index.html

Questions

1. A patient with a history of alcohol use states that he consumes a 12 pack of beer a day. On assessment using the CIWA-Ar tool, the patient is given a score of 12. Which of the following would be the most appropriate intervention at this time?

   A. Administer an ethanol infusion to manage the current DTs
   B. Continue to monitor, no treatment is required at this time
   C. Administer a benzodiazepine to prevent AWS
   D. Discontinue using the CIWA-Ar since the patient is no longer at risk for AWS

2. When obtaining a history from the family, it is noted that the patient is allergic to lorazepam and soybean. Which of the following infusions should be avoided in this patient?

   A. Cardizem
   B. Morphine
   C. Esmolol
   D. Propofol

3. A patient with known alcohol dependency is admitted to the ICU. The physician orders thiamine and multivitamins. What syndrome is thiamine used to prevent?

   A. Wernicke–Korsakoff syndrome
   B. Syndrome of inappropriate antidiuretic hormone
   C. Myelodysplastic syndrome
   D. Metabolic syndrome

4. Which of the following has been shown to decrease the number of ventilator days and length of ICU stay?

   A. Light levels of sedation
   B. Strict glycemic control
   C. Promote sleep
   D. Daily chest x-ray

5. A 76-year-old patient with a history of congestive heart failure (CHF) is in the ICU for 3 days. She is demonstrating a decrease in awareness of her surroundings and is beginning to have hallucinations. Which of the following is the most likely cause of her mental changes?

   A. Anxiety
   B. Agitation
   C. Delirium
   D. Dementia

6. Which of the following statements is the most accurate regarding acute pain?

   A. Men have greater pain following a cardiac surgery than women.
   B. Pain cannot be assessed in an intubated, nonverbal patient.
   C. Pain is frequently remembered after discharge and can cause PTSD.
   D. Chest tube placement is a painful procedure that requires preemptive analgesia but removal of chest tube is well tolerated without analgesia.

7. A behavioral tool is used in nonverbal patients to assess pain and determine the need for analgesics. In which of the following patients is a BPS not as reliable?

   A. Elderly patient
   B. Brain-injured patient
   C. Burn patient
   D. Patient with psychiatric disorder history

8. Which of the following sedatives provides some control of pain in addition to the sedation?

   A. Dexmedetomidine
   B. Propofol
   C. Haloperidol
   D. Diazepam

9. An 84-year-old patient with a history of dementia has an increased risk of developing sundowners' syndrome and falling. Which of the following would be the best nursing intervention to lower the risk?

   A. Place restraints on patient in the evening
   B. Increase the dose of sedation in evenings
   C. Require the family to provide a sitter through the night
   D. Turn on lights well before sunset and close the curtains at dusk

10. A patient with cancer has been admitted to the ICU with a Mallory–Weiss tear that occurred during vomiting resulting from his chemotherapy treatment. He tells you he has been experiencing unrelenting pain and does not want any of his family to visit him. Which of the following would be the greatest concern for this patient at this time?

   A. Depression
   B. Suicide
   C. Psychosis
   D. FTT

Professional Caring and Ethical Practice

In this chapter, you will review:

- Synergy model
- Advocacy and moral agency
- Caring practice
- Collaboration
- Systems thinking
- Response to diversity
- Facilitation of learning
- Clinical inquiry

SYNERGY MODEL

- *According to the synergy model, what drives the characteristics or competencies of the nurses?*
- **Patient and family needs**

The needs of patients and families drive the competencies of the nurses. Synergy occurs when the nurse's competencies match the characteristics and needs of the patient. Optimal outcomes occur when the nurse and the patient are in synergy. Patient and nurse work together, synergistically, toward a common goal.

> **> HINT**
> The emphasis of the synergy model for clinical practice is that the patient's needs always come first.

- *Following onset of sepsis, an intensive care unit (ICU) patient develops acute kidney injury (AKI) and acute respiratory distress syndrome (ARDS). Which patient characteristic is the greatest concern at this time?*
- **Complexity**

Patients and families all have similar needs but each person brings unique characteristics to the current situation. Individualization of care focused on the patient's needs or characteristics depends on where the patient is on the continuum of health and illness. Patient characteristics can evolve or change over time and are based on a continuum. Complexity is the intricate entanglement of two or more systems. A patient with sepsis and multiorgan dysfunction is a high-complexity patient because of the influence of each system's failure on the other (see http://ajcc.aacnjournals.org).

> ❯ HINT
>
> The higher acuity patients will tend to have greater complexity. All patient characteristics are intertwined and cannot be viewed alone.

■ **What level of expertise does a nurse have who has been practicing for 25 years in the ICU and is able look at the whole picture and make decisions based on her experience and knowledge?**

■ **Expert (Level 5)**

The level of competency of a nurse depends on her experience, knowledge, desire to learn, and to meet the patient's needs. Competencies may range from novice to expert in each of the nurse characteristics. The goal of nurses should be to practice at the highest level of competency.

> ❯ HINT
>
> Level 5 is the highest level or level of an expert and should be the goal for ICU nurses (see http://ajcc.aacnjournals.org). The professional and caring practice questions are based on the patient and nurse characteristics.

ADVOCACY AND MORAL AGENCY

■ **What occurs when two or more unattractive courses of action are possible and either course opposes the other?**

■ **Ethical or moral dilemma**

Ethics encompasses all aspects of life, including our conduct, behavior toward ourselves, toward others, and toward the environment. Ethical dilemmas exist when two or more unattractive courses of action are possible but neither have an overwhelming rationale choice. Equally compelling alternatives and a moral argument can be made for and against each alternative.

> ❯ HINT
>
> Ethical dilemmas in hospitals have been increasing in frequency and intensity (Box 10.1).

Box 10.1 Common Ethical Dilemmas in the ICU

Contradictory beliefs (patient, family, health care providers)	Removal of life-sustaining therapies
Lack of clear clinical or legal guidelines	Assisted suicides
Futility issues	Scarce resources for allocation
Do-not-resuscitate (DNR) issues	Increased costs for new technology and patient care

■ *What occurs when the nurse believes that she knows the ethically correct action in a situation but a different action is occurring?*

■ **Moral distress**

Moral distress is common in the health care environment with the complexity of ethical dilemmas that occur. Moral distress occurs when the nurse believes that she knows the ethically correct action to take in the situation but a conflicting action is being pursued due to other members of the health care team or family members. ICU nurses need to be aware of their own personnel beliefs and to be aware of the differences in professional and personal values. The optimal is allowing the nurse to practice in a manner that maintains her own sense of self-respect while maintaining the dignity of the patients.

> ❯ HINT
> The American Association of Critical Care Nurse (AACN) views moral distress as a key issue for critical care nurses (Box 10.2).

Box 10.2 AACN's Four "A"s in Moral Distress

Ask
Affirm
Assess
Act

Source: AACN (www.aacn.org).

■ *What are frequently used to determine the "right" actions in an ethical dilemma?*

■ **Ethical principles**

Ethical principles, professional guidelines, and ethical processes are used to determine the "right" action. Moral principles are approaches used in ethics to determine what is right and wrong. There are certain ethical principles more commonly used in health care ethical dilemmas.

> ❯ HINT
> Remember, ethical decisions are not absolute in what is right and wrong, and reasonable people can still disagree with the action. That is why it is called a dilemma.

■ *What is the ethical principle of an obligation to maximize benefits and minimize harm?*

■ **Beneficence**

Beneficence is the obligation to promote the welfare of others by maximizing benefits and minimizing harm. Beneficence is frequently used in ethical dilemmas in the hospital and refers to the health care practitioner's responsibility to benefit the patient, usually through acts of kindness, compassion, and mercy.

> **HINT**
>
> This is the principle often used to analyze futile care and withdrawal of life support (Box 10.3).

Box 10.3 Ethical Principles

Utilitarianism	It is based on the following two principles: 1. The greatest good for the greatest number 2. The end justifies the mean The situation determines whether the act is right or wrong
Deontology (formalistic)	This principle is based on moral rules and unchanging principles. Morality is defined by the act, not the outcome. The principles are: 1. People should be treated as ends and never as a means 2. Human life has value 3. One is to always tell the truth 4. Above all, do no harm 5. All people are of equal value
Justice	This principle is that every person is to be treated similarly, avoiding discrimination on the basis of age, sex, perceived social worth, financial ability, or cultural/ethnic background Incorporates ideas of fairness and equality
Beneficence	Refers to the health care provider's responsibility to benefit the patient, usually through acts of kindness, compassion, and mercy Action maximizes the benefit and minimizes the harm
Nonmaleficience	This principle requires that actions do not inflict harm The definition of harm becomes crucial when applying this principle
Autonomy	The belief is that the competent patient has the right to determine his or her own care The right to refuse therapy It recognizes that each person has worth as an individual and the capacity to choose The patient's values and wishes should be upheld unless they impose unfair burden on health care providers or institutions
Paternalism	Based on the belief that health care professionals have a duty to benefit the patient, outweighing the right of independent choice The principles include: 1. Benefits provided outweigh autonomy 2. Patient's condition severely limits ability to choose autonomously 3. Intended action may be universally justified in relevantly similar circumstances
Fidelity	Duty to be faithful to others by keeping promises and fulfilling contracts and commitments. Moral obligation of the nurse to have a duty to his or her patients
Veracity	Duty to tell the truth and not to lie or deceive others

■ **What ethical principle is being used when the health care team obtains informed consent for a procedure?**

■ **Autonomy**

Decision making in the ICU has been divided into paternalism and autonomy. The goal has been toward autonomy, encouraging patient and families to make their own decisions regarding health care. During times of crisis, using a pure autonomy model for decision making may put undue stress on family. The family may require more assistance from health care providers in making critical decisions. A newer model of shared decision making may help patients and families in critical situations to make a more informed decision with less anxiety and more appropriate input from physicians in some cases. This has been found to improve collaboration between health care providers and families.

> **HINT**

Family members may be required to take sole responsibility for decision making regarding end of life with limited information or understanding. Nurses play an important role in assessing the family's level of knowledge and in providing an education for the family.

■ **When an ethical dilemma occurs in the ICU, what is the first step in resolving the dilemma?**
■ **Data collection**

Many decisions made in the ICU have an ethical component. Decisions need to be made based on a learned skill not just an emotional response. Making such decisions should involve using a systematic process and ethical principles to provide direction. Without guidance, the decisions are made on emotions, intuitions, or fixed policies. Data collection is the first step in resolving a moral or ethical dilemma. It involves gathering of medical facts, including the prognosis, alternatives, and assessment of patient/family knowledge. Social facts are also collected, including the living environment, family and significant others, economic concerns, and current or previously stated wishes.

> **HINT**

Steps of resolving an ethical dilemma are similar to the nursing process (Box 10.4).

Box 10.4 Steps in Determining Ethical Dilemma

Step 1: Data collection	Gather medical facts, including the prognosis, alternatives, and assessment of patient/family knowledge Gather social facts, including the living environment, family and significant others, economic concerns, current or previously stated wishes
Step 2: Identify the conflict	Weigh the values and determine where they conflict or compliment, determine who and what are involved in the conflict State the family's, patient's, and health care provider's ethical position
Step 3: Define the goals	Are goals patient-centered, realistic, achievable, and collaborative? Examples are the goal of prolongation of life, relief of pain, maximum recovery
Step 4: Identify ethical principles	List the principles and rank order them to identify the primary principle. There may be conflicting principles.
Step 5: Review alternative courses of action	Compare the alternatives to the goals, predict possible consequences of the alternatives, and prioritize acceptable alternatives.
Step 6: Choose the course of action	This is the alternative that breaks the fewest ethical principles.
Step 7: Develop and implement a plan of action	Following determination of action, a plan is developed to determine how to carry out the action and is performed.
Step 8: Evaluate the plan	Follow up after the action is implemented to determine if pre-set goals were reached. If not, determine what could have improved the action to meet the goals.

■ *When a patient is in an irreversible coma and the physicians have declared that treatment can not cure or improve quality of life that would be satisfactory to the patient, what is it called?*

■ **Futile care**

Futile care is any clinical circumstance in which the physician and his or her consultants, consistent with the available medical literature, conclude that further treatment cannot, within a reasonable probability, cure, ameliorate, improve, or restore quality of life that would be satisfactory to the patient (Box 10.5).

> ❯ HINT
> Examples of futile-care situations include an irreversible coma or persistent vegetative state or terminall illness, where application of life-sustaining procedures would serve only to delay the inevitable.

Box 10.5 Criteria Used to Determine Futility of Care

Severity of illness	Expected long-term outcomes
Comorbidities	Duration of therapy
Life expectancy	Cost of treatment
Predicted quality of life	

■ *What is a legal document, that identifies someone who will have the power to make medical treatment decisions in the event the patient is unable?*

■ **Durable power of attorney**

The Patient Self-Determination Act (PSDA) went into effect in 1991 requiring all health care facilities receiving Medicare or Medicaid funds to provide written information to the adult patient about his or her rights according to the state law to make treatment decisions and execute advanced directives. A durable power of attorney is a legal document, which identifies someone who will have the power to make medical treatment decisions in the event the patient is unable. This is initiated at a time when the patient loses the capacity to participate in the decision-making process (Box 10.6).

> ❯ HINT
> Advanced directives were developed to ensure a patient's right for autonomy and to provide high-quality care at the end of life.

Box 10.6 Common Reasons for Not Having a Power of Attorney

Reluctance to talk about death
Patient waiting for physician to initiate the conversation
Difficulty in completing the required forms
Unaware of power of attorney
Nurses unaware or do not initiate conversation

CARING PRACTICE

- **What do patients experience in the ICU because of constant noise, alarms, and hearing unfamiliar voices?**
- **Sensory overload**

Patients in the ICU experience sensory overload due to constant noise and alarms. Sensory overload contributes to sleep deprivation, anxiety, agitation, and delirium in ICU patients. Other negative experiences reported by patients in the ICU include fear, anxiety, sleep deprivation, lack of privacy, pain, and discomfort (Box 10.7).

> **❯ HINT**
> Patients experience a more positive outcome in ICUs that incorporate natural lighting, soothing sounds, meaningful stimuli, and pleasant views.

Box 10.7 Causes of Sensory Overload

Frequent alarms	Constant stimulation
Blinking lights	Bright lights
Unfamiliar sounds	Unpleasant smells
Machinery sounds	Multiple lines and tubes
Unfamiliar voices	Restraints
Clinicians talking at the bedside	Hurried pace in crowded space

- **What are two of the most disruptive noises patients report hearing in the ICU?**
- **Talking and alarms**

Noise is an environmental hazard that causes patient discomfort. Loud conversation by health care providers is one of the most frequently reported noises the patient recalls after being in an ICU. Nurses do not realize sometimes how loud they are when talking to each other in the unit and at the patient's bedside. This is reported to be disruptive to patients. Alarms are also frequently reported as being disruptive (Box 10.8).

> **❯ HINT**
> Nurses are not always aware of their loudness in conversation and should take an objective assessment of the ICU environment. Noisy environments can lead to sleep deprivation, psychosis, and delirium (Box 10.9).

Box 10.8 Causes of Loud Noises

Staff conversations	Telephones ringing
Alarms going off all the time	Televisions on all of the time
Banging doors	Noisy machines and equipment (i.e., intra-aortic balloon pump , ventilators)

Box 10.9 Adverse Effects of Noisy Environment

Sleep disruption	Vasoconstriction
Activation of sympathetic nervous system	Hyperarousal
Impaired wound healing	Delirium

■ *What do patients in the ICU commonly perceive as a loss that creates anxiety?*

■ **Loss of control**

Patients in the ICU commonly experience a loss of control that creates anxiety. Providing order and predictability can create an illusion of some control by the patient. This is called anticipatory guidance that keeps the patient from being surprised at a routine. Once the patient is able to make simple decisions, allow the patient to make small choices. Give some control back to the patient in areas in which he or she can make decisions. Other common causes of anxiety in the ICU include a loss of function or self-esteem, sense of isolation, and a fear of dying.

> ❯ **HINT**
> Allowing small choices can assist the patient's coping with larger procedures in which little choice is present (Box 10.10). Patients should also have the right to make decisions about visitors; who can visit and for how long.

Box 10.10 Examples of Patient Choices

Do you want a bath now or in 20 minutes?
At what angle do you want your head of bed?
Do you want to turn to your right or left side?
Do you want your pain medication now or in 20 minutes?

■ *What do families typically express in regard to their feelings while their loved ones are in the ICU?*

■ **Helplessness**

The suddenness of injury or illness may cause family members to have uncertainty about the situation. They may approach the ICU nurse with multiple questions and concerns. The family is thrown into a whirlwind of activity and commonly experience feelings of helplessness. They are often unprepared for the whole impact of the injury or illness. Frequently, families experience a "roller coaster" of emotions during the ICU stay. They may be happy that their loved one is alive but upset about the injury or losses; there are good days and bad days with many ups and downs.

> ❯ **HINT**
> Family members may ask "unanswerable" questions and usually do not expect an answer. It shows their deep and inner fears (Box 10.11).

Box 10.11 Family Member Reactions to Illness

Shock	Distrust
Anxiety	Guilt
Denial	Remorse
Hostility/anger	Depression

■ *What is a common coping mechanism that family members have following a critical illness or injury in order to regain some control?*

■ **Vigilance**

The initial emotional reaction of fear, shock, or panic is sometimes followed by irrational acts and demanding behaviors. Vigilance becomes a coping mechanism by family members in an attempt to regain some control of the situation. Family members commonly want to be at the bedside or in the ICU waiting room 24 hours a day. They may express concern about being gone because:

1. What if something happens?
2. They may miss meeting with the physician.
3. Their loved one may "wake up" while they are gone.

Vigilance includes constantly seeking information to ensure that tasks are being carried out (i.e., "I thought they were going to CT this morning?" "Has she had dinner yet?").

> ❯ **HINT**
> Establishing a trusting relationship immediately relieves some of the anxiety, then family members are more likely to feel comfortable enough to leave the hospital (Box 10.12). Explain to the family that this is more a "marathon" than a "short sprint" and they need to save energy for when the patient leaves the ICU or hospital.

Box 10.12 Interventions for Families

Obtain correct phone numbers and keep at bedside	Show interest in how the family is doing
Take initiative and call family frequently with updates	Be courteous
Teach about what to expect while in ICU	Allow family members to express negative feelings
Set up physician and family visits or conferences	Ask what the family needs
Establish a trusting relationship	Do not give false reassurances
Follow through with tasks	Allow family members to assist in providing
Provide honest information about the condition of the patient	basic aspects of care (brush teeth, comb hair, assist with bath, help with meals)
Explain why things are done the way they are	Provide consistent information to family

■ *What intervention can an ICU nurse do to decrease the number of calls about the status of a patient?*

■ **Establish a contact person**

A common issue ICU nurses encounter is constant calls from family and friends seeking updates. Setting up a contact person from the family for the health care providers to provide updates will decrease the number of calls into the ICU. Remember, frequent calls to the immediate family can increase their stress and time spent updating other relatives and friends (Box 10.13).

> **HINT**
Encourage immediate family members to have down time; "allow" them to screen their calls.

Box 10.13 Recommendations for Frequent Calls With Family

Establish chain of calls to deliver information to larger number of people
One person will make outgoing calls when an update is given
Develop an updated outgoing message on phone daily
Develop a website for updates, information, and progress
Establish a guest page
E-mail updates as a group e-mail

■ *What should families be told about bedside conversations in the patient's room?*

■ **Avoid talking about the patient's medical condition**

Family members and health care providers should avoid talking beside the patient's bed about the patient's medical condition. Patients may be able to hear even if they are not responding or appear to be disoriented. Families frequently do not know what to say to the patient or what to talk about at the bedside. Some families just stand at bedside and are afraid to touch their loved ones because of all of the lines and tubes. ICU nurses can encourage them to talk to the patient directly and touch their loved ones (Box 10.14).

> **HINT**
Patients report increased anxiety and fear when overhearing conversations about procedures at the bedside.

Box 10.14 Interventions to Encourage Conversations With Patients

Encourage family and friends to normalize conversations
Talk about daily happenings at work and home
Encourage families to keep a diary at home and then talk to the patient from the diary
Avoid talking only about the illness, injury, or treatments
If patient is unresponsive, talk about her hobbies, likes, or favorite activities
Avoid talking beside the patient's bed about the patient's medical condition

■ *What is the most common need or priority of family members in the ICU?*

■ **Need for information**

The number one identified need of the family members is the need for information. Family members frequently ask for lab results, vital signs, or watch monitors. They may fixate or focus on certain things such as blood pressure, heart rate, or temperature. Families experience increased frustration when they get different information from different health care providers. Continuity of nursing assignments provides consistency for patients and families. The nurse is more aware of family needs and better able to reinforce teaching already provided to family. Nurses need to create an atmosphere of understanding, concern, and empathy with the family (Box 10.15).

> **> HINT**
>
> Most families do not want "sugar-coated" answers; they want to be told the truth. Honesty and full disclosure of prognosis are recommended. Hope is not just avoiding death but being pain free or hoping for a dignified death.

Box 10.15 Common Needs of Families

Need to feel hope	Need for honesty
Need to receive information about the patient on a daily basis	Need to see the patient frequently
	Need to know the patient is comfortable and without pain
Need to feel the nurses and physicians care about the patient	Need for support from the health care personnel
Need to know the prognosis	Consistency in nurses and physicians

■ *What visitation policy can offer a more healing environment and family-focused care?*

■ **Flexible (open) visitation policy**

The ICU environment is becoming more of a family-focused care culture. Allowing a more open visitation policy provides families with a greater feeling of being welcome to be with their loved ones. Increasing the visitation times can strengthen the relationship between the family and the nurse. Research has also shown benefits of allowing families to remain at the bedside based on the patient's physiological responses (decrease anxiety, intracranial pressure). There is a need for less restrictive and individualized visitation in ICUs (Box 10.16).

> **> HINT**
>
> Advocate the adjustment of visitation hours to meet the needs of family members. Novel visitation policies include allowing young children to be accompanied by adults and pet-assisted therapy in the ICU.

Box 10.16 Advantages of Open Visitation

Families feel more assured about the care that their loved ones are receiving	Allows ability to regain sense of control
More aware of any changes that occur with their loved one	Improves family coping skills
Not knowing what is happening on the "other side" of the doors produces anxiety	Strengthens relationships with the nurses
Provides a sense of direction	

■ *Family presence during resuscitation may benefit the family member. What is an important aspect to success of family presence during resuscitation?*

■ **Support person remains with family member**

In family presence during resuscitation programs, usually one family member is allowed to remain in the room during resuscitation. Success of the program depends on the ability to keep a support person with the family member to explain what is happening, provide emotional support, and evaluate the person's response. This program originally started in trauma resuscitation and has expanded to resuscitation in cardiopulmonary arrests in the hospital (Box 10.17).

Box 10.17 Benefits of Family Presence During Resuscitation

Family members observe the efforts of the health care providers	The mystery of activities behind "closed doors" is reduced
Family members can provide comfort and words of encouragement to the patient	Assist with decision making about code versus DNR (family may halt code)
Ability of the family to have closure	Facilitation of bonding between patients' family members and health care providers
Acceptance of the outcome is facilitated	
Families perceive that they are actively involved in the resuscitation of their loved one	Holistic approach is fostered
	Lowered legal malpractice suits

> **HINT**
> Families allowed to remain in the room during resuscitation typically express feelings that they know the health care staff did everything possible to save their loved one. Most concerns have been unfounded in research involving family presence during resuscitations (Box 10.18).

Box 10.18 Identified Fears of Staff in Family Presence

Fear of increased stress of health care personnel involved	Fear of litigation
Uncertainty of helpfulness of family member during the procedure or resuscitation	Long-term effects on family's emotional status; posttraumatic stress disorder
Fear that the family member will interrupt/disrupt the resuscitation	Violation of patient's privacy
Family members may be offended and potentially engage in negative behaviors	Lack of the family member's understanding of tasks and procedures being performed
Staff might feel inhibited from performing necessary tasks	Increased required number of staff involved in the code

COLLABORATION

■ *What negative effect on patient outcomes has been found when nurses practice in an unhealthy work environment?*

■ **Medication errors**

An unhealthy work environment can lead to increased medication errors and poor patient-care delivery. Errors in delivering patient care will negatively affect outcomes for patients. There is a link between healthy work environments, excellent nursing care, and patient outcomes. A healthy work environment should be focused on safety, caring, and respect for each other, including all health care providers, patients, and families (Box 10.19).

Box 10.19 Negative Effects of an Unhealthy Work Environment

Medication errors
Poor delivery of care
Patient-care errors
Stress to health care professionals
Higher nurse turnover

■ *What is the biggest underlying issue found in an unhealthy work environment?*

■ **Poor communication**

Each bad situation relates back to poor communication and ineffective relationships among health care providers. Health care providers need to improve working relationships and communicate on a more professional level. Outbursts and disruptive behavior may prevent a nurse from calling a physician to report patient changes or question an order. This may lead to medication or patient-care errors. According to the AACN, a healthy work environment has six standards that must all be instituted to establish a healthy work environment and improve patient outcomes (Box 10.20).

Box 10.20 Six Standards for a Healthy Environment by the AACN

Skilled communication	Appropriate staffing
True collaboration	Meaningful recognition
Effective decision making	Authentic leadership

■ *When engaged in skilled communication, what is an important aspect the nurse must have to ensure the mutual respect of their colleagues?*

■ **Listen to the other individual's perspectives**

It is important to treat others with respect and to develop a mutually respective relationship. Listening to other health care professionals' perspectives during the discussion will improve the skilled communication and assist with the development of mutual respect.

> **HINT**
> The focus is not on to "win" but to find an agreeable solution with a desirable outcome (Box 10.21).

Box 10.21 Aspects of Skilled Communication

Health care organization should provide education on skilled communication	Use mutual respect
	Congruence between word and action
Focus is to find solutions and desirable outcomes	Zero tolerance for abuse and disrespectful behavior
Protect and advance professional relationships	
Listen to all relevant perspectives	

■ *What is a common time for breakdown of communication between nurses to occur?*

■ **Shift change**

Shift change is a common time for breakdown of communication to occur. This was quoted to be the "single largest source of medical error" with errors ranging from administering wrong medication to resuscitating a DNR patient. A significant amount of information is passed along among nurses during period of report and change of patient care from one nurse to another. Ensuring important information regarding the previous shift events and future care is important to ensure continuity and to avoid missing important changes in the patient's status.

> **❯ HINT**
> Communication during shift report may be inadequate if nurses are tired and stressed (Box 10.22). Distraction is a significant cause of medication errors. Assuring a "quiet zone" while obtaining and administering medications is important to prevent medication errors.

Box 10.22 Use of Mnemonic "I PASS the BATON"

Introduction	Introduce self (if needed)
Patient	Name, identifiers, age, sex, location, physicians involved in care
Assessment	Presenting chief complaint, vital signs, current system review, symptoms, and diagnosis
Situation	Current status, circumstances, including code status, recent changes, responses to treatment
Safety	Critical lab values, reports, allergies, fall risk, isolation
Background	Comorbidities, previous episodes, current medications, family history
Actions	What actions were taken or required?
Timing	Level of urgency and explicit timing, prioritizing of actions
Ownership	Who is responsible?
Next	What will happen next? Anticipated changes, what is the plan?

■ *What is the standardized framework for members of the health care team to communicate about a patient's condition?*

■ **SBAR (Situation, Background, Assessment, Recommendation)**

SBAR is a standardized framework for members of the health care team to communicate about a patient's condition. SBAR was originally used by nuclear submariners during exchange of command. It frames a conversation and facilitates communication with physicians. It has been found to lower adverse events (Box 10.23).

Box 10.23 Barriers of Communication Among Health Care Providers

Language barriers (accents differ even in English-speaking people)	Conflict with personalities
Varying communication styles	Workload
Distraction	Stress

■ *What needs to be considered in planning family conferences in regard to health information privacy regulations?*

■ **Determining those approved for medical information**

When planning a health care conference to discuss the patient's clinical status and treatment plans, ensure that the family members involved have the patient's approval to obtain health care information regarding the patient. During family meetings, open-ended questions are used to determine what the family understands about their loved one's condition. Repeating or reflecting what the family said will allow a chance for them to correct any misunderstandings. Hearing all the family members' thoughts and opinions before making a decision can facilitate a consensus even if the final decision may be against their own beliefs.

> **HINT**
> Reflection is a good technique when determining patients' or family members' understanding about the illness or treatments.

■ *When making decisions regarding end of life and withdrawal of life support, whose perspective or opinion should be considered?*

■ **The patient's**

In situations when the patient is unable to make decisions regarding life support, the family will make those decisions. The decision should still be made based on the wishes of the patient. A living will may indicate the extent of life support the patient would want. Without a living will, sometimes asking the family, "What do you think your loved one would want in this situation?" will encourage them to make decisions based on what they think their loved one would want.

SYSTEMS THINKING

■ *Holistic nursing care is healing oriented and is centered on which relationship?*

■ **Relationship with patient**

Holistic nursing is patient-centered care directed toward healing, not diseases. It protects, promotes, and optimizes healing while attempting to alleviate suffering. It is comprehensive and recognizes the totality of the patient by interconnecting the body, mind, spirituality, energy, culture, relationships, and environment. It promotes comfort, empowerment, healing, and the well-being of the patient.

> ❯ HINT
> Holistic nursing emphasizes self-care and autonomy. A role of a holistic nurse is to ensure that the patient is aware of alternatives and the implication of treatment options.

■ *What is a complementary intervention used to manage anxiety?*
■ **Deep-breathing exercises**

Managing anxiety in ICU patients includes instructing them in deep-breathing exercises. Other exercises may include relaxation or imagery techniques. Holistic nurses incorporate both conventional and complementary/alternative/integrative modalities (CAM) into practice (Boxes 10.24 and 10.25).

Box 10.24 Complementary Techniques to Manage Anxiety/Pain

Deep-breathing exercises	Aromatherapy
Relaxation techniques	Massage
Guided imagery	Pet therapy
Deep-muscle relaxation	Humor
Music therapy	

Box 10.25 Examples of CAM

Natural products	Practice of traditional healers
Mind–body medicine	Energy therapies (i.e., magnet therapy, light therapy)
Spinal manipulation	Homeopathy
Movement therapies and massage	Acupuncture and acupressure

■ *What effect does frequent sleep interruptions have on rapid eye movement (REM) sleep?*
■ **Decreases REM sleep**

Little to no REM sleep occurs in ICU patients because of frequent stimulation and awakenings. They experience shorter amounts of sleep than reported at home and frequently perceive quality of sleep as poor (Boxes 10.26 and 10.27).

> ❯ HINT
> Self report of sleep quality is the best assessment if the patient is able to communicate. Poor sleep patterns may already be experienced by elderly patients who are exacerbated being in the ICU.

Box 10.26 Adverse Effects of Sleep Deprivation

Altered cognition	Muscle weakness or fatigue
Lowered seizure threshold	Delayed wound healing
Decreased ability to wean from ventilator	Suppressed immune system

Box 10.27 Interventions to Promote Sleep in ICU Patients

Avoid unnecessary baths between hours 2:00 and 5:00 a.m.	Position patient for comfort
	Manage pain and anxiety
Back massage	Turn down lights during sleep time
Sleep promotion protocols	Turn televisions off or down
Observed quiet time or blocked sleep time	Turn alarms down during quiet or sleep time
Obtain a routine chest x-ray and labs either at 10:00 pm or 5:00 a.m. (avoid hours between 2:00 and 4:00 a.m.)	Perform basic p.m. tasks similar to routine at home
	Allow family member to stay with the patient
Provide large clocks easily visible by patient	Post sign on door "Sleeping, please be quiet"
Provide ear plugs for patients at night	
Music therapy or background of comforting sounds (i.e., ocean sounds)	Close doors during sleep time
	Use relaxation or imagery techniques
Aromatherapy	

■ **What is the quest to discover the ultimate meaning and purpose of one's life called?**

■ **Spirituality**

Spirituality is the culmination of a person's quest to discover the ultimate meaning and purpose of his or her life. Spirituality reflects the essence and substance of that person. Religion is the belief in and worship of a superhuman controlling power, especially a personal God. Religion can impact the development of spirituality and provides some answers to spiritual questions. ICU nurses should assess spiritual issues while reassuring patients there is no pressure on them to discuss issues they do not want to discuss. Active listening is sometimes the best intervention to help a patient clarify his or her wishes, hopes, and beliefs (Boxes 10.28 and 10.29). Religion may provide support to patients and their families and can be a significant part of their coping mechanism. Health care providers will want to explore the patient's contact with formal religious institutions, as well as informal spiritual beliefs. Knowledge of a patient and his or her family's religious beliefs are particularly important for health care professionals whose patients are struggling with serious illnesses.

> **❯ HINT**
> Spirituality is a part of the holistic care. The ICU nurse can provide support, solace, spiritual strength, and presence. Prayer has been found to be a powerful tool to help patients cope with critical illness and impending death.

Box 10.28 Common Spiritual Issues

Desire for forgiveness	Need for affirmation of a person's value/meaning
Need to forgive	Hope for a peaceful and painless death
Desire for closure	Concern for loved one's left behind

Box 10.29 Spiritual Questions Commonly Encountered in ICU

Why me?	What will the last hours be like?
Is my illness a punishment?	Is there a God?
Why was I placed on Earth?	What happens after death?
Is there hope?	Will I be punished for my sins?
How can I be forgiven?	Will I be alone?
How can I forgive?	Will I be remembered?

■ *What is a common issue in caring for an awake and alert patient on a mechanical ventilator?*

■ **Communication**

Effective communication is known to assist with establishing a trusting relationship. Effective communication with intubated patients on mechanical ventilation is a challenge to critical care nurses. Slowing down, demonstrating patience, and allowing time for the intubated patient to communicate is a large step in improving effective communication (Box 10.30).

Box 10.30 Communication Adjuncts for Intubated Patients

Nonverbal signals
Writing tablets
Communication boards

RESPONSE TO DIVERSITY

■ *During the admission assessment, the family states that the patient is from a tribe in Africa. What is the nurse's initial priority in providing care that is compatible to the patient's cultural beliefs?*

■ **Perform a cultural assessment**

Cultural sensitivity often begins with a cultural assessment that includes finding information on the patient's cultural beliefs, views, and cultural norms. Individuals can vary within a particular culture with regards to beliefs or norms so the patient should be recognized as an individual within a cultural context. Identifying how the patient has responded to an illness in the past and exploring what effect the critical injury or illness will have on the patient is essential to determine the patient's perceptions. Health care beliefs regarding chronic illness, seeking medical attention, and death and dying may vary among cultures and ethnic backgrounds (Box 10.31).

> ❯ HINT
> Determine whether there is anything the nurses should or should not do when providing care that is sensitive to the individual's values and beliefs. Awareness and acceptance are at the heart of cultural sensitivity.

Box 10.31 Components of Cultural Assessment

Place of birth	Health beliefs and practice
Number of years in the United States	Who is the primary decision maker?
Primary and secondary language	View on death and dying
Religious practices	Role in the family

■ *What is it called when one practices patient-centered care while understanding the patient's needs from the patient's perspective?*
■ **Cultural competence**

Cultural competence is not knowing or having a complete understanding of all ethnic and cultural beliefs and world viewpoints but the ability to assess and determine the individual patient's beliefs and needs. Open-ended questions may assist with determining the person's beliefs that influence his or her understanding of their illness and health care.

> ❯ **HINT**
> Chaplains and social workers may also be resources to collaborate with to understand particular ethnic or cultural belief systems (Box 10.32). The custom in several cultures is for the family to be informed of the poor prognosis and allow the family to decide whether the patient should be told, whereas American health care providers put strong emphasis on patient's rights (Box 10.33).

Box 10.32 Challenges in the ICU

Cultural or religious diets	Self-inflicting injuries (i.e., rubbing coins on body to create welts)
Religious belief against use of blood transfusions	
Stoicism or vocal responses to pain	Sacred threads or jewelry
Particular practices involving end of life and death	Herbal or complementary treatments
Safety risks	Interpretation of eye contact
Patriarchal cultures and the Health Insurance Portability and Accountability Act (HIPAA) laws	Interpretation of touch or hands-on care
	Male nurses caring for female patients

Box 10.33 Examples of Potential Compromises With Cultural Beliefs

Challenges	Potential Remedies
Lighting candles under bed	Use of flashlights instead of candles
Belief that one should die facing east	Physically move bed to accommodate belief
Sacred threads on wrist	Tape to avoid need to remove before surgery

■ *What is it called when one believes that all Hispanic women are vocal when in pain?*
■ **Stereotyping**

Stereotyping is making the assumption that everyone within a certain ethnic background or culture will have the same beliefs and reactions to certain situations. There is a difference between stereotyping and generalization. Generalization is the recognition of a cultural pattern (i.e., Hispanic women are vocal when in pain) that requires follow-up to assess whether this individual follows that pattern. Generalization is a starting point and can benefit the care provided to the patient and family. Stereotyping, on the other hand, can lead to undue stress, decreased quality of care for patients and their families, and should be avoided. Stereotyping could lead to undertreating pain in Hispanic women. Individual assessment of a typical pain response will avoid overgeneralization based on culture.

> ❯ HINT
> Be aware of beliefs and differences in cultures but ensure individualized assessment and care.

■ **What is frequently a significant barrier between different ethnic backgrounds?**

■ **Language**

Frequently, language is a significant barrier between health care providers and patients of a different ethnic background. Patients may be relatively new to America and speak very little English. Using medical interpreters will facilitate communication and improve a trusting relationship. Children of the patient may be more fluent in English but should not be used as an interpreter in the health care setting. Exposure of the child to sensitive health care information and role reversal can cause undue stress and adverse effects. Other concerns are the accuracy of the interpretation, especially the medical terminology, competency, and potential conflict of interest that may exist. Competent translators require knowledge of two different languages, medical terminology, and maintain ethical and professional practice standards.

> ❯ HINT
> Provide written patient education materials in other languages besides English.

■ **A Spanish-speaking patient is scheduled for surgery in the morning. What would be an important step in obtaining a signed consent for surgery?**

■ **Use hospital translator**

It is recommended that an interpreter be used when obtaining signed consent forms from a patient or family member with limited or no English-language abilities. Consent forms can be translated into multiple languages, but an interpreter should still be used to assist with obtaining a signed consent, assess the patient's understanding, and assist in translating questions that the patient may have regarding the procedure. Cultural beliefs may impact their understanding of the procedure and the use of a translator allows for facilitation of dialogue between the patient and health care providers, and allows for patient/family to ask questions and express concerns about the scheduled surgery or procedure (Box 10.34).

> ❯ HINT
> Nurses need to know how to access language services in their hospital. This may be an in-house person or via telephone or video. Remember

deaf and hearing-impaired patients or family members may require sign-language interpreters.

Box 10.34 Strategies When Using Translator

Provide background information to translator before session	Avoid medical jargon
Explain purpose of session to translator	Look directly at the patient/family and not at the interpreter
If possible, have interpreter talk to patient/family before session begins	Observe patient's/family's facial expressions and body language (nonverbal language) in response to the discussion
Develops a trusting relationship	
Able to determine individual beliefs, not stereotyping	Be patient
Speak in shorter sentences and avoid long explanations	Have family repeat back to the interpreter to verify understanding

■ *Besides language interpretation, what else may translators be able to assist with?*

■ **Understanding cultural beliefs**

Different cultures have different rules of behavior. Interpreters fluent in the language are frequently from the same cultural background and can function as a cultural broker as well as perform interpretation. Cultural brokers are a resource when patient's cultural beliefs affect patient care. Hospitals are increasingly being staffed by people from different countries with diverse cultural backgrounds. These health care providers can also function in the role of a cultural broker.

> ❯ HINT
>
> These cultural differences in health care providers, however, can also create conflict and misunderstanding, which can result in tension among the staff and affect patient care.

■ *A septic patient is of the belief that he is ill because his soul was stolen and he wants a shaman to come in to find the soul. Should he receive antibiotics, the shaman, or both?*

■ **Both**

The mind is very powerful and can help heal the body. If the patient's belief is that the soul is stolen and he will not get better until it is recovered, he may not get better with medical management alone. The treatment of allowing the shaman to find the patient's soul will benefit the patient along with the antibiotics. Treatment should be appropriate to etiology and benefit the patient by treating his beliefs. The nurse needs to increase the effort of understanding how the patient views the illness, allowing interventions to be tailored to those beliefs.

> ❯ HINT
>
> Do not allow ethnocentrism to interfere with caring for a patient. Who knows which belief is either right or wrong?

FACILITATION OF LEARNING

■ *When teaching a patient or family member, what should be avoided or used sparingly?*

■ **Medical terminology**

Avoid or limit the use medical terminology. Health care providers are perceived as "speaking a different language." Physicians tend to either use short answers or answers full of medical terminology and nurses frequently adopt the role of "interpreter." Nurses should regularly attend patient/physician conferences or rounds to assist with interpretation and clarification. Plain language should be used in both verbal and written information provided for the patient and family.

> **〉 HINT**
> Families are more likely to ask questions of the nurses than the physicians.

■ *When assessing learning needs of a patient in the ICU, what is an important factor to determine?*

■ **Readiness or ability to learn**

In critically ill patients, a significant component of the learning assessment is to determine whether the patient is ready and able to learn. If sedated and ventilated or unable to respond, they may not be ready for learning. Families, however, may become the focus of the education in the ICU (Box 10.35).

Box 10.35 Assessment Components of Patient/Family Education

Who needs to be taught?	Health literacy
What needs to be taught?	Identify factors that may impede learning
How does it need to be taught?	Identify interventions to address these factors
Readiness to learn	

> **〉 HINT**
> Health literacy is a common issue that impedes learning. Written material is more effective if written at sixth- to eighth-grade levels.

■ *When teaching, should basic information be provided first or should the more pertinent complex information be provided at once?*

■ **Basic information**

Knowledge expands on basic understanding and previous knowledge. Teaching or development of learning materials should be organized from basic to complex information. The simple ideas and understandings are introduced first, followed by more complex or harder concepts. Teaching a complex motor skill is facilitated by taking the total skill and breaking it down into simple steps.

> **〉 HINT**
> It takes practice to become proficient at performing skills.

■ **What is the primary principle of an adult learner that needs to be considered when teaching patients or family in the ICU?**
■ **Need to know**

Adults need to know why it is important to learn something new. If the knowledge is perceived as important, greater effort will be committed to learning it. The learner needs to be aware of his or her deficiencies in knowledge. Adults are also self-directed learners and are responsible for their own decisions regarding learning (Box 10.36).

Box 10.36 Principles of the Adult Learner

Need to know	Orientation to learning
Self-directed	Internal motivation to learn
Influence of learner's life experience	Use active participation in learning
Progress from known to unknown	Require reinforcement of behavior
Readiness to learn	

> **HINT**
Life experiences shape values, beliefs, and attitudes that influence learning.

■ **What are the two important aspects for providing education to patient and families?**
■ **Simplicity and reinforcement**

Keeping instruction and education simple with minimal medical jargon facilitates understanding and learning. A good technique is to begin teaching sessions with open-ended questions used to evaluate current level of understanding. Medical topics can be complex and intimidating to teach. Keeping it simple can assist the teacher and learner with difficult topics. Choose three or four essential concepts of a given topic to teach. Reinforcement is the concept of repeating the information multiple times during the session. Provide written material to reinforce learning sessions.

> **HINT**
Frequently, informal teaching at the bedside is the best opportunity to provide education ("teachable moments"). Patient care and patient education are inseparable.

■ **What frequently interferes with the ability of a patient and family to concentrate and learn?**
■ **Anxiety and stress**

Anxiety can markedly decrease the ability of the patient or family to concentrate and learn. Frequently, family members repeat questions even after answers and explanations are provided, due to stress and anxiety. This affects their readiness to learn (Box 10.37).

Box 10.37 Barriers to Learning

Stress or anxiety	Presence of pain
Lack of support systems	Literacy and health literacy
Lack of time	Language barriers
Lack of confidence by nurse	Cultural differences
Lack of motivation by patient/family	

■ *What can the ICU nurse do to facilitate the transfer of the patient from the ICU to a lower acuity area?*

■ **Education**

Critical care nurses need to prepare the patient and family for the eventual transfer from the ICU to a lower acuity area. This is a milestone in recovery but may be viewed by the patient or family as being stressful. They may experience relief and joy about the transfer if they believe the patient has improved but if they believe the patient still requires close monitoring, the transfer may trigger fear of an inadequate level of monitoring. This may produce resistance to the transfer by family. The patient and family will experience less stress if the ICU nurse has spent time educating them about the step-down or floor routines, staffing patterns, and visiting hours. Reassure the patient and family of the competency of the nurses even if the level of monitoring has changed.

> **HINT**
> Acknowledge the anxiety of the transfer and emphasize the transition is a positive sign of recovery.

■ *What should occur after the patient or family is taught a new concept or medication?*

■ **Evaluation of learning**

Evaluation of learning is important in determining the effectiveness of the education. Evaluating learning can indicate need for further reinforcement of key concepts. Questions to the learner regarding the information reviewed provides immediate feedback as to the effectiveness of the instruction. When evaluating the learning of a motor task, use return demonstration.

CLINICAL INQUIRY

■ *What is it called when practice is based on the best available research data from well-designed studies?*

■ **Evidence-based practice (EBP)**

EBP is the use of the best available research data to guide practice and develop guidelines. EBP uses one's expert level of knowledge and experience to apply the data to clinical situations. Patient's and family's preferences are combined with this knowledge to individualize the plan of care. EBP optimizes patient's outcomes and assists nurses with keeping up with frequent changes in health care. EBP demonstrates a change from the historical practice based on authoritative opinions to emphasize findings from research and studies (Boxes 10.38 and 10.39).

> **HINT**

Use of protocols, clinical pathways, and algorithms facilitate incorporating EBP to the bedside. Review the "Practice Alerts" posted on the AACN website for EBP recommendations by the AACN.

Box 10.38 Barriers to Implementation of EBP

Lack of knowledge	Changing behavior met with resistance
Inability to understand statistical analysis	Change is a slow process
Lack of time	Lack of management commitment
Heavy patient assignments	Lack of organizational support
Lack of skills/resources	Large amounts of research and data available

Box 10.39 Research Terminologies

Qualitative	Research that seeks to provide understanding of human experience, perceptions, motivations, intentions, and behaviors based on description and observation
Quantitative	Traditional scientific methods, which generate numerical data and usually seek to establish causal relationships between two or more variables, using statistical methods to test the strength and significance of the relationships
Randomized controlled trials (RCTs)	Prospective, randomized, experimental studies using control groups
Meta-analysis RCT	Summary of relevant RCT

> **HINT**

Randomized controlled trials (RCTs) are considered the most reliable form of evidence. RCTs and meta-analysis of RCTs are considered level I evidence (the highest).

- **What is the first step to using EBP in the hospital?**
- **Identify knowledge gaps**

Knowing that there is a knowledge gap between research and actual practice is the first step in initiating change based on EBP. Critical and continuous evaluation of practice is the best opportunity to identify gaps or needed changes in practice (Box 10.40).

Box 10.40 Steps to Evidence-Based Practice

Identify knowledge gap	Determine validity of research study
Formulate questions	Apply research findings to patient care
Conduct literature searches	Appropriately involve patient in decision making

> **HINT**

EBP training can benefit nurse's competency in initiating EBP and increase participation in EBP activities.

■ *What framework can be used when a nurse performs a clinical inquiry on a clinical practice issue?*

■ **Patient, intervention, comparison, outcome (PICO)**

The PICO framework assists the nurse in formulating the question regarding the clinical practice issue. Some clinical questions may be simple, whereas others are more complex. Once the question is formulated, then the next step is to review the literature (Box 10.41).

Box 10.41 PICO

PICO	Example
P = Patient/Population/Disease	Patients ready to be weaned from ventilator
I = Intervention	Pressure support
C = Comparison	Other weaning methods: continuous positive airway pressure (CPAP), flow-by, synchronized intermittent mandatory ventilation (SIMV)
O = Outcome	Safety, effectiveness, and number of ventilator days

> **HINT**
> PICO may be used as a first step to assist with literature review (Box 10.42).

Box 10.42 Steps of Clinical Inquiry

Identify the knowledge gap	Determine how findings relate to practice
Formulate the question	Apply the findings in practice
Review literature	Evaluate the change in practice (i.e., outcomes, compliance)

■ *What are patient-centered, multidisciplinary plans of care that use EBP?*

■ **Clinical practice guidelines (CPG)**

CPGs are patient-centered, multidisciplinary, multidimensional plans of care that help the health care team to move toward EBP and improve the process of how care is delivered. It involves collaborative practice groups working with developing CPG (Box 10.43).

> **HINT**
> Clinical interventions must be based on strong evidence demonstrating improved outcomes or benefit to the patient.

Box 10.43 Benefits of CPG

Improves practitioner accountability	More cost effective
Increases coordination of care	Greater ability to evaluate care is provided
Decreases unnecessary variations in practice	Improves transition through health care settings
Improves quality of care	

■ *What is the tool used in the clinical setting that guides care in a specific clinical problem?*
■ **Clinical pathway**

Clinical pathways (also called critical pathways or clinical maps) are document-based tools that provide a link between evidence and practice. They are structured, multidisciplinary plans of care that detail essential steps and provide a timeline. They detail the steps in the course of treatment (algorithms, protocols) and evaluate variances from the pathway. A variance is an omission of an action, an inappropriate action, or an action that did not occur according to the timeline (usually late). Clinical pathways may be better suited for patients who are more predictable.

> ❯ **HINT**
> Critical areas of the clinical pathway can be highlighted to guide nurses in the important steps found to improve outcomes (Box 10.44). Reviewing the variance record can be used to improve the quality of care, make changes in practice to improve outcomes, and provide a means of continuous quality improvement.

Box 10.44 Components of Clinical Pathway

Timeline
Steps of care or interventions
Intermediate and long-term goals
Variance record

■ *What is a common goal when using EBP medicine?*
■ **Quality improvement**

EBP, CPG, and clinical pathways all strive to improve patient outcomes and maximize clinical efficiency. They also help to reduce variance in care by promoting standardization and provide care according to accepted standards of care.

> ❯ **HINT**
> Remember, guidelines are guidelines and should not be viewed as "prescriptive" but can be overridden by good clinical judgment.

BIBLIOGRAPHY

AACN Certification Corporation, The AACN Synergy Model of Patient Care (www.certcorp.org)

American Association of Critical Care Nurses (AACN). (2005). Standards for establishing and sustaining healthy work environments. Retrieved from http://www.aacn.org

American Association of Critical Care Nurses Certification Corporation: General information regarding certification. Retrieved from www.certcorp.org

Becker et al. (2006). Activities Performed by Acute and Critical Care Advanced Practice Nurses: American Association of Critical Care Nurses Study of Practice, *American Journal of Critical Care. 15*, 131–133, The American Association of Critical Care Nurses.

Wilson-Stronks., A., & Glavez, E. (2007). *Hospitals, language and culture: A snapshot of the nation.* Washington, DC: The Joint Commission.

Questions

1. During a discussion with the physician regarding an order for the patient, the focus of the skilled communication for the nurse is to

   A. Agree with the physician to avoid a disagreement
   B. Threaten to initiate the chain of command
   C. Advocate only for the patient
   D. Find a solution that achieves the desirable outcome for the patient

2. Patient C has been in the ICU for 5 days following a drug overdose. The patient is not responding, exhibits no reflexes but does overbreathe on the ventilator. The physician is continuing to order hemodialysis daily to treat the metabolic acidosis. The nurse caring for the patient is frustrated and believes that the physician should talk to the family regarding a DNR status. Which of the following is the most correct statement?

   A. The nurse is correct and needs to initiate the conversation with the family
   B. The nurse is experiencing moral distress
   C. The physician is the final decision maker regarding medical interventions
   D. This situation should be immediately brought to the ethics committee for review

3. A nurse, being a moral agent, should emphasize which of the following principles?

   A. Natural law
   B. Justice
   C. Paternalism
   D. Autonomy

4. Patient M is 2 days post–cardiac surgery. He is extubated, weaned off all vasoactive infusions, and has adequate pain control. Mr. M is being assessed for transfer to the progressive care unit. It has been noted that no family has been in to see him following the surgery. He is awake and alert and has been following commands. Which of the following characteristics is the primary concern of the nurse caring for this patient at this time?

   A. Vulnerability
   B. Complexity
   C. Participation in care
   D. Resource availability

5. A nurse, working with the family of a patient in a coma due to intracranial hemorrhage, approaches the family regarding end of life and removal of life support. The family refuses to terminate life support even with the presence of a living will in which the patient stated that the patient did not want to live on life support. Which of the following ethical principles is commonly used to justify removal of life support in terminally ill patients?

   A. Beneficence
   B. Paternalism
   C. Justice
   D. Deontology

6. In the admission assessment an ICU nurse determines that the patient does not have a durable power of attorney for health care decisions. Which of the following actions by the nurse would demonstrate that the nurse is being a moral agent for the patient?

   A. Flag the chart for the physician to talk to the patient about a power of attorney
   B. Respect the patient's wishes not to talk about death
   C. Tell the patient it is required by law to have a power of attorney
   D. Initiate the discussion with the patient regarding power of attorney

7. A patient in the ICU is agitated and pulling on lines. Which of the following would be the most appropriate intervention?

   A. Dim the lights and limit loud conversations around the patient
   B. Restrain the patient to prevent self-injury
   C. Administer sedation to decrease the agitation
   D. Ask the family members not to visit the patient because of the agitation

8. A patient is admitted to the ICU following a motor vehicle collision (MVC). The patient is unresponsive and on a mechanical ventilator. The family has expressed a need to stay with the patient or remain in the waiting room 24 hours a day to be available for their loved one at all times. Which of the following would be the best response by the ICU nurse?

   A. Reassure the family that the physician is the best and their loved one will be okay
   B. Tell the family there is nothing they can do to help and should not remain in the waiting room all day
   C. Explain to the family that they also need to get rest to be more prepared for when their loved one may require more of their care
   D. Encourage the family member to stay with the patient 24 hours a day

9. A patient from India is in the ICU following a diabetic ketoacidosis (DKA) crisis due to newly diagnosed diabetes. The family wants to bring food to the patient but it does not meet the prescribed diet for diabetes. What is the best intervention by the nurse?

   A. Inform the physician of the problem and set up a physician/family conference
   B. Allow the patient to eat the food they bring to encourage autonomy
   C. Teach the family about diabetic diet and determine what might be appropriate for the patient to eat
   D. Tell the family the patient can only eat the food provided by the hospital

10. A Hispanic woman in the ICU requires immediate surgery and the physician states that he will be there shortly to obtain the consent from the patient. Being aware of cultural differences, the nurse knows Hispanic women typically view their husbands as the decision maker. Which of the following would be the most appropriate intervention?

    A. Call the husband to come to the ICU to meet with the physician and his wife
    B. Encourage the patient to make her own decisions
    C. Suggest the physician use a two-doctor signature for the consent form
    D. Delay the surgery until the conflict can be resolved

11. A Japanese male is in the ICU following stroke. It is noted by the nursing staff that his wife is very involved in the patient's care and is not encouraging the patient to do things for himself. On assessment, the nurse discovers that the patient does not value independence but is of the belief that his wife should take care of him. Which of the following is the most appropriate intervention?

    A. Discuss the issues of the need for independence and self-care with the wife
    B. Allow the wife to continue to care for the patient
    C. Ask the wife to limit her visits until the patient has recovered and ready to be transferred
    D. Notify the physician and set up a physician/family conference

12. A female patient from Saudi Arabia is admitted for acute coronary syndrome. Her husband has accompanied her to the ICU and is upset because a male nurse is attempting to perform an assessment. Which of the following is the most appropriate response to the situation?

    A. Explain to the husband that the male nurse is a professional and it is his assignment
    B. Call security to de-escalate the situation
    C. Ask the husband to leave the room while the assessment is being performed
    D. Change the assignment to a female nurse to accommodate the husband's wishes

13. A patient is brought to the ICU following an MVC. He is requiring a second emergency surgery and a consent form needs to be obtained. His wife has limited English knowledge but their 15-year-old son speaks fluent English. Which of the following is the most appropriate action?

    A. Allow the son to translate to obtain the consent
    B. Ask other nurses in the ICU whether they speak the language and could help with the interpretation
    C. Use the telephone translator services to obtain the consent
    D. Leave it to the physician to obtain the consent

14. A patient is ready to be transferred to the floor. She has a history of cardiovascular disease. The patient does not exercise and eats unhealthy food. Which of the following would be the best focus for patient education at this time using the holistic nursing approach?

    A. Harmful effects of alcohol
    B. Smoking cessation
    C. Family support groups
    D. Lifestyle changes

15. Allowing a patient to make decisions will assist with providing control back to the patient and lowering anxiety. Which of the following would be an appropriate decision to assist with preventing loss of self-control?

    A. Whether the patient wants to be turned or remain supine
    B. Which of the family members can visit and for how long

C. Whether the patient wants an IV or not

D. Whether the patient wants to remain in the ICU or transfer to the progressive care unit

16. A family arrives in the ICU to see their loved one for the first time. They are asking questions and becoming more agitated. Which of the following best explains the behavior of this family?

A. Feelings of helplessness

B. Guilt feelings

C. Poor coping skills

D. Denial

17. Which of the following is the primary goal of implementing evidence-based practice (EBP) into the clinical setting?

A. Decreases nursing time required at the bedside

B. Facilitates communication between physicians

C. Improves patient care and outcomes

D. Provides patients with a plan of care

18. Which of the following is an important step in providing family-oriented care in the ICU?

A. Written information regarding expectations in the ICU

B. Open visitation policy

C. Encourage patients to become involved in self-care

D. Allow autonomy of the patient

19. Which of the following would be considered an environmental hazard in the ICU?

A. Visiting family

B. Noise

C. Cardiac monitor

D. IV infusions

20. A patient has been noted to have problems sleeping at night in the ICU. Which of the following nursing interventions would be most beneficial for the patient to assist with sleeping at night?

A. Administer sedative at 10:00 p.m.

B. Turn television on for background noise

C. No visitors after 8:00 p.m.

D. A 5-minute back rub

21. An intubated patient is attempting to communicate with the nurse. He is becoming frustrated. Which of the following would be the best response by the nurse?

A. Reassure the patient that this is a short-term problem

B. Administer sedation to calm the patient

C. Use a communication board to facilitate communication

D. Explain the difficulty of lip reading to the patient

22. A patient is scheduled for a surgery in the morning. The patient has been "acting out" all day and is becoming hostile. Which of the following would be the most appropriate response by the nurse?

    A. "I will have to restrain you if you continue being so hostile."
    B. "The physician will be in soon, so you need to be calmer to talk with him."
    C. "What are you feeling right now?"
    D. "Tell me why you are so angry."

23. A group of night nurses have noticed that lab draws ordered for 2:00 a.m. interrupts sleep patterns. Which is the best strategy for addressing this issue?

    A. Refuse to obtain routine labs at 2:00 a.m.
    B. Assemble a work group to research best practice and determine the best policy
    C. Perform a survey of nursing opinions regarding the current policy
    D. Request physicians to develop a committee to address the problem

24. A patient experiences a near-death experience and wants to talk to the nurse about the experience. What is the best response by the nurse?

    A. Encourage the patient to talk about her experiences and listen actively
    B. Explain to the patient the hallucinations are due to the pain medications
    C. Reorient the patient to the actual events of the resuscitation
    D. Tell the patient it is important to talk to her family about the issue

25. A preceptor observes that the new orientee is performing a task using a different method than the preceptor has used. What is the appropriate response by the preceptor?

    A. Tell the orientee he is doing it incorrectly and needs to perform the task as taught by the preceptor
    B. Survey other nurses in the unit on their method of performing the task
    C. Perform a literature review to determine whether the orientee's method is appropriate
    D. Ignore the difference and assume the orientee is aware of the correct method

26. During visitation, the nurse observes the wife of the patient is just standing at the patient's bed. She is not talking to him or touching him. What would be the most appropriate response by the nurse?

    A. Recognize the wife's discomfort and do not force her to touch the patient
    B. Encourage the wife to touch the patient and talk to him
    C. Notify the physician of a potential conflict of interest with the wife
    D. Ask the physician for a psychological consult to work with the wife

27. What has been found to be the most common reason for a medication or treatment error?

    A. New drugs
    B. Inadequate resource available to nurses
    C. Lack of knowledge
    D. Communication problem

28. Laughter has been found to have which positive effect?

A. Improve patient's spirituality
B. Lower risk of strokes
C. Decrease pain
D. Reorient patient

29. While teaching the patient, the nurse uses a real or simulated example to demonstrate the importance of the lesson. This is using which of the following adult learning principles?

A. Need to know
B. Learner's self-concept
C. Internal motivation to learn
D. Life experiences

30. Following a hemorrhagic stroke, a patient is unresponsive and has a poor prognosis. A family conference is scheduled to talk about end-of-life care. Which of the following is the most appropriate response of the nurse to the family?

A. Your loved one may improve, don't give up hope. You never know, he may respond.
B. Your loved one has no chance of survival and we need to stop providing him care at this time.
C. Everything will be fine with your loved one. We just need to talk about your feelings and wishes at this time.
D. Your loved one has a severe injury and has a very low chance of survival. At this time, we can provide him comfort and pain management to help him at the end of life.

31. To help a patient develop a sense of self-control, which of the following would be the best intervention?

A. Offer choices to the patient as much as possible
B. Explain the rules of the ICU
C. Ask the patient how he or she feels about being in the ICU
D. Ask the family to stay with the patient and provide emotional support

32. Which of the following is the most effective method to establish learning needs of a family member?

A. Literacy assessment to determine level of education
B. Informal assessment with open-ended questions
C. Formal assessment tools with questions about health beliefs and learning styles
D. In-depth interview to determine learning styles

33. The ICU nurse provides information to the family regarding anticoagulation therapy, including indications and complications. Which of the following would ensure that the family member understands the education about anticoagulation therapy?

A. Determine the family member has a college degree
B. Observe the family looking through the educational material

    C. Ask the family member to explain to you the purpose and complications of antico-
       agulation therapy

    D. Provide written information at the fifth-grade reading level to the family member

34. While teaching the patient to perform a dressing change, which of the following evaluations will determine the effectiveness of the learning?

    A. Do not ask for a demonstration if it embarrasses the patient

    B. Patient states the steps of performing a dressing change

    C. Patient states his wife can do the dressing change

    D. Patient demonstrates critical elements of the dressing change

35. A family is requesting to stay at the bedside during resuscitation of their loved one.
Which of the following is a benefit of family presence during resuscitation?

    A. Family member will see that everything was done for their loved one

    B. Staff will try harder to resuscitate the patient

    C. Resuscitation time will be shorter with the family member present

    D. Physician will interact with staff better during the resuscitation

36. Which of the following is a component of family-oriented palliative care after the death
of the patient?

    A. Preparing the body

    B. Funeral arrangements

    C. Bereavement care

    D. Family conferences

37. During a family conference, which of the following statements is the best way to introduce bad news and the poor prognosis to the family?

    A. "Your sister has a very poor prognosis, do you want us to do everything for her?"

    B. "Your sister's blood pressure is a problem. It is very low and she is already on the
       maximal amount of support but it is still low."

    C. "What are your feelings about removing life support?"

    D. "We would like to call the organ donation team to come evaluate your sister for
       organ retrieval."

38. At the end of life, pain management is an important aspect of patient care. The principle of double effect typically refers to which of the following situations?

    A. Disagreement between family members in regards to removal of life support

    B. Stopping tube feeds but maintaining IV hydration

    C. Removal of life support even if the patient is awake

    D. Administration of opioids for pain even though they may cause respiratory
       depression

39. A physician orders a medication that the ICU nurse feels may be contraindicated.
Which of the following would be the most appropriate initial action of the nurse?

    A. Refuse to administer the medication

    B. Notify the charge nurse and supervisor of the order

C. Call and discuss the medication order with the ordering physician

D. Administer the medication as ordered

40. Orders have been received to get a bariatric patient out of bed and sitting in a chair. The patient weights 450 pounds. The chair in the ICU for patients has a weight limit of 400 pounds. Which of the following would be the most appropriate response by the nurse?

A. Discuss purchasing chairs for bariatric patients with the management

B. Obtain an order to get a specialty bed company to bring a bariatric chair

C. Refuse to get the patient out of bed because of the weight of the patient

D. Use the chair available since there is only a 50-pound difference

Adult CCRN® Review Answers and Rationale

CHAPTER 1. CARDIOVASCULAR SYSTEM REVIEW

1. C

Right precordial leads aid in the diagnosis of RV involvement. Elevation of the V_{3R} and V_{4R} would indicate an RV MI. Extending the left precordial chest leads assists with the diagnosis of a posterior–lateral MI, and posterior leads may be used to diagnose a posterior wall MI. Measurement of QTc interval is important in critically ill patients, not just inferior wall MI patients.

2. A

Troponin levels can elevate in conditions other than acute MIs. Acute cardiomyopathy can elevate troponin levels and could account for the patient's syncopal episode. Sepsis has also been reported to elevate troponin levels indicating myocardial dysfunction and poor outcome, but would not fit this scenario, nor would the cardiomyopathy. Scleroderma and glioblastoma (brain tumor) do not typically elevate troponin levels.

3. B

Brugada's syndrome is a condition that causes disruption of the heart's normal rhythm. Specifically, this disorder can lead to uncoordinated electrical activity, ventricular arrhythmias, and ST-segment elevation that mimics STEMI. If untreated, the irregular heartbeats can cause syncope, seizures, difficulty breathing, or sudden death. These complications typically occur when an affected person is resting or asleep. Hypothermia, dilated cardiomyopathy, and mitral regurgitation do not typically elevate the ST segment.

4. A

BMS and DES coronary artery stents are both used in PCI for a variety of indications, including stable and unstable angina, acute MI, and multiple-vessel disease. But BMS is indicated in patients who are scheduled or who need elective noncardiac surgical procedures soon after stent placement, or in patients with bleeding disorders. BMS requires a minimum of 4 to 6 weeks of antiplatelet therapy, whereas DES requires a minimum of 12 months. The patient in this question is not experiencing a STEMI so he does not require thrombolytic therapy. There is no indication for a CABG. Uncomplicated two-vessel disease is managed with percutaneous coronary intervention (PCI).

5. B

Once proper lead placement has been determined, mark skin electrode placement with indelible ink. Do not alter the location of the skin electrodes during monitoring as this can create false-positive ST-segment changes. If the ECG patches were removed and not replaced in the same location following the bath, this might account for the increase in ST elevation. A 12-lead ECG may be obtained to verify the ST-segment elevation. The physician needs to be notified of the presence of a new ST-segment elevation but does not necessarily have to prepare for cardiac catheterization. It is not normal to have an increase in ST segment after stent placement, which can indicate a reinfarction. It is not appropriate at this time to ask the patient whether he wishes to be resuscitated.

6. **A**

Concurrent use of clopidogrel plus a PPI is associated with a significant increase in risk of an adverse cardiovascular event in patients with ACS. Calcium channel blockers, antihistamines, and β-blockers do not interfere with the efficacy of clopidogrel.

7. **B**

People with a reduced function CYP2C19 allele (may be as high as 30% of people) have significantly lower levels of the active metabolite of clopidogrel and less platelet inhibition from clopidogrel therapy. Restenosis is a risk after stent placement but is not considered a "very common" complication. The patient may have been noncompliant with taking home medications, but the CYP2C19 deficiency is a better answer without further information in the scenario regarding the patient's compliance. A CABG procedure is not required after a stent restenosis.

8. **A**

The use of a β-blocker in cardiogenic shock will worsen myocardial contractility, cardiac output, and hypotension. Patients with stable CHF have been shown to improve outcomes with β-blocker therapy following an ACS. Elderly patients are often managed with β-blocker therapy in the presence of cardiovascular disease. Chronic lung disease is not contraindicated if the patient is without active bronchospasm.

9. **C**

Inspra (eplerenone) is an aldosterone blocker. An aldosterone causes the reabsorption of sodium and the excretion of potassium. An aldosterone blocker causes loss of sodium and reabsorption of potassium. Close monitoring of potassium levels is required to prevent complications of hyperkalemia. Eplerenone should be held if the potassium levels are > 5.0 mEq/L.

10. **D**

RV infarction can be associated with an inferior wall MI. As the RV dilates, it bulges into the LV, compromising the filling and function of the LV. This results in decreased LV stroke volume and hypotension. CHF is LV failure causing pulmonary congestion and crackles on auscultation. A dilated cardiomyopathy may involve the LV and RV. Septal wall infarction results in changes in the anterior leads (V_1 and V_2).

11. **D**

NSAIDs can cause sodium retention and vasoconstriction. They can also lower the effectiveness and enhance renal toxicity of diuretics and ACE inhibitors. Antidepressants, anticonvulsants, and opioids are not contraindicated in patients with a history of CHF.

12. B

Creatinine should be < 2.5 mg/dL in men and < 2.0 mg/dL in women, and potassium should be < 5.0 mEq/L when administering an aldosterone antagonist. An aldosterone antagonist will cause the kidneys to hold on to the potassium and excrete sodium. Aldosterone antagonists may worsen renal failure in patients with elevated creatinine levels.

13. A

The prolonged QRS complex indicates abnormal cardiac conduction and may be causing dyssynchronous ventricular contraction. This may result in suboptimal ventricular filling and contraction. A low EF is a common finding caused by the dyssynchronization. Electrical activation of both the LV and RV in a synchronized manner can be accomplished with a biventricular pacemaker device. This is called cardiac resynchronization therapy.

14. D

The administration of a dual antiplatelet therapy prior to or during PCI is recommended. The combination of an ASA and a thienopyridine drug is commonly used. Prasugrel should not be given to a patient with a history of stroke. The combination of an ASA and clopidogrel can be administered though. Fondaparinux, as a sole anticoagulant, is not recommended to support primary PCI because of the higher risk of catheter thrombosis.

15. B

Captopril is an ACE inhibitor. Once a patient develops angioedema from an ACE inhibitor, it is contraindicated to further prescribe ACE inhibitors. Lisinopril is an ACE inhibitor. An ARB is the next class of drug that is used to manage HF in patients who are intolerant to ACE inhibitors. Losartan is an ARB. Eplerenone is an aldosterone blocker and is frequently used in addition to an ACE inhibitor and a β-blocker when a patient continues to have an EF ≤ 40%. Nesiritide is a BNP.

16. A

Pericardial tamponade is commonly caused by a penetrating trauma to the chest. A flail chest, bronchial tear, and an aortic dissection are caused by a blunt mechanism of injury. Patients with pericardial tamponade frequently insist on sitting bolt upright, become confused and agitated, and may demonstrate signs of air hunger. A flail chest may have signs of increase in work of breathing and paradoxical chest wall movement but not necessarily air hunger. A bronchial tear typically presents with unresolved pneumothorax and subcutaneous air. An aortic dissection causes hypotension and chest pain.

17. D

Ultrasonography is one of the most important tools used to assess pericardial tamponade. The FAST technique is a more rapid assessment performed at the bedside in patients with chest trauma and is used to assess for pericardial fluid. CXR is obtained in patients with chest trauma and may demonstrate a widened mediastinum, but its reliability is not as good as an ultrasonography. CT scan and MRI are not recommended initially to locate an injury because of the need to transport the patient, who may be unstable.

18. **A**

Increased central venous pressure will present as an increased jugular distention. The pressure surrounding the heart limits the ability of the ventricles to fill with blood, thus the pressure in the venous side elevates. Patients are typically agitated but this is not a component of the Beck's triad. Hypotension, not hypertension, is another sign of the Beck's triad. The heart sound changes are muffled heart sounds, not the development of a gallop.

19. **D**

The heart appears to "swing" in the pericardium with a pericardial tamponade and is considered a classic finding. An ultrasonography may also find pseudohypertrophy of the ventricle wall and collapsing of the ventricles during diastole. Pericardial tamponade does not cause a dilated ventricle, dyskinesia, or a new-onset mitral regurgitation.

20. **B**

The "swinging" of the heart in the pericardium following a pericardial tamponade produces the pulsus alternans found on the ECG and arterial waveforms. This is a phenomenon of alternating strong and weak beats. An auscultatory gap is frequently found in hypertensive patients. A Water Hammer's sign is found in aortic regurgitation patients, whereas a Levine's sign indicates chest pain caused by myocardial ischemia.

21. **D**

Avoiding intubation and positive pressure ventilation is recommended if possible. The positive pressure ventilation causes a decrease in venous return and worsens filling volumes of the ventricles. If intubation and ventilation may not be avoided, minimize the amount of PEEP utilized. BiPAP also increases positive pressure in the chest in turn affecting venous return.

22. **B**

Tachycardia is the most common arrhythmia following a myocardial contusion. The patient's identified injuries do not result in significant blood loss, so hypovolemic shock is not the highest suspicion. The patient does not have any signs of pericardial tamponade. Septic shock is not typically present on admission to the ICU following a trauma. There are no other signs for septic shock in this scenario.

23. **A**

The hint in this scenario is the widened mediastinum on CXR associated with a left hemothorax. Patients with a traumatic thoracic aortic injury may present with a cyclic hypotension, which responds to fluids. Myocardial contusion, pericardial tamponade, and tension pneumothorax can also cause hypotension but the scenario does not provide any other data leading to the other diagnoses.

24. B

Maintaining systolic BP less than 120 mmHg will lower the risk of rupture following an aortic injury. Administering large amounts of fluid or increasing venous return with the passive leg raise procedure may actually increase the risk of rupture of the aorta. Dopamine would increase BP and heart rate, thus increasing the risk of rupture of the aorta.

25. C

One of the causes of a restrictive cardiomyopathy is a history of mediastinal irradiation. The radiation treatment causes fibrosis of the myocardium and endocardium, slightly thickening the ventricle walls, and creating a noncompliance of the ventricle for filling. The high pressure in the ventricles creates a backward flow of blood and signs of LV dysfunction and pulmonary congestion.

26. D

A β-blocker is the first-line management of HF in hypertrophied cardiomyopathy, titrated to a heart rate of 60 to 65 bpm. This is used to treat angina or dyspnea. Verapamil (an L-type calcium channel blocker) may also be helpful but is typically used only if the β-blockade is not effective. Nifedipine or other dihydropyridine calcium channel blockers and digitalis in the absence of AF or any positive inotropes are all potentially harmful to patients with hypertrophic cardiomyopathy.

27. D

A hypertensive crisis includes both hypertensive emergencies and hypertensive urgencies. A hypertensive crisis is a systolic BP greater than 180 mmHg and/or a diastolic greater than 110 mmHg. But the BP range does not define whether it is a hypertensive emergency or a hypertensive urgency. The presence of organ dysfunction is used to define hypertensive emergency. The BP of a patient with hypertensive urgency is titrated down slower, over a 24- to 48-hour time period. The most common cause of hypertensive crisis, either urgency or emergency, is the history of chronic unmanageable hypertension.

28. B

A continuous infusion of esmolol would be the most appropriate order for a patient presenting with hypertensive crisis emergency. The IV continuous infusion route and titrating the dose to the goal BP is the most preferred method. Sublingual and oral route of administering nifedipine is potentially dangerous and should be avoided for hypertensive emergencies. ACE inhibitors and clonidine are long acting and poorly titratable, and so are not recommended for hypertensive emergencies. An ACE inhibitor may be used with hypertensive urgencies.

29. B

The metabolism of esmolol is by rapid hydrolysis of ester linkage by RBC esterases. It is not dependent on the liver to metabolize or on the kidneys to excrete the drug. It may be used in hepatic and renal dysfunction. The half-life is 10 to 20 minutes and can be administered IV or as a continuous infusion. It is a nonselective β-blocker, so it may lower the heart rate. It does not cause reflex tachycardia.

30. A

Fenoldopam is mixed in a solution containing metabisulfate and can cause an allergic reaction in patients with sulfite hypersensitivities.

31. D

Nicardipine, a calcium channel blocker, vasodilates the cerebral vasculature and is frequently used in neurological patients to control BP. Nipride may increase intra-cranial pressure and should be avoided in neurological patients with an increased risk of cerebral hypertension. Nitroglycerin reduces both preload and afterload and may compromise cerebral blood flow. Nimodipine is used to prevent ischemic injuries in vasospasms following a subarachnoid hemorrhage but is not indicated for treating acute hypertension.

32. B

Clevidipine, a calcium channel blocker, is a milky white, lipid emulsion. It is contrain-dicated in patients with allergies to soy products, eggs, and egg products, similar to Diprivan. Nimodipine and nicardipine are also calcium channel blockers but are not mixed in a lipid emulsion. Sodium nitroprusside is also not prepared in a lipid solution so an allergy to soy would not be contraindicated.

33. D

The initial treatment goal in hypertensive emergency is to reduce MAP by no more than 25% with a targeted systolic BP of 160 mmHg and a diastolic pressure of 100 mmHg. Aim for 25% reduction in mean arterial BP within minutes to 1 hour. Then, if the patient is stable, reduce BP to 160/100–110 mmHg over 2 to 6 hours and normal-ize within 24 to 48 hours. Exceptions include stroke (unless BP is lowered to allow thrombolytic agents to be used) and dissecting aortic aneurysm (target systolic BP is < 100 mmHg if possible).

34. D

Esmolol (Brevibloc) has a quick onset and a shorter duration, making the drug easily titratable. It also produces a slowing of the heart rate and contractility. This is beneficial in managing aortic dissections because the propagation of the dissection is dependent on both the BP and the velocity of LV ejection. Even though Nipride has a quick onset and a shorter duration (and has been used in thoracic dissections), it is a direct vasodi-lator, which results in reflex tachycardia and an increase in ejection velocity. If used, it should be in combination with a β-blocker. Hydralazine is longer acting with a half-life of up to 10 hours. It is not titratable and should be avoided to prevent a sudden and prolonged period of hypotension. Nicardipine also has a longer half-life (1 hour) and may not be as titratable as esmolol.

35. A

Perioperative β-blockers are the first-line drug for managing high-risk cardiac compli-cations. The target is to lower BP to within 20% of the patient's baseline pressure.

36. A

β-blockers should be avoided in acute cocaine toxicities. The drug of choice is an α-antagonist, which is a direct arterial vasodilator. This will lower BP first. Only after the α-blocker can a β-blocker be administered to assist with BP management, if needed.

37. C

β-blockers are negative chronotropic agents and are frequently used to manage mitral stenosis. The narrow orifice of the mitral valve delays the filling time of the LV. Tachycardia can worsen symptoms of mitral stenosis. Administering agents that decrease heart rate will increase the filling time and allow for more complete filling of the LV. Agents frequently include β-blockers and rate-control calcium channel blockers. Digitalis is not indicated unless there is RV or LV dysfunction. Although diuretics are used in patients with mitral stenosis, they manage pulmonary congestion. Alpha-antagonists should not be administered because of the side effect of reflex tachycardia.

38. B

The level of occlusion influences the symptoms of the patient. Femoropopliteal arterial obstruction results in the presence of a femoral pulse and diminished or absent pulses in the popliteal and distal arteries. Claudication is typically in the calf. Aortoiliac level of occlusion may result in buttock, thigh, or calf claudication and erectile dysfunction in men. In the more distal arteries, femoropopliteal pulses are present but the dorsalis pedis is weak to absent.

39. B

ABI is used to determine the severity of obstruction of flow in the lower extremities. It can be used to screen symptomatic patients before signs of limb ischemia occur. A normal ABI is 1.00 to 1.40. If greater than 1.40, it indicates that the artery is noncompressible. A lower ABI value indicates a more severe obstruction. An ABI of less than 0.40 is considered severe and often indicates a need for an intervention.

40. D

An arteriogram is recommended prior to angioplasty/stent intervention or bypass surgeries. Doppler ultrasonography is used to determine pressure gradients and may be used in the initial evaluation. This patient is admitted for an intervention. The physician is already aware of the severity of the obstruction. An arteriogram is needed at this time to evaluate the location of the obstruction. Cardiac catheterization is not required unless the patient presents with signs of CAD in addition to the claudication. This scenario did not provide any signs of CAD. MRI would not be helpful at this time.

41. C

Watershed strokes primarily occur during periods of hypoperfusion. A watershed area of the brain is between two major cerebral vascular territories. Surgeries using CPB may have hypoperfusion because of the nonpulsatile flow. Lacunar strokes are due to chronic hypertension damaging the smaller diameter vessels of the brain. Vasospasms of cerebral vessels occur after subarachnoid hemorrhages. Aneurysm ruptures are the most common cause of subarachnoid hemorrhage.

42. A

Phenylephrine is the only vasoconstrictor that is an α-agonist only. Because of the patient's history of hypertrophic cardiomyopathy, drugs that have β-agonist effects should be avoided. Norepinephrine, dopamine, and epinephrine all have both α- and β-agonist effects.

43. C

Epoprostenol is an inhaled prostacyclin that has been found to decrease pulmonary vascular resistance and lower the resistance of RV. Inhaled epoprostenol decreases mean pulmonary artery pressure but does not have the same effect on mean arterial BP. Nitroglycerin should be avoided in RV failure because of its venodilation effect. Venous pooling decreases RV preload and may worsen RV contractility. Nipride is an arterial and venous vasodilator that may worsen right HF. Nicardipine does not have significant vasodilation effects on the pulmonary vasculature.

44. C

Administration of recombinant factor VIIa has been used to manage refractory bleeding disorders, but there is a potential risk of arterial thromboembolic events.

45. A

A new RBBB after cardiac surgery is not uncommon and is usually temporary and of little clinical significance. Associated shifts of the axis are considered benign and usually do not require intervention. It does not indicate the need for external pacing or placement of a biventricular pacemaker.

45. B

ST elevation in two or more contiguous leads in the territory of the grafted artery indicates graft failure. ST-segment monitoring in the leads of the territory of the grafts is recommended to assess for this acute complication. ST elevation in all the leads would indicate pericardial inflammation or pericarditis. ST elevation in all the anterior leads may indicate LIMA spasm, if the LIMA was grafted to the LAD.

47. B

Repositioning a patient on her side after a cardiac surgery may cause drainage of a pre-existing collection of old blood that has pooled in the thoracic cavity. Old blood is of a darker color, whereas bright-red blood would indicate fresh bleeding. Continue monitoring the patient for any signs of hemodynamic instability. If it was fresh blood and especially preceded by hypertension, the correct answer would be to page the physician stat and be ready to take the patient back to the OR. Stripping mediastinal chest tubes would be indicated if there was a sudden cessation of output instead of an increased output.

48. D

The hint in this question is the administration of protamine. A sudden change in a patient's condition immediately following the administration of a drug should be closely looked at for the cause of the change. A protamine reaction causes pulmonary hypertension, hypoxia, and systemic hypotension. The other answers are potential complications but the information provided in the scenario did not lead toward the other answers.

49. C

A CXR can identify the types of leads, the number of leads, and their positions. The shape of the pacemaker and manufacturer can assist with further identifying the type of pacemaker. A 12-lead ECG or ECG monitoring can identify pacer spikes with P waves or QRS complexes (atrial or ventricular pacing) if pacing, but does not differentiate accurately between DDD and VVI or AAI. An echocardiogram is used to evaluate the mechanical response of the heart, not the electrical activity.

50. B

A patient with a second-degree Mobitz Type II heart block requires pacing below the level of the block. This patient currently has an atrial pacemaker (AAI). An external pacemaker should be applied and the patient must be prepared for replacement of the AAI with either a VVI or a DDD. A second-degree Mobitz Type I heart block would not require a pacemaker and would just be watched for any progression to a greater degree of heart block. Placing a magnet over the AAI pacemaker does not improve the situation of needing to pace below the level of the block.

51. A

A pacing threshold is the minimum electrical stimulus needed to consistently capture the heart outside of its own refractory period. Once the pacemaker and leads are implanted, there is a maturation process. Thresholds, initially following implant, are low. Within a week, the threshold peaks and becomes its highest. This is because of tissue reaction and edema. Once the tissue reaction diminishes, the threshold will decrease to a steady plateau, slightly higher than the original threshold but below the peak. Other problems, such as a fracture, kink, or loss of lead contact, can also interfere with the ability to capture, but the most likely cause is the normal process of lead maturation because of the timing of 1 week after placement.

52. B

The goal in managing a dissecting aorta is to lower BP and HR. Esmolol is a β-blocker; it will lower BP and decrease HR. Nipride is also an antihypertensive, but it will have a reflex tachycardia. This patient's HR is already at 108, so it needs to be lowered to 60 to 80 bpm before a vasodilator may be administered. Levophed is a vasoconstrictor and would be contraindicated in this patient. Dobutrex is an inotropic agent. Increasing myocardial contractility will increase the stress on the aortic wall and will potentially extend the dissection.

53. C

If VO_2 increases after there is an increase in supply, this indicates an oxygen debt. The DO_2 was not sufficient for the demands of the tissue, and the tissues were hypoperfused. This is an example of supply dependence (not independence). It does not indicate a miscalculation of either VO_2 or DO_2.

54. A

The patient is hypothermic with a temperature of 35.0°C. This can trigger the shivering reflex, which increases oxygen demand and consumption. A larger amount of oxygen consumed will decrease the amount returned to the right side of the heart, thus lowering SvO_2. Agitation, anemia, and hypoxia can also lower SvO_2, but in this case there was no clue to the presence of agitation and the patient had adequate hgb/hct and oxygenation.

55. B

In a hypotensive, cardiogenic shock patient, the first-line therapy is an inotropic agent. Dobutamine is typically the preferred inotrope over dopamine because of the potential vasoconstriction effects of dopamine. Even though the patient is hypotensive, vasoconstrictors are not typically used early because of high SVR associated with cardiogenic shock. The greater resistance on the heart results in a more severe LV failure. IABPs are frequently used in patients with hypotensive cardiogenic shock, but in this case, the patient was diagnosed with aortic insufficiency. IABP is contraindicated in aortic insufficiency.

56. C

The IABP is positioned in the aorta just proximal to the renal arteries. If the balloon migrates, it can cause obstruction of the renal arteries resulting in decreased urine output. A balloon rupture would have blood present in the balloon tubing. Timing issues of early inflation during systole would demonstrate a significant worsening of HF. The patient may still be hypoperfused and developing renal failure, but the potential complication of migration of the balloon should be first ruled out.

57. B

Passive raising of the legs has been proven clinically to act like a "self-volume challenge" to indicate the patient's status on the Frank–Starling curve. This determines the patient's responsiveness to fluids. It is not a direct measurement of preload (CVP and presence of hypovolemia). Jugular venous distention is determined with the patient's head of the bed elevated.

58. A

A Stage B classification for HF is structural heart disease but without signs or symptoms of HF. The drugs indicated include ACE inhibitors and/or β-blockers. Ramipril is an ACE inhibitor. Digoxin is not indicated in this patient because of an EF of 55%. Digoxin, Isordil, and Lasix are not usually indicated until at Class II HF (Stage C).

59. B

Hypertrophied cardiomyopathy is a cause of diastolic HF. Calcium channel blockers are typically prescribed to decrease myocardial contractility resulting in ventricular relaxation with improved filling of ventricles. Inotropic agents are contraindicated because they decrease the chamber size and further limit filling during diastole. Lasix would also not be indicated because of its effect on preload.

60. **C**

BNPs are like endogenous renin–angiotensin inhibitors released from overstretched ventricles during HF. BNPs increase glomerular filtration rates (GFRs), inhibit release of renin, decrease Na^{++} reabsorption, and increase blood flow to the kidneys. An increase in BNP levels indicates HF.

61. **D**

Hypertrophied cardiomyopathy has a normal to increased EF due to the thickened muscle. Contractility is not a problem with a hypertrophied heart but it is filling the heart due to a small chamber size. The other cardiomyopathies result in a decrease in EF/CO/CI.

CHAPTER 2. PULMONARY SYSTEM REVIEW

1. **D**

Normally, as the minute ventilation (MV) increases, the $PaCO_2$ should decrease. The normal pattern is an inverse relationship. In dead space, the alveolar ventilation decreases even as the respiratory rate increases. This results in an increase in CO_2 and an abnormal relationship between MV and $PaCO_2$. The patient has respiratory acidosis, not metabolic acidosis. It is not a normal blood gas for a patient with COPD because the pH is abnormal. There is no indication in this scenario that this would be an upper airway obstruction.

2. **C**

VQ shunting is perfusion without ventilation. A compensatory mechanism for the VQ shunt is pulmonary vasoconstriction to redistribute blood flow to ventilated alveolar units. In VQ shunts, patients increase their respiratory rate, causing an increase in minute ventilation. Bronchoconstriction occurs with dead space in an attempt to shunt ventilation to perfused alveoli. An increase in cardiac output can occur in response to tissue hypoxia but is not considered a compensatory mechanism for a pulmonary shunt.

3. **A**

An obstructive airway disease causes a decrease in FEV1 with a relatively normal FVC resulting in a decrease in the FEV1/FVC ratio. A normal ratio is 75% to 80%. The lower the ratio, the greater the obstruction of airflow. This test is used to assess asthma patients during bronchodilator treatments. A normal FEV1/FVC ratio would indicate a restrictive airway disease.

4. **D**

To calculate, take the PaO_2 from the ABG and divide by the FiO_2 the patient was on when ABG was drawn. The PaO_2 of 82 divided by 0.4 equals 205.

5. **D**

According to the Berlin definition of ARDS, a PaO_2/FiO_2 ratio less than 100 is considered to be a severe oxygenation impairment. Moderate is 100 to 200 and mild is 200 to 300. Normal PaO_2 ratio is greater than 300.

6. **C**

Atelectrauma is injury caused by the repeated cycles of recruitment and derecruitment during mechanical ventilation of an ARDS patient. Barotrauma is injury to the lungs due to high ventilatory pressures, and volutrauma is caused by high volumes. Biotrauma is related to release of mediators in the lungs.

7. **A**

The inspiratory volume is determined by the preset inspiratory pressure limit. When the upper pressure limit is reached, the ventilator stops delivering the breath in a pressure-controlled mode. To increase the amount of volume delivered, the pressure limit would need to be increased. Increasing PEEP will improve the PaO_2/FiO_2 ratio and oxygenation. Decreasing respiratory rate will not increase the TV and would actually further decrease the minute ventilation. Decreasing flow rate will not increase TV and may worsen dyspnea.

8. **A**

In the APRV mode of ventilation, there are three ways to increase oxygenation. One is to increase the FiO_2. In this patient, the FiO_2 was already 100%. The other ways are to increase the high pressure (P high) or to prolong the time in high pressure (T high). This increases the mean airway pressure and oxygenation.

9. **D**

Frequency is measured in hertz (Hz) on an HFOV. By lowering the frequency, the tidal volumes increase, thus increasing the elimination of CO_2. Increasing the power would also be a change that can increase CO_2 elimination (not decreasing the power). Increasing the mPaw and FiO_2 affects the oxygenation, not CO_2 elimination.

10. **B**

A 2/4 twitch correlates to about 80% block of the neuromuscular junctions. A TOF of 4/4 twitches is 0% to 75%, 1/4 twitch at least 75% block, 3/4 twitches is 90%, and 0/4 twitches correlates to almost 100% block. Frequently, the TOF is ordered to maintain between 1 and 2 twitches.

11. **D**

Paradoxical breathing indicates diaphragmatic fatigue, impending ventilatory failure, and respiratory arrest. The patient requires ventilatory support at this time due to the ventilatory fatigue. Hypercapnia and sputum production occur chronically in a COPD patient and by themselves are not indications for ventilation. Inspiratory wheezing needs to be managed in a COPD patient but does not necessarily indicate the need for ventilation.

12. **C**

Oxygen should be administered to COPD patients to maintain oxygen saturation greater than 90% to 92% but with the lowest FiO_2 possible to reach the goals. High levels of FiO_2 can increase dead space and worsen hypercapnia.

13. **D**

Patients with COPD have chronic respiratory acidosis (hypercapnia) compensated with an elevation of bicarbonate levels. This corrects the pH to normal. A respiratory acidosis without a normal pH (acidosis) indicates an acute on chronic respiratory failure. The decision to intubate from an ABG is based on the pH, not the $PaCO_2$ levels. A $PaCO_2$ of 64 mmHg, PaO_2 of 60 mmHg, and saturation of 90% may be found on a chronic ABG without acute changes.

14. **B**

Auto-PEEP can develop in patients breathing at ventilator breath rates, especially on assist control (AC). Unexplained hypotension in a mechanically ventilated patient may indicate presence of auto-PEEP. The best treatment of auto-PEEP is to decrease the total inspiratory time, usually accomplished by decreasing the respiratory rate. In this situation, just decreasing the rate will not necessarily improve the auto-PEEP because the patient is breathing faster than the set rate. Sedation and neuromuscular blocking agents will decrease the spontaneous breaths with better control of the total minute ventilation. Decreasing the TV is effective but less efficient and, in this particular situation, it is not excessively high but the rate is the issue with the minute ventilation. Increasing the flow rate does not effectively decrease the inspiratory time unless set inappropriately to begin with.

15. **C**

The severity of the asthmatic attack is determined by the degree of dyspnea. A patient experiencing dyspnea that interferes with daily activities is considered a moderate severity and will usually be treated and sent home. A patient with such severe dyspnea that results in an inability to speak is considered life-threatening asthma and is more likely to be admitted to the ICU for monitoring and treatment. Wheezing may or may not be present in acute asthma and does not determine the severity. In fact, the absence of wheezing may indicate a "silent" chest and is considered life threatening. Corticosteroid treatment for airway inflammation can be prescribed on an outpatient basis with the oral route.

16. **D**

Administering an inhaled β_2 agonist to control the bronchospasm is the initial pharmacological management of a severe asthma attack. An inhaled anticholinergic may be used in combination with a β_2-selective agonist drug to improve responsiveness and outcomes but is not recommended as the first-line drug. Leukotriene receptor antagonist and Heliox are not recommended in the management of acute asthma.

17. **D**

A small pneumothorax (< 2 cm) in an asymptomatic patient may be observed unless on positive pressure ventilation. If the patient is on CPAP or mechanically ventilated, a chest tube would be indicated even in an asymptomatic patient with a small pneumothorax. The positive pressure can increase the size of the pneumothorax. If the pneumothorax is large (> 2 cm), a chest tube is indicated.

18. **D**

One of the clinical signs that the pneumothorax has resolved is the cessation of bubbling in the chest drainage system. A chest x-ray should be obtained to verify the reinflation of the lung. Intermittent bubbling indicates that the pneumothorax is still unresolved and that the chest tube system needs to remain in place. Subcutaneous emphysema does not determine the discontinuation of the chest tube system. A drainage tube placed for the purpose of a pneumothorax may not drain more than 50 mL in a 12-hour period but it does not indicate that the pneumothorax has resolved.

19. **B**

The minimal endotracheal tube cuff pressure recommended to prevent aspirations of secretions pooled above the cuff is 20 cm H_2O. Below 20 cm H_2O pressure aspiration of secretions is likely. The recommended cuff pressure is 20 to 30 cm H_2O. A pressure greater than 30 cm H_2O can increase the risk of trauma to the trachea and should be avoided.

20. **A**

Idiopathic pulmonary hypertension involves the precapillary pulmonary vasculature. This involves the pulmonary arterial system and is called PAH. Left ventricular failure, COPD, and PE involve both the precapillary and postcapillary pulmonary vasculature (arterial and venous circulation). PAH is a subcategory of pulmonary hypertension (PH).

21. **B**

Administration of a vasodilator to determine reactiveness in the pulmonary artery (vasodilator reactivity test) is performed on all PAH patients to determine whether long-term calcium channel blockers will benefit them. A decrease in mPAP by more than 10 mmHg or an absolute reduction of mPAP to less than 40 mmHg without decrease in cardiac output indicates responsiveness to arterial vasodilation. Fluid challenges and stress testing do not determine effectiveness of a calcium channel blocker in the long-term management of PAH.

22. **A**

The RSBI is used to predict success of weaning and extubation. It is calculated by dividing the respiratory rate by the TV. An RSBI of fewer than 80 bpm/L is predictive of successful weaning, between 80 and 100 predicts that the patient may or may not be ready, and more than 100 predicts unsuccessful weaning and extubation.

23. **B**

Initial interventions for the management of laryngospasm include turning the patient to a lateral position to drain secretions and administering 100% oxygen. Racemic epinephrine is administered to open the airway. If the patient continues to have airway difficulties, the option of administering a small dose of succinylcholine or reintubation is indicated. Heliox treatment is used primarily with airway edema but it can also be used in laryngospasms if the initial treatment fails.

24. **B**

The obstruction from the embolus induces a pressure load on the right ventricle (RV) resulting in RV decompensation and increased distensibility. This shifts the septal wall toward to the LV. The decrease in blood flow to the LV as a result of RV failure and the smaller LV chamber size due to the septal wall shift results in a decrease in LV filling or preload. A PE causes a decrease in the coronary perfusion gradient of the RV. The coronary perfusion gradient is calculated by taking the MAP minus the RV end-diastolic pressure (RVEDP). A decrease in MAP and an increase in RVEDP due to a PE can cause an ischemic injury of the RV.

25. **D**

Pulmonary embolism (PE) causes an obstruction in the lungs resulting in RV failure. This elevates the CVP. Less blood is going forward to the LV so the PAOP is normal to low. In pulmonary edema, both the CVP and PAOP are elevated. Atelectasis and pneumonia do not necessarily affect the preload of the RV or LV.

26. **A**

The $S_1Q_3T_3$ pattern is considered to be the classic ECG finding of cor pulmonale or a PE. Another common finding is the anterior T-wave inversion and has been found to correlate with severity.

27. **B**

Intracranial hemorrhage is an absolute contraindication to receiving anticoagulation or antithrombolytic therapy. Hypertension should be managed prior to initiation of anticoagulation therapy. Uncontrolled hypertension is a relative contraindication and can increase the risk of bleeding. Postoperative patients may receive anticoagulation therapy to prevent or manage a VTE unless actively bleeding or determined to be at a higher risk of bleeding. Anticoagulation therapy should be held at least 12 hours before or after placement of an epidural catheter.

28. **A**

In spontaneous ventilation, inspiration causes a negative pressure within the thoracic cavity. Stronger respiratory muscles will cause a greater negativity during initiation of a breath. The NIP is the maximal inspiratory pressure and is used to assess muscle strength. An NIP value of less than -20 to -25 cm H_2O is predictive for successful weaning. VC, MV, and spontaneous TV are weaning parameters and are used in determining the readiness of the patient for extubation but the answer that correlates best to respiratory muscle strength is the NIP.

29. **C**

The RSBI is a calculated number used to predict success of weaning. It is calculated by taking the respiratory rate (RR) and dividing it by the TV. A score of 80 or more predicts successful weaning, 80 to 100 means weaning may or may not be successful, and a score of 100 or more predicts weaning is unsuccessful. Even though this patient is determined to have an unsuccessful weaning at this time, it does not indicate the need for sedation and paralysis. This patient is not ready for immediate extubation.

30. **C**

The hint in this question is the patient is 24 hours post blunt chest trauma. Pulmonary contusions are a result of a blunt chest injury and typically become symptomatic within 24 to 48 hours. The presentation is very similar to ARDS but there is no sign of sepsis in the presentation of this patient. Volume overload during resuscitation can worsen pulmonary contusions, but again, there is no indication in this scenario of an aggressive resuscitation. Hospital-acquired pneumonia (HAP) does not present within 24 hours of hospitalization (considered to be HAP if it develops 48 hours after admission).

CHAPTER 3. ENDOCRINE SYSTEM REVIEW

1. **B**

Fluid administration is considered to be the first-line treatment in managing hyperglycemic emergencies (DKA, HHNS). Fluid is used to correct the significant water depletion that occurs with severe hyperglycemia and establishes reperfusion of the kidneys. The administration of fluid begins to correct the hyperglycemia and can decrease serum glucose concentrations by up to 50 mg/dL. Insulin replacement should be initiated after initial fluid resuscitation is given. Sodium bicarbonate is not usually recommended in the management of DKA/HHNS. Electrolyte replacement is a component of treatment but fluids are still initiated before Mg^+ replacement.

2. **D**

Initiation of insulin should be delayed until potassium is administered, if potassium levels are less than 3.5 mEq/L initially. Once potassium is above 3.5 mEq/L, IV fluids and insulin infusions may be initiated. Administration of insulin, either bolus or continuous infusion, will drive the potassium back into the cells causing an even greater decrease of potassium and an increase in arrhythmias.

3. **A**

DI is a neuroendocrine disorder that presents with large amounts of diuresis. It is caused by a lack of ADH either being produced from the hypothalamus or released from the pituitary. The diuresis results in hemoconcentration and hypernatremia. SIADH and CSWS both cause hyponatremia. DM does not necessarily affect sodium levels.

4. **B**

Hypoglycemia is the most significant complication of obtaining an intensive strict glycemic control of 80 to 110 mg/dL. Hypoglycemia can negatively affect outcomes and should also be avoided. American Association of Clinical Endocrinologists (AACE) and the American Diabetic Association (ADA) recommend IV insulin therapy in persistent hyperglycemia to be treated if greater than 180 mg/dL with a goal of maintain glucose between 140 and 180 mg/dL in most critically ill patients. This will help avoid the complication of hypoglycemia. The glucose level and amount of insulin required to lower glucose levels in stress-induced hyperglycemia does not typically result in cerebral edema. Hyponatremia is not a complication of insulin therapy. Hypokalemia, not hyperkalemia, may be a complication of insulin therapy.

5. **D**

Cognitive impairment is the symptom most commonly associated with hypoglycemia in critically ill patients. Hypoglycemia can also result in seizures and death. The subtle signs of hypoglycemia are not always recognized in the intensive care unit (ICU) setting and include fatigue, headache, and impaired judgment. Hypoglycemia may cause small tremors but not typically muscle twitching. SVT is not a commonly associated sign of hypoglycemia. The patient may develop sinus tachycardia but is typically not SVT.

6. **C**

Patients with noninsulin-dependent diabetes typically present with HHNS. They have minimal production of insulin, enough to control the ketones but not enough to control the glucose. Patients with NIDDM develop a hyperglycemic, hyperosmolar state without a significant increase in ketones and ketoacidosis. Patients with DKA become sicker sooner than those with HHNS because of the ketones. The osmolality level does not play a role in fatty acid oxidation and ketone production. The kidneys do not play a role in the prevention of ketoacidosis in patients with HHNS.

7. **C**

Both CSWS and SIADH cause hyponatremia (DI causes hypernatremia). In CSWS, the hyponatremia is caused by loss of sodium in the urine, whereas SIADH is dilutional sodium. In this scenario, the urine output is normal to high, serum osmolality is normal, and urine sodium is elevated. This indicates a loss of sodium, not dilutional sodium. DM can also produce a dilutional hyponatremia but serum glucose and serum osmolality are not elevated, as would be the case in DM.

8. **B**

Administration of a hypertonic solution too fast can cause a rapid shift in serum osmolality to a hyperosmolar state. This results in irreversible demyelination of the neurons in the brain, particularly in the pons. This is called central pontine myelinolysis (CPM). Fluid shifts into the vascular space when administering a hypertonic solution, not into the extravascular space, which would result in cerebral edema, ACS, or ARDS.

9. **D**

DI is associated with abnormally large urine output, typically more than 250 mL/hr; this commonly occurs in patients who are neurologically injured. DM can also cause a hyperglycemic diuresis, but the scenario does not have any information leading toward being concerned for significant hyperglycemia. Volume overload and over use of Lasix can also cause diuresis but fluid shifts tend to have a gradual increase in urine output (not sudden increase as in the question) and there is no indication that Lasix was given.

10. **B**

Patients with DI will lose large amounts of fluid with the diuresis. The urine is dilute and therefore would have low urine osmolality and specific gravity. Serum osmolality would be high with hypernatremia because of hemoconcentration.

CHAPTER 4. HEMATOLOGY/IMMUNOLOGY SYSTEM REVIEW

1. **D**

   LMWH does not typically require monitoring but in certain situations of increased risk or potential interference with the drug's effectiveness or risk of bleeding, an anti-Xa assay may be used to monitor LMWH. The aPTT and PT with INR does not alter with the administration of LMWH so is not be used to monitor effectiveness. Platelet aggregometry is used to monitor effectiveness of antiplatelet drugs.

2. **C**

   Vitamin K and FFP are used to reverse bleeding or potential bleeding complications with Coumadin. Protamine sulfate is used to reverse any adverse effects of heparin. Oral vitamin K may be used in patients with high INR but with no signs of bleeding. Signs of bleeding require vitamin K to be administered via IV for more rapid reversal. The oral route is slower but safer. The IV route, however, has a small risk of anaphylaxis.

3. **D**

   DIC is the only coagulopathy in which the patient clots first and then bleeds. The formation of clots in the microcirculation causes activation of the thrombolytic system and breakdown of the clots. The D-dimer measures the byproducts (fibrin degradation products) of the clot. There are multiple coagulopathies that can elevate aPTT and/or PT with INR. Fibrinogen levels can decrease in DIC, following massive blood transfusions.

4. **B**

   The hallmark sign of HIT is a significant decrease in platelet count (> 50%) over a 24-hour period without any other known causes for thrombocytopenia within 4 to 14 days after starting heparin. The peak incidence occurs 5 to 10 days after initiation of heparin. The other sign of HIT in this scenario is the diagnosis of a DVT even after being on heparin for prevention. DIC and ITP can decrease platelet count, but they are not the best answers because the scenario indicates that the patient is on heparin and has a newly developed DVT within 7 days of the initiation of heparin. This leads to the answer of HIT.

5. **A**

   Cryoprecipitate is used to manage actively bleeding patients with low fibrinogen levels in combination with FFP. It can be used to reverse anticoagulation overdoses but is not the blood product of choice. FFP contains more coagulation factors, and reversal of anti-coagulants is faster than cryoprecipitate. Correcting thrombocytopenia requires administration of platelets. Hemolytic anemia requires packed red blood cells (PRBC) therapy.

6. **B**

   This patient has developed DIC as a complication of abruptio placenta. Widespread clots formed in the microcirculation results in microvascular occlusion. The microvascular occlusion that occurs in DIC results in the conversion of aerobic to anaerobic metabolism with the elevation of lactate levels and metabolic acidosis. Troponin is more specific to cardiac muscle but would elevate after organ dysfunction. Myoglobin elevates with muscle injury. Thrombin time measures the amount of time it takes to form a clot. It is elevated in DIC but indicates bleeding abnormality, not microvascular occlusion.

7. **C**

Nonheparin anticoagulation should be initiated promptly to limit thrombosis complications. Heparin is replaced with either a direct thrombin inhibitor (DTI) or fondaparinux. Stopping the heparin only without the initiation of anticoagulation therapy can increase the risk of developing thrombosis. Direct Coomb's (antiglobulin) test is used to diagnose blood transfusion reactions. Platelets are typically only administered if the patient is actively bleeding with a really low platelet count. Heparin should not be restarted even if there is an increase in platelet count. Circulating antibodies to heparin remain for at least 100 days.

8. **C**

ITP is also called immune thrombocytopenia. It is a complex syndrome that involves both humoral and cellular immunity causing the destruction of platelets and also a decrease in production. Oral corticosteroids are considered the initial treatment for ITP. This includes oral prednisone or high-dose dexamethasone (Decadron). Heparin and fondaparinux are anticoagulants that can worsen the bleeding potential in ITP. Acyclovir is an antiviral medication and is not indicated in ITP.

9. **B**

All of the listed transfusion reactions can cause death, but TRALI is the most commonly found transfusion reaction. TRALI is a form of noncardiogenic pulmonary edema. Presentation occurs usually within 6 hours with fever, hypotension, and hypoxia. AHTR occurs due to ABO incompatibility and is almost exclusively related to clinical errors. Hospital policies requiring two nurses checking the blood at beside and newer scanning methods have lowered this risk significantly. TTD is rare in the United States due to improved donor screening and development of specific tests for the diseases. ATR occurs in patients who are IgA-deficient and is a rare reaction.

10. **A**

Direct antiglobulin (Coomb's) test is used to detect antibodies or proteins that are bound to the transfused red blood cells (RBCs) causing agglutination and hemolysis. Other laboratory tests include sending a new hemoglobin, type, and crossmatch, and urine to assess hemoglobinuria. Myoglobin is nonspecific and measures muscle damage. Enzyme-linked immunosorbent assay (ELISA) is a general lab method used for testing multiple antibodies. The PT and aPTT are bleeding times and are not used to verify a hemolytic blood transfusion reaction.

CHAPTER 5. NEUROLOGICAL SYSTEM REVIEW

1. **B**

Benzodiazepines are used as a first-line drug during a seizure. They potentiate GABA, which is an inhibitory neurotransmitter. Even though diazepam is also a benzodiazepine and can be used first for a seizure, it has a shorter antiepileptic effect than lorazepam. Lorazepam is considered the preferred first-line antiepileptic agent to treat a seizure. Phenytoin is recommended as a second-line antiepileptic. It works by inhibiting the sodium channels, preventing depolarization. Phenobarbital can also be used but is typically given to patients who have failed third-line antiepileptic agents.

2. **C**

The Brain Trauma Foundation's recommendation for antiepileptic prophylaxis is 7 days following a TBI, if no seizure occurs in the interval. This is the same recommendation for supratentorial postcraniotomy patients. The use of prophylactic antiepileptic therapy after ischemic strokes is not recommended but intracerebral hemorrhagic strokes have a higher incidence of seizures and may require short-term prophylaxis.

3. **C**

Based on some recent studies, some stroke centers extend the window of opportunity to administer IV tPA in an ischemic stroke to 4.5 hours. There is additional exclusion criteria used for the 3- to 4.5-hour time interval. These include: (a) history of both stroke and diabetes, (b) patients receiving oral anticoagulation therapy regardless of INR, (c) patients older than 80 years of age, and (d) baseline NIH Stroke Scale greater than 25.

4. **A**

Current American Stroke Association guidelines recommend allowing systolic BP to elevate for perfusion if the patient is not a candidate for tPA. The recommendation is to treat the BP if systolic BP is greater than 220 mmHg or diastolic BP greater than 120 mmHg. If the patient is a candidate for thrombolysis, the BP is treated if systolic pressure is greater than 180 mmHg and diastolic pressure is higher than 105 mmHg to lower risk of bleeding.

5. **B**

Fever is clearly associated with infarct expansion and worsening of cerebral edema. The mechanism is probably due to an increase in cerebral metabolic rate and oxygen consumption. Currently, the recommendation is to achieve normothermia after acute ischemic strokes. Hyponatremia and hyperglycemia are other metabolic abnormalities that have been shown to worsen infarcts and neurological outcomes following strokes.

6. **C**

Hyperosmolar therapy is commonly used to manage an increased ICP. Mannitol or HS can be used as hyperosmolar therapy. Monitoring serum sodium and osmolality levels is recommended during treatment, as is holding hyperosmolar therapy if serum osmolality is higher than 320 mOsm/kg. The concern for sodium with hyperosmolar therapy is the development of hypernatremia, not hyponatremia. Urine output is typically high during mannitol treatment because of its osmotic diuretic effects. An ICP greater than 20 mmHg would actually be an indication to administer hyperosmolar therapy.

7. **C**

During the first 24 to 48 hours after an aneurysm rupture, the primary goal of treatment is to prevent a rebleed. Antihypertensive therapy is used to maintain lower BP to prevent a rebleed. SAH precautions recommend keeping the room dark, administering analgesics and sedation, limiting stimulation, and preventing Valsalva maneuvers. Administering PRBCs and albumin will increase blood volume and BP, which may increase the risk of a rebleed. A vasoconstrictor would elevate BP and significantly increase the risk of rebleeding.

8. B

The diagnosis of cerebral VS is suspected with neurological changes and variations in the transcranial Doppler studies. The gold standard for the diagnosis of VS is angiography. This may be performed by arteriogram or CT angiography. MRI without angiography does not provide information on the cerebral vasculature.

9. A

The triple H therapy is commonly used to manage cerebral VS following an SAH. This includes hypertension, hypervolemia, and hemodilution. The mechanism of triple H therapy is to maintain high circulating blood volume and pressure to increase cerebral blood flow through the narrowed vessels. The goal is to prevent ischemic injuries from the VS. Hypovolemia would worsen cerebral blood flow. Hypothermia is currently not recommended in treating stroke patients. Hyperosmolar therapy does not benefit VS.

10. B

The preferred induction for RSI in patients with increased ICP is a short-acting agent such as propofol or etomidate. Midazolam is a longer acting sedative and may interfere with neurological assessment. A paralytic agent may be added but should also be a short-acting nondepolarizing agent. Succinylcholine is short acting but is a depolarizing NMB agent. It can cause hyperkalemia, malignant hyperthermia, and increased ICP in patients with intracerebral lesions. A short-acting nondepolarizing agent is rocuronium. Vecuronium is a longer acting NMB agent with a potential for prolonged paralysis.

11. D

When maintaining a lower BP to manage hemorrhagic strokes, the most commonly used antihypertensives are β-blockers and calcium channel blockers. Alpha-blockers, such as Nipride, can cause significant vasodilation of the cerebral vessels, resulting in an increase in cerebral edema and ICP. Continuous infusion of antihypertensive agents would indicate the need to use shorter acting, more titratable drugs such as nicardipine or esmolol. Labetalol is commonly used as an IV prn medication to lower BP in neurological patients.

12. C

CPM is a complication that results from increasing serum sodium levels too rapidly. This increases serum osmolality. Serum sodium levels should not be increased more than 12 mEq/L over a 24-hour period. Frequent sodium-level checks should be followed during the infusion of 3% NaCl. Cerebral edema, coma, and cerebral herniation are potential complications when serum osmolality is lowered too rapidly, causing fluid to shift out of the vascular space into the tissue.

13. **D**

In an MG patient, both a myasthenia crisis and a cholinergic crisis can result in respiratory weakness and failure. The hint in this question is that the patient was taking double his dose of pyridostigmine, which is an anticholinesterase inhibitor. Cholinergic crisis is a result of exaggerated cholinergic activity and is characterized by respiratory failure, bradycardia, urinary retention, and increased oral secretions. Myasthenia crisis is typically a result of failure to take medications or ineffectiveness of the medications.

14. **A**

Rapid treatment with IVIG or plasmaphoresis is comparable in efficacy but in hemodynamically unstable patients, plasmaphoresis is contraindicated. Rapid intervention with IVIG is the most appropriate intervention. Concomitant administration of steroids may be given but steroids alone have been found to exacerbate muscle weakness within 5 to 10 days. Anticholinesterase inhibitors are typically held during a myasthenia crisis due to aggravation of secretions and can be restarted when the patient has improved clinically.

15. **C**

In penetrating brain injuries, especially gunshot wounds, metal fragments, or bullets, may remain within the cranium. An MRI has the risk of moving the metal objects or creating heat because of the high magnetic field. Reminding the physician of the patient's mechanism of injury would be the most appropriate response. An MRI actually provides a greater structural detail than a CT. There was no indication in the scenario indicating the patient needed to be taken emergently to surgery.

16. **A**

The dilated, nonreactive pupil is on the left side indicating that the mass lesion, such as a hematoma, would also be on the left side. Uncal herniation is a lateral transtentorial herniation and results in ipsilateral pupil dilation. In bilateral cerebral edema, the herniation would be a central herniation resulting in bilateral pupillary dilation.

17. **B**

Cerebral edema tends to peak 2 to 3 days after a TBI. Close monitoring and sedation are typically performed on severe injuries for several days following the trauma. ICP is monitored typically longer than 24 hours and the greatest risk period for neurological deterioration is within 3 to 4 days post injury.

18. **D**

Permissive hypercapnia is a technique used to manage ARDS by manipulating ventilators based on hypoxia only and not treating hypercapnia. This can worsen ICP in a neurological patient due to the cerebral vasodilation effect of hypercapnia. Even though aggressive hyperventilation is no longer recommended, hypercapnia should be avoided. The use of PEEP can be used to assist with oxygenation in a neurological patient with ARDS but caution should be exercised as to the amount of PEEP. Increasing intrathoracic pressure with high levels of PEEP can cause a decrease in venous drainage from the brain with an increase in ICP. The other modes of ventilation are acceptable in the management of neurological patients with ARDS.

19. D

Long-term or high-dose use of propofol has been found to cause propofol infusion syndrome. Symptoms include metabolic acidosis, hyperkalemia, rhabdomyolysis, renal failure, and myocardial failure. The use of exogenous steroids can result in Cushing's syndrome but does not typically present with metabolic acidosis or hyperkalemia. Sepsis identifiers are tachycardia, fever, leukocytosis, and tachypnea. LNCD may be caused by the presence of delirium and use of sedation but is a complication experienced after the ICU and does not present with metabolic acidosis or hyperkalemia.

20. B

During an apnea test used to determine brain death, hypercapnia and respiratory acidosis are expected and part of the criteria. The complication of hypercapnia and respiratory acidosis is hypotension and arrhythmias. The patient should be on a cardiac monitor and BP must be monitored closely. Hemodynamic instability is an indication to stop the apnea test before completion. Bradycardia can occur, but the patient will typically become hypotensive, not hypertensive. A decrease in oxygen saturation can occur and supplemental oxygen is frequently administered during the test but the risk of aspiration is not increased during apnea testing.

21. C

CN IV and V are responsible for the gag and swallow reflex, whereas CN XII is responsible for tongue movements and strength. A swallow evaluation needs to be performed on all patients with neurological injuries prior to eating and drinking. CN III, IV, and VI are responsible for extraocular eye movement. CN V, VII, and VIII are responsible for facial sensory and motor movement as well as hearing.

22. A

The P1 component of the ICP waveform has the highest amplitude, followed by P2 then P3. When the P2 component is greater than the P1 component, it indicates brain noncompliance. An ICP reading of 15 mmHg is on the high side of normal but is not considered an increased ICP at this time.

23. C

Following brain death, pituitary hormones are not released resulting in low levels of thyroid-stimulating hormone and T_3/T_4 levels. There are also low levels of cortisol and insulin due to loss of function of the pituitary gland. Brain-dead patients become hemodynamically unstable because of deficiency of hormones, development of DI, and loss of sympathetic tone. The administration of thyroxine though replaces the deficient hormone. It does not increase catecholamines, reverse DI, or improve sympathetic tone through the ANS.

24. A

The aqueduct of Sylvius is located between the third and fourth ventricles. It forms a narrow passage for CSF to flow through from the supratentorial (cerebral cortex) to the infratentorial (brainstem) portion of the brain and is easily obstructed. It is the most common site due to the narrowness of the aqueduct. The foramen of Monro is an opening located between the lateral ventricles and the third ventricle. It is the anatomical landmark used to level the ICP transducer and is not as commonly obstructed. The foramen of Magnum is the opening in the cranium for the spinal cord.

25. D

Anoxic brain injuries result in cytotoxic cerebral edema, which is intracellular swelling. Administering hyperosmolar therapy, such as mannitol or HS, is not effective in treating cytotoxic cerebral edema. Steroids have not been found to be effective in the management of anoxic brain injuries. Therapeutic hypothermia is the most effective in managing anoxic brain injuries, such as post–cardiopulmonary resuscitation (CPR). TBIs, brain tumors, and other brain injuries frequently have primarily vasogenic cerebral edema. This is swelling in the interstitial space and is more amendable by hyperosmolar treatment.

CHAPTER 6. GASTROINTESTINAL SYSTEM REVIEW

1. B

Early intubation should be performed for any signs of respiratory distress or failure in a patient with an upper GI bleed. Airway and breathing are always a priority and in this case, the risk of aspiration is great and requires that the airway be protected. Fluids need to be administered to manage the blood loss and an endoscopy will probably be performed but an airway needs to be established prior to endoscopy. A central venous access may be required at some point but is not a priority of care at this time.

2. C

Pitressin is a vasoconstrictor of the splanchnic vascular bed but will also vasoconstrict coronary arteries, causing myocardial ischemia. Administration of nitroglycerin is frequently used concurrently with pitressin to prevent myocardial ischemia. Vasopressin can also cause hypertension and cardiac arrhythmias. Terlipressin is an analog of pitressin but has fewer vasoconstrictive effects on coronary arteries. Octreotide is also a vasoconstrictor of splanchnic vasculature but does not cause coronary or renal vasoconstriction. Magnesium citrate is not a vasoconstrictor. It is used to purge the bowel of blood and fecal matter to prevent absorption of ammonia.

3. D

Typically following a splenectomy, there is a significant increase in platelets and WBCs due to the loss of the spleen's ability to remove platelets and WBCs from the circulation. This usually peaks in 7 to 20 days and will return to more normal levels. The thrombocytosis can increase the risk of venous as well as arterial thrombosis. Hydroxyurea may be used to lower the platelet count if thrombotic complications occur. Postsplenectomy patients will have a leukocytosis, not a leukopenia. Concentrated hematocrit or hyperkalemia are not common findings following a splenectomy or exploratory laparotomy.

4. A

Verifying the position of feeding tubes by x-ray should be done prior to feeding patients. Ausculatory methods to determine correct placement are often inaccurate. Misplacement of a feeding tube can result in inadvertent feeding into the lungs or pleural space. Aspiration from feeding tubes may be difficult especially with small-bore tubes, which collapse easily, making pH assessments more difficult. The assessment of pH and bilirubin to determine placement is more cost-effective and relatively effective but not as accurate as a radiograph.

5. D

Prealbumin levels have a shorter half-life and so have been found to be a greater predictor of protein malnutrition and outcomes. The half-life is 2 days compared with a 20-day half-life of albumin. Weight loss and muscle weakness are nonspecific and are not the best assessments of protein malnutrition.

6. A

A concentrated hematocrit in a pancreatitis patient indicates third spacing of fluids, demonstrating a more severe episode of pancreatitis. Amylase and lipase levels may be elevated in pancreatitis but the degree of elevation does not indicate the severity of the pancreatitis. Potassium levels typically decrease in pancreatitis, and do not increase.

7. B

Stage II hepatic encephalopathy demonstrates marked asterixis and deterioration in hand writing. Stage I presents with behavior changes and mild confusion. Stage III marks confusion and combativeness. In Stage IV, the patient is unresponsive, in a coma.

8. C

Following abdominal trauma and surgery, the patient develops an increase capillary permeability and third space their fluids. The bowel becomes edematous and fluid shifts into the abdominal compartment. This causes pressures within the peritoneum to increase thereby developing intra-abdominal hypertension. The increased pressure within the peritoneum can interfere with the diaphragm and cause respiratory failure. This can mimic an ARDS. ARDS can be a complication but is typically seen 48 to 72 hours after insult or injury. There is no indication in the scenario that the patient was at risk for CHF or is presenting with a dilated cardiomyopathy.

9. A

Following an esophagectomy, the presence of subcutaneous air around the chest and neck region indicates a rupture of the anastomosis. The patient may also have associated tachycardia, tachypnea, or signs of peritonitis. This can lead to sepsis and death if unrecognized. This is not a normal finding with this surgical procedure. A pneumothorax or ruptured bleb can cause subcutaneous air but the risk is less common than leaking at the anastomosis.

10. D

Pancreatitis can be classified as edematous or hemorrhagic pancreatitis. Hemorrhagic pancreatitis involves pancreas necrosis. The necrosis is either infected or noninfected.

A patient with a noninfected pancreatitis is typically observed and followed, but if it develops into an infected necrosis surgical debridement is required. Pancreatic fistula and pseudocysts are typically medically managed. Edematous pancreatitis is less severe than hemorrhagic pancreatitis and is managed medically.

CHAPTER 7. RENAL SYSTEM REVIEW

1. **D**

   Oliguria, in adults, is defined as urine output less than 0.5 mL/kg/hr for 6 consecutive hours. Infants are less than 1 mL/kg/hr. Acute kidney injury is defined as either serum creatinine (SCr) absolute increase by 0.3 mg/dL or a relative increase in SCr to 1.5- to twofold, or oliguria despite fluid resuscitation.

2. **D**

   ESRD is defined as a complete loss of function requiring replacement therapy for longer than 3 months. Chronic renal failure is defined as a complete loss of function for longer than 4 weeks. A threefold increase in creatinine or decrease in GFR by 75% is criteria for acute renal failure.

3. **D**

   ACE inhibitor blocks the conversion of angiotensin I to angiotensin II. This inhibits the vasoconstrictive effects of angiotensin II on the efferent arterioles in the glomerulus, lowering GFR. NSAIDs block prostaglandins, which play a role in vasodilating the afferent arterioles. This can decrease GFR in volume-depleted or hypoperfused patients. Contrast medium and aminoglycosides cause intrarenal failure.

4. **A**

   Rhabdomyolysis is caused by breakdown of muscle, elevating myoglobin levels that can damage the renal tubules. Tea colored or "Coke"-colored urine is characteristic of rhabdomyolysis. Other renal failures result typically in dark amber urine. White cell casts in the urine indicate interstitial nephritis. Tubular epithelial casts in the urine are caused by acute tubular necrosis (ATN).

5. **B**

   ATN is a type of intrarenal failure. During intrarenal failure, the kidneys lose the ability to concentrate the urine, which results in a decrease in urine osmolality or dilute urine. The urine specific gravity will also be low, reflecting dilute urine. The kidneys also lose the ability to reabsorb sodium, resulting in high urine sodium levels. Prerenal failure has the elevated BUN:creatinine ratio. Renal failure causes hyperphosphatemia.

6. **C**

   Ultrafiltration is used to manage volume overload. Water moves across a semipermeable membrane by pressure gradient. It does not pull off solutes. Diffusion is the movement of solutes from an area of higher concentration to an area of lower concentration. The concentration gradient is maximized by running countercurrent dialysate to blood flow. Smaller molecular-weight solutes are cleared efficiently but larger molecular-weight solutes are not. Convection occurs by combining ultrafiltration with a pressure gradient and dragging both small and large molecular-weight solutes across the semipermeable membrane.

7. A

Continuous renal replacement therapy (CRRT) frequently results in hypophosphatemia. Adding phosphate into the replacement fluid or dialysate solution can prevent this complication of CRRT. Hypophosphatemia may prolong respiratory failure due to effects of respiratory muscle weakness. Azotemia is an elevated BUN and is not related to the hypophosphatemia. Mechanical ventilation may increase release of antidiuretic hormone, causing dilutional hyponatremia but does not significantly affect the phosphate. Calcium has an inverse relationship with phosphate but potassium does not typically affect phosphate levels.

8. C

Hypomagnesium symptoms are similar to hypocalcemia. Low magnesium causes an increase in muscle tone, deep tendon reflexes, muscle tremors and spasms, and positive Chvostek and Trousseau's signs. It may also result in seizures. Hypophosphatemia and hypercalcemia both cause muscle weakness and decrease of deep tendon reflexes. Potassium abnormalities may cause some muscle weakness and apathy.

9. A

Dilutional hyponatremia is one of the most common causes of low sodium in an ICU patient. This condition is a result of excessive water retention or fluid intake and not due to an actual loss of sodium. Serum chloride levels may be used to assist with differentiation of hemodilution versus loss of sodium. If the patient has an excess of water in relation to normal sodium, the chloride will also be normal. If the hyponatremia is due to a true loss of sodium, the chloride will also be low.

10. D

Hypophosphatemia causes muscle weakness, including weakness of the diaphragm and other ventilatory muscles. Low phosphate has been found to be associated with failed weaning from the ventilator. Potassium abnormalities cause ventricular arrhythmias. Magnesium plays a role in skeletal muscle and regulation of other electrolytes. Sodium primarily influences intravascular osmotic pressure.

CHAPTER 8. MULTISYSTEM REVIEW

1. B

A spinal cord–injured patient develops an atonic bladder early after injury during the period of spinal shock. Initially, due to fluid resuscitation, the patient may require an indwelling catheter but the goal is intermittent catheterization. An indwelling catheter increases the risk of catheter-related urinary tract infection and urosepsis. This complication can increase length of stay in the acute care facility and the risk of mortality. Spinal cord–injured patients will typically have an inability to empty the bladder completely so an external catheter is not effective in these patients. Urethral stents are being used in some patients with bladder outlet obstruction.

2. **A**

Sepsis is an inflammatory response to a known infection and SIRS is an inflammatory response to a clinical insult. Both sepsis and SIRS use the same criteria to diagnose; the difference is that sepsis has a known infection (including positive blood cultures), whereas in SIRS it is not possible to locate an infection (negative blood culture). At this time, Ms. J meets the criteria for an inflammatory response but no culture results or potential locations are provided in the scenario. It could be either sepsis or SIRS because of the elevated WBC count, fever, tachycardia, and tachypnea. To meet the criteria for severe sepsis, her systolic BP would have been less than 90 mmHg and/or lactate levels elevated greater than 4 mmol/L. Septic shock is hypotension and hypoperfusion despite adequate resuscitation. The scenario for Ms. J does not indicate the presence of organ dysfunction.

3. **A**

It is recommended by the Sepsis Campaign that antibiotics be initiated within 1 hour of recognition of sepsis. This patient meets the criteria for sepsis. The recommendation to resuscitate and correct hypotension and hypoperfusion is within 6 hours. This patient does have indicators for antibiotics because he meets the criteria for sepsis.

4. **B**

Initial fluid bolus for severe sepsis or sepsis-induced hypoperfusion should be a crystalloid (normal saline [NS] or lactated Ringer's). There is no known benefit of albumin over crystalloids in the initial fluid bolus and albumin is more expensive. If the patient requires substantial fluid to maintain hemodynamic parameters, it is recommended to administer albumin in addition to NS. Hetastarch is not recommended and may actually increase mortality. PRBCs may be given at some point in the resuscitation to maintain oxygen delivery but are not recommended as the initial fluid.

5. **C**

Corticosteroid therapy is recommended in septic shock patients who are hypotensive despite adequate fluid resuscitation and vasopressor therapy. Administration of 200 mg/24 hours of hydrocortisone is recommended to improve BP and perfusion to the tissues. Cortisol levels and ACTH test are not recommended to guide steroid therapy in septic shock patients. The lack of responsiveness to treatments is thought to be due to a cortisol resistance, not an actual adrenal insufficiency. Organ dysfunction or failure is not required before the initiation of steroids.

6. **D**

Hyperglycemia and hypernatremia are two common side effects of corticosteroid administration. Glucocorticoids decrease utilization of glucose in the peripheral resulting in hyperglycemia. They cause an increase in the excretion of potassium by the kidneys with an increase in the reabsorption of sodium. This results in hypokalemia and hypernatremia. Glucose, sodium, and potassium should be closely monitored during treatment.

7. **C**

Norepinephrine increases MAP through vasoconstriction with little to no effect on HR and less increase in stroke volume. Norepinephrine has been found to improve MAP and outcomes in sepsis over dopamine. Dopamine increases CO and MAP primarily by increasing stroke volume and has significant tachycardic effects on the heart. Dopamine also causes a greater risk for the development of arrhythmias. Vasopressin is not recommended to be used alone as the initial treatment for septic shock. It has been found useful in refractory hypotension as a secondary vasoconstrictor. Phenylephrine is not recommended in sepsis even though it has the least effect on heart rate. This is because of a potential decrease in stroke volume.

8. B

Shellfish and fish are common foods responsible for an IgE-mediated anaphylaxis reaction. The airway edema, wheezing, nausea, and vomiting are all signs of either anaphylaxis or an anaphylactoid reaction but since the most obvious cause is a food allergy due to the scenario of the patient eating in a seafood restaurant, the correct answer is anaphylaxis. Food allergies cause an IgE-mediated reaction. Anaphylactoid is a non-IgE-mediated hypersensitivity reaction. This indicates angioedema but is probably related to a food allergen rather than to a drug. The cause cannot be food poisoning because of wheezing and airway edema.

9. A

A cholinergic overdose presents with "wet" symptoms of increased salivation, lacrimation, urination, and emesis. An anticholinergic overdose presents with urinary retention, hyperthermia, tachycardia, and mydriasis. A sedative overdose presents with a decreased LOC and hypotension. An overdose of β-blockers will show bradycardia and hypotension.

10. B

Lorazepam infusions can lead to an accumulation of propylene glycol toxicity. High doses over 3 days will produce the highest incidence. Common symptoms of propylene glycol are anion-gap metabolic acidosis and increased osmolal gap. Other symptoms include renal dysfunction, hemolysis, cardiac arrhythmias, and CNS depression. Ketones are produced during metabolism of some alcohols when metabolized but are not found in propylene glycol toxicity. Thiocyanate toxicity is caused by the use of Nipride for extended periods of time. Lactic acid is produced during anaerobic metabolism. The anion-gap metabolic acidosis in this situation is caused by the addition of propylene glycol, not lactic acid.

11. C

Intravascular cooling has been found to be the fastest method of induction to the goal of TH. Surface cooling devices, ice packs, and cooling blankets are all methods of surface cooling or external cooling and may take longer to achieve the goal of hypothermia.

12. D

Blowing warm air across the face or body is called surface warming and can decrease or prevent the shivering response to cooling. Other methods may include covering the hands and feet. Covering the patient with warm blankets would generate heat and be counterproductive to the induction of hypothermia. Thorazine and anticonvulsants are not considered first-line therapy in managing shivering when inducing hypothermia.

13. B

Near-drowning victims sustain anoxic brain injuries. These are global injuries causing cytotoxic cerebral edema. The best management for global anoxic injuries is TH. She is not brain dead. She still has gag and cough reflexes as well as brainstem reflexes. Anoxic brain injuries are likely to have vasogenic cerebral edema (cytotoxic edema) and monitoring of ICP pressure has not been found to be effective. The most important complication at this time is her neurological injury. She does have the potential for pulmonary complications as well.

14. B

The goal for the maintenance phase of TH is 32°C to 34°C. This lowers metabolism and has been shown to improve neurological outcomes with fewer complications from the hypothermia. A range of 34°C to 36°C would be considered maintaining normothermia with less benefit of neuroprotection but a lower complication rate of hypothermia. Less than 32°C causes more shivering and is associated with greater complications of hypothermia.

15. C

BSAT is a common assessment tool used to determine severity of shivering. Shivering in the neck and chest area (score of 1) then progresses to gross movement of the upper extremities (score of 2). If shivering involves gross movements of the trunk and upper and lower extremities, it is considered severe (score of 3). No shivering scores a 0.

CHAPTER 9. BEHAVIORAL/PSYCHOLOGICAL REVIEW

1. C

CIWA-Ar is a tool used to determine the severity of AWS and guide therapeutic intervention. A score of less than 9 means the patient must be observed. If the score is greater than 9, a benzodiazepine should be administered. Score assessment is then repeated each hour until less than 10 and dosing of benzodiazepine is continued until less than 9. At this point, scoring can be every 8 hours then discontinued when score is less than 6 on four consecutive assessments.

2. C

Propofol is dissolved in a 10% lipid emulsion containing egg lecithin and soybean oil. This can precipitate allergic reactions if a person has an allergy to either eggs or soybeans. Morphine, Cardizem, and esmolol infusions would not be a problem with this patient's allergies.

3. A

Wernicke–Korsakoff's syndrome is a result of thiamine deficiency that occurs in alcohol-abuse patients. Administration of IV thiamine is used routinely to prevent Wernicke–Korsakoff's syndrome. Syndrome of inappropriate antidiuretic hormone involves antidiuretic hormone being overproduced in the brain. Myelodysplastic syndromes are types of cancer affecting bone marrow production of cells. Metabolic syndrome is a set of risk factors for cardiovascular and cerebrovascular disease.

4. **A**

Maintaining a light level of sedation is associated with improvements in clinical outcomes of ICU patients. These improvements include shorter ICU stays, shorter overall hospital days, fewer ventilator days, and complications from mechanical ventilation. Strict glycemic control is no longer recommended in all ICU patients because of complications of hypoglycemia. Promoting sleep may decrease the incidence of delirium but has not specifically been found to decrease the number of ventilator days. Daily CXR does not necessarily decrease ventilator or ICU days.

5. **C**

Delirium is a syndrome characterized by acute onset of cerebral dysfunction with a change of fluctuation in baseline mental status, inattention, and either disorganized thinking or an altered LOC. The cardinal signs of delirium are a disturbed LOC and a change in cognition, such as hallucinations and delusions. Anxiety is a subjective feeling of uneasiness or apprehension associated with a real or perceived threat. Agitation is an excessive, purposeless, cognitive and motor activity or restlessness, usually associated with a state of tension or anxiety. Dementia is a progressive syndrome characterized by the development of multiple cognitive dysfunctions.

6. **C**

Pain is frequently remembered after discharge from ICU and contributes to PTSD. Women have greater pain following a cardiac surgery when compared to men. Pain assessment is recommended even in intubated or nonverbal patients. Motor pain scales are frequently used to assess pain upon observation. Chest-tube placement and removal require preemptive analgesia to control the pain. The removal of a chest tube has been found to be a painful procedure.

7. **B**

A brain-injured patient's motor movement and behaviors may not indicate pain or lack of pain. Patients in a coma or locked-in syndrome may not be able to move but can experience pain. Other brain-injured patients may be very agitated but the agitation is not due to pain. Elderly patients can be assessed for pain by self-report or observation tools like any other adult. Patients with a psychiatric disorder may show signs of increased delirium but BPSs are frequently used.

8. **A**

Dexmedetomidine is a selective α-receptor agonist. It is different from other sedatives because it has been found to have analgesic effects and may allow for a lower dose of the opioid. Propofol and diazepam have sedative, amnesic, and hypnotic effects but do not have analgesic properties. Haloperidol is an antipsychotic drug without analgesic effects.

9. **D**

Sundowning is a type of agitation that occurs with older patients and patients with dementia. In the evenings or during the night, these patients become more disoriented and agitated. This agitation can frequently contribute to patient falls in the hospital.

Turning on lights well before sunset and closing the curtains at dusk will minimize shadows and may help diminish confusion that occurs with sundowning. Increasing sedation and placing restraints may actually increase the disorientation and agitation of sundowner's syndrome. A sitter is not necessarily required for all elderly patients with dementia.

10. **B**

In critically ill or injured patients, coping skills that normally have been functional may not be effective. The illness is frequently seen as being overwhelming and feelings of hopelessness become more common. Most in-hospital suicides are impulsive, without apparent planning. Unrelenting pain and refusing to see family and friends are two warning signs of suicide. Ask at least once a shift regarding suicidal intent in patients with warning signs. Depression and FTT are concerns as well but the greatest concern is potential of suicide. Psychosis is not necessarily a potential concern in this patient.

CHAPTER 10. PROFESSIONAL CARING AND ETHICAL PRACTICE

1. **D**

Skilled communication should have the focus of finding a solution to the situation that achieves the desirable outcome for the patient. The nurse is a patient advocate, but the question centered on a skilled communication interaction with the physician. Agreeing with the physician to avoid a disagreement may lead to harm of the patient. This has been associated with medical errors and is not recommended. The chain of command may be used if the skilled communication does not accomplish its goal of finding an appropriate solution. Threatening to use the chain of command is not representative of a skilled communication.

2. **B**

Moral distress occurs when the nurse believes that he or she knows the ethically correct action to take in the situation but a conflicting action is being pursued due to other members of the health care team or family members. There is more than one option to an ethical dilemma; with each option having an equally compelling alternative, the a moral argument can be made for and against each alternative. A discussion or conference with the physician and the family would be indicated before the issue is sent to the ethics committee. The physician does not have final decision making against the patient's or family's wishes.

3. **D**

Autonomy is considered a very important principle when working as a moral agent for the patient or family. The nurse should respect and not interfere with choices and decisions made by the autonomous individual (patient and/or family member). Paternalism is the principle used when physicians overrule family or patient's wishes for the patient's own welfare. This principle is appropriate in certain situations but is not the primary principle of moral agents for patients. Justice is fairness to everyone and is used frequently in cases of scare resources. Natural law means actions are morally right when they are in accordance with the end purpose of human nature and goals. Natural law is higher than man-made laws and is not a commonly used principle with ethical dilemmas in health care.

4. D

Patient M has been weaned from the ventilator, extubated, and off all vasoactive infusions. This indicates that he is less vulnerable and complex than immediately following the cardiac surgery. He is awake, alert, and follows commands, so is likely to be able to participate in his own care. He has had no family members visiting him since his surgery. This indicates that the area of concern is resource availability. He has minimal to no personal, psychological supportive resources or social system resources.

5. A

Beneficence refers to health care's responsibility to benefit the patient, usually through acts of kindness, compassion, and mercy. This means balancing between benefit and harm and determining which action maximizes the benefit and minimizes the harm. This is the principle used to analyze futile care and withdrawal of life support. Paternalism is based on the belief that the health care professional has the duty to benefit the patient with their decision outweighing the right of independent choice. This principle may be used in pediatric patients, in which medical professionals believe that a treatment would benefit the patient but family refuses the treatment (i.e., blood transfusions). Justice incorporates ideas of fairness and equality and is used frequently in determining distribution of scarce resources.

6. D

The nurse should initiate the discussion of the purpose and importance of a durable power of attorney. Just because the patient does not have a power of attorney does not necessarily mean that the patient does not want to talk about death. Lack of knowledge regarding the Patient Self-Determination Act and durable power of attorney is the most common reason for not completing the form. It is not required by law for all patients to actually have a power of attorney, but state laws require health care facilities receiving Medicare or Medicaid funds to provide written information to the adult patient about his or her rights according to the state law to make treatment decisions and execute advanced directives. The conversation can be initiated by any health care provider and does not require waiting for a physician to discuss it with the patient.

7. A

The initial intervention for a patient who is starting to become agitated may be to decrease the environmental stimulation. Sensory overload is a common cause of agitation in the ICU. Dimming the lights and limiting conversations around the patient has been found to decrease agitation. Restraints can be used to prevent self-injury but should not be an initial intervention. Sedation may also be an option but has been found to increase ICU length of stay. Family members at the bedside may actually help the agitation by allowing the patient to hear familiar voices.

8. C

Family members frequently react with a need for vigilance following a critical injury or illness. Encourage the family to leave the hospital at times to take breaks and get some rest. Explaining to them that they need their rest to be prepared to assist with the care when their loved one is ready will sometimes help the family understand the process. Reassuring the family that the patient will be okay is a false reassurance and can lead to issues with trust. Telling the family there is nothing they can do fosters the feelings of helplessness. There is always something the ICU nurse can find for the family to do to assist with patient care, even if it is prayer in a religious family. Allowing a less restrictive visitation in the ICU has been found to benefit both the patient and family members but encouraging a family member to remain 24 hours a day will lead to exhaustion of the family member.

9. **C**

Family members want to feel involved in caring for the patient and frequently want to bring in meals they have cooked. If the patient is on a special diet and the food they bring does not meet the specifics of the diet, then the most appropriate intervention is to teach the family about the diet. The family can bring food to the patient but the food needs to meet the specifics of the diet. Telling them they cannot bring food can create stress and further feelings of helplessness. Allowing the patient to eat the food that does not meet the diet may worsen the patient's condition and does not facilitate lifestyle changes that may be required after discharge. Informing the physician and setting up a physician/family conference should not be the initial intervention. If the family continues to disregard the request of the staff, even after teaching and reinforcing the instructions, then a conference may be considered.

10. **A**

The nurse is demonstrating patient advocacy by taking the initiative to call the husband and arrange for him to meet with the physician and his wife to discuss the surgery and obtain a consent form. This keeps with the cultural belief system of the patient and family, and facilitates care. Encouraging the patient to make her own decisions may delay the required surgery. A two-doctor signature is not required in this situation. The patient has the legal and ethical right for information about the proposed surgery and the ability to make her own decisions. To delay the surgery while attempting to resolve the conflict may cause complications and poor outcomes if the patient requires immediate surgery.

11. **B**

Different cultures have different values and beliefs. In American hospitals, independence and self-care are considered important values. But other cultures may not view this as important and actually place the value on family support and care. Cultural sensitivity includes not imposing our beliefs on other cultures when it is not necessary for recovery. Allowing the wife to continue to care for her husband demonstrates cultural sensitivity. Attempting to stop the wife through discussions, limiting visitation, or physician conferences is an attempt to force the values of independence and self-care on the patient and family.

12. **D**

Changing the assignment to allow a female nurse to care for the patient demonstrates cultural sensitivity and competency. In the Arab culture, female purity and maintaining gender segregation are valued. This belief system involves extreme modesty for women and would require the women to be kept completely covered if a male enters the room. Explaining to the husband about professionalism would not correct the situation of a male exposing the women to perform an assessment. Requiring the husband to leave the room or calling security would escalate the situation and might interfere with patient care and well-being.

13. **C**

It is recommended that an interpreter be used when obtaining signed consent forms from a patient or family member with limited or no English-language ability. Using the telephone translator is an appropriate response to the situation and would not delay obtaining the consent. A child of the patient may be more fluent in English but should not be used as an interpreter in the health care setting. Exposure of the child to sensitive health care information and role reversal can cause undue stress and adverse effects. Other concerns are the accuracy of the interpretation, especially the medical terminology, competency, and the potential conflict of interest that may exist. Competent translators require knowledge of two different languages, medical terminology, and maintain ethical and professional practice standards. Nurses may have some knowledge and ability to speak the language but may not be competent in translating for a consent form. Leaving it to the physician may delay the surgery.

14. **D**

Holistic nursing focus on lifestyle changes, prevention, and overall well-being. The scenario gave the information that the patient does not exercise and eats unhealthy food. This indicates a need for lifestyle changes to improve her health and prevent further complications of cardiovascular and cerebrovascular disease. Education on smoking and alcohol can also benefit patients, but there was no indication in this scenario that the patient was a smoker or used alcohol. Family support groups are important but the focus of this scenario was on the patient.

15. **B**

Patients in the ICU commonly experience a loss of control that creates anxiety. Once the patient is able to make simple decisions, allow the patient small choices. Give some control back to the patient in appropriate areas. Patients should have the right to make decisions about visitors, who can visit, and for how long. Patients need to be turned to prevent pressure sores. Giving them the choice of which side they would like to be turned to is appropriate, but not whether they want to be turned or not. An IV is also a safety issue. The patient may assist by stating which arm he or she prefers but not whether to have an IV. When a patient is ready to be transferred to PACU, he or she may require reassurance but is not given the choice to remain in the ICU.

16. **A**

Families may experience all of the feelings—helplessness, guilt, and denial—but the best answer, according to the presentation of the family, is feelings of helplessness. The suddenness of injury or illness may cause family members to have uncertainty about the situation. They may approach the ICU nurse with multiple questions and concerns. The family is thrown into a whirlwind of activity and commonly experiences feelings of helplessness. Asking questions and becoming agitated during the initial visit following a sudden illness or injury does not necessarily indicate poor coping skills. Family members are often unprepared for the whole impact of the injury or illness.

17. C

EBP is the use of the best available research data to guide practice and develop guidelines. EBP uses one's expert level of knowledge and experience to apply the data to clinical situations. The goal of EBP is to improve patient care and outcomes by implementing the most current guidelines. It does not necessarily decrease nursing time caring for patients. It can facilitate communication between health care providers and may be used as a plan of care but these are not the primary goals.

18. B

ICUs have been changing to become more family oriented. An important step is to allow family more time at the patient's bedside. Facilitation of family-oriented care and visitation should be encouraged and not strictly limited as has been the previous practice in the ICU. Written information regarding the ICU is appropriate but is not the main focus of changing policies to focus more on families. Encouraging the patient to be more involved in self-care and allowing autonomy are encouraged in the ICU but these practices are not focused on the family.

19. B

Noise is an environmental hazard that creates discomfort to the patient and can negatively affect outcomes. The two most common sources of noise in the ICU are voices (typically of staff) and alarms. Noisy environments cause sleep disturbances, anxiety, impaired wound healing, and activation of the sympathetic nervous system. Family visitors are not considered environmental hazards. Cardiac monitors and IV infusions are a part of the ICU care of a patient and are not considered environmental hazards.

20. D

Studies have found that a 5-minute back rub may increase sleep by 1 hour. Administering sedatives or hypnotics may actually decrease rapid eye movement sleep, which has the most benefit for the patient. Allowing visitors to stay with the patient at night may actually improve the patient's sleep by having a familiar person with them. Noise is one of the contributing factors for inability to sleep. Turning on the television will just increase the noise level unless the patient states that his or her normal routine at night is to fall asleep with the television on.

21. C

Inability to effectively communicate while intubated and mechanically ventilated creates stress and anxiety in the patient. Using sign language, lip reading, or communication boards can facilitate communication with nonverbal patients. Just reassuring the patient or explaining the problem to the patient without attempting to improve the communication just creates more anxiety. Administering a sedative is not indicated in a situation of communication issues.

22. C

Asking an open-ended question allows for exploration of possible meaning behind the patient's behavior. Threatening to restrain the patient or bargaining in regard to the physician's visit are inappropriate responses to acting-out behavior of the patient.

Asking the patient to tell you why he or she is angry can put the patient on the defensive and does not facilitate exploration of his or her feelings.

23. **B**

The first step to determining best practice is to be aware of the problem. In this situation, the problem identified was sleep disruption of critical care patients to obtain labs. The next step is to assemble a work group to research current literature and studies regarding the formulated problem. Once the best practice is identified, then presenting a plan for changing current practice is received better than just refusing to follow a particular practice. Obtaining other nurses' opinions is not basing the practice on research. This is not a situation or time in which the physicians should be requested to form committees to institute change.

24. **A**

Allowing the patient time to talk about an experience helps the patient to work through thoughts and emotions regarding the event. The nurse should listen actively to the patient. Downplaying a patient's experience as a hallucination or attempting to reorient the patient to the actual events is not beneficial to the patient and may actually be counterproductive. Referring the patient to talk to her family instead of the nurse may cause the patient to lose trust in the health care provider.

25. **C**

Professionalism includes mentoring others as well as being mentored. The preceptor is mentoring and teaching the orientee but can learn from the orientee as well. If there is a difference in methods for performing a procedure, perform a literature review to determine best practice. There is more then one way to do some procedures and one way is not always the best way. Stating that the orientee is wrong, without appropriate research, does not acknowledge the nurse as having a base of knowledge and skills. Surveying other nurses can be done in certain circumstances but is not the best answer in this scenario. Ignoring the identified problem does not allow for growth in either the preceptor or orientee.

26. **B**

Patients may be able to hear even if they are not responding or appear to be oriented. Families frequently do not know what to say to the patient or what to talk about at the bedside. Some families just stand at bedside and are afraid to touch their loved ones because of all of the lines and tubes. ICU nurses can encourage them to talk to the patient directly and touch their loved ones. This behavior does not indicate a conflict of interest in the wife making decisions for the patient. It is a common response and does not require psychological workup.

27. **D**

Most medication or procedure errors relate back to poor communication and an ineffective relationship among health care providers. Health care providers need to improve working relationships and communicate on a more professional level. Outbursts and disruptive behavior may prevent a nurse from calling a physician to report patient changes or question an order. This may lead to medication or patient care errors.

Resources are typically available in the ICU, including drug resource websites or books. New drugs can also be looked up and reviewed before being administered. Lack of knowledge can contribute to medication errors, but the most common reason is communication problems.

28. **C**

Laughter has been found to lower pain even up to 15 minutes after laughing. It has been reported by oncology patients to be the best self-prescribed pain management. Laughter increases the release of endorphins, the body's endogenous opioid. Laughter has not been found to lower the risk of strokes or affect patient orientation. Spirituality is a person's sense of belonging and belief in a higher being. Laughter has not been shown to affect spirituality.

29. **A**

One of the most important principles of adult learning is the need to know what is being taught. By giving real or simulated examples pertinent to the patient, the nurse is providing the patient with why he or she needs to know what is being taught. Learner's self concept is the self-motivation to learn and can be facilitated by providing more self-directed learning material. Internal motivation to learn is based on a person's internal desire to learn or become motivated to improve quality of life. Adult education should also be focused on the patient's life experiences. This would be facilitated initially by asking questions about the patient's current knowledge or skill level.

30. **D**

Honesty with the family regarding the severity of injury and prognosis fosters a trusting relationship and has been shown to be important to family members. Explaining the severity of the injury and the prognosis without discouraging all hope is the most appropriate response. The hope is their loved one will have comfort and pain management at the end of life. Telling the family in this situation "not to give up hope" is not being honest about the patient's prognosis. Discouraging the family by stating "we need to stop providing care" is inappropriate and leads the family to believe that their loved one will not be cared for appropriately. Falsely reassuring the family "everything will be okay" does not establish a trusting relationship between the family and health care providers.

31. **A**

Offering choices about small issues can help the patient when there are no choices about a bigger issue. Allow the patient to make decisions about which direction he or she wants to turn, when he or she wants a bath, and so on. Explaining the rules of the ICU may actually contribute to feelings of loss of control. Allowing patients to express their feelings and having family presence for support are both good responses of the ICU nurse toward the patient but do not affect the loss of self-control issues experienced in the ICU.

32. **B**

An informal assessment of learning needs using open-ended questions is the best method to determine learning needs. It may also be used to validate understanding of concepts being taught. For example, "What is your understanding of your loved one's condition?" Formal assessment tools use generic questions regarding health beliefs and learning styles and are not individualized for the learner. Talking with the family and asking open-ended questions provides an informal assessment of the patient's education and literacy level. This assessment requires sensitivity because adults will try to hide illiteracy. In-depth interviews to determine learning styles do not provide the information needed to provide education to family members. Informal, short sessions at the bedside may be the most effective teaching method.

33. C

Asking the learner to tell you about what was taught, in his or her own words, assists with determining his or her understanding of the learned topic. This assesses the learner's comprehension and not just ability to repeat what was taught. Although a person may have a college degree, he or she may have a low level of health literacy. Health literacy is the ability of the person to understand basic health information. Observing the person looking through the literature provided does not ensure the person can read or comprehend the literature. The nurse should read the information in addition to providing it in a written format. Preparing the educational material at the fifth- to eighth-grade reading level still does not assure that the person can read.

34. D

When teaching a psychomotor skill, following verbal and written instructions regarding the steps, the patient needs to perform the skill so knowledge can be evaluated. Critical elements of the skill need to be identified and those need to be demonstrated by the patient when performing the skill. Just stating the steps of a skill does not demonstrate proficiency in actually performing the skill. Stating that the wife can do the dressing change does not evaluate any learning, either of the patient or wife. Learning a new skill can be difficult and requires encouragement by the nurse; avoid embarrassing the patient but do not avoid a return-demonstration for fear of embarrassing the patient. Learning has to be evaluated.

35. A

Family presence during resuscitation has shown benefit for the family. One of the commonly expressed benefits is the family member is able to see everything that could be done for their loved one was done, instead of being on the other side of the door not knowing what was happening. Family presence should not make the staff try harder, improve physician interactions, or the resuscitation time shorter (which may not be a benefit in many cases).

36. C

Family-oriented palliative care is centered around four major cornerstones—open visitation, family conferences, family presence during resuscitation, and bereavement care. After the death of a loved one, support of the family should be provided. Providing information about funeral arrangements may be a component of support but will depend on the family's past experiences. Bereavement care may include allowing the family time at the patient's bedside after death. Family conferences are a part of palliative care while the patient is alive.

37. **B**

Introduce the bad news by identifying the symptoms that are indicating a poor prognosis. It gives family a chance to see what the health care professionals are already seeing. Then, if the need arises to talk about withdrawal of life support, the family is more prepared for the conversation. Asking whether they want "everything done" for their loved one sets up a "yes" answer. Clarifying what "everything" means and ensuring care is still provided although they will not be resuscitated is more appropriate. When discussing the issue of withdrawal, a better question is to ask what the patient would have wanted, not what the family's feelings are about it. Even if a patient is brain dead or a potential organ donor, the focus of the family conference is poor prognosis. Organ donor organizations typically will initiate the conversation about organ donation with the family.

38. **D**

The principle of double effect is commonly applied to the administration of opioids for pain management at the end of life. The principle refers to an action having two effects, one good and one bad. Providing analgesics controls pain but opioids can cause respiratory depression. If the primary goal is to control pain, even though the patient develops respiratory depression, this is ethically okay. Disagreements between family members in decision making and stopping tube feeds while maintaining hydration are not considered a double effect. Life support may be removed even if a person is awake. Removal of life support can be considered to have a good and bad effect but the hint in the question is the sentence regarding pain management.

39. **C**

Discussing the order with the ordering physician typically will allow the physician to explain the justification of the order. It is the most appropriate first response when questioning an order. If this does not clear up the issue regarding the order, then following the hospital protocol for using the chain of command should be initiated. This may include notifying the charge nurse and supervisor. If the ICU nurse still feels that the order may harm the patient after discussing it with the physician, refusing to administer the medication is an appropriate action. Administering a medication when it may be harmful to the patient is not appropriate without further discussion and additional steps.

40. **B**

Obtaining a bariatric chair that has an appropriate weight limit would be the best response of the nurse. Refusing to get the patient out of bed would not benefit the patient. The nurse needs to be an advocate for the patient. Discussing the need to purchase chairs for bariatric patients is a good response but will not benefit this patient at this particular time. Using a chair that is not approved for the patient's weight is an inappropriate answer. The nurse would be legally liable for any injury incurred if the chair broke and the patient was injured.

Index

Printed in the United States
By Bookmasters